Psychiatric Intensive Care

Psychiatric Intensive Care

Edited by

M Dominic Beer
MD MRCPsych MA (Oxon)

*Snr Lecturer (Guy's, King's St. Thomas' & Institute of Psychiatry) and
Honorary Consultant Psychiatrist in Challenging Behaviour
and Intensive Care Psychiatry (Oxleas NHS Trust
Bexley Hospital, Bexley, Kent, UK)*

Stephen M Pereira
MD MRCPsych DPM MSc

*Consultant Psychiatrist and
Honorary Snr Lecturer in Psychiatry Guy's, King's and
St Thomas' School of Medicine
Pathways, Psychiatric Intensive Care Unit
Goodmayes Hospital
Essex, UK*

Carol Paton
BSc Dip Clin Pharm MRPharmS

*Chief Pharmacist
Oxleas NHS Trust
Bexley Hospital
Bexley, Kent, UK*

CONTENTS

Section 2: Forensic and Risk Issues

Section 3: Structure and Management

CONTRIBUTORS

Zerrin Atakan MRCPsych
Consultant Psychiatrist
Honorary Senior Lecturer (Guy's,
King's and St Thomas' Medical
School)
South Western Hospital
London, UK

James Anderson MRCPsych
MRCP
Consultant Forensic Psychiatrist
Bracton Centre
Bexley Hospital
Bexley
Kent, UK

M Dominic Beer MD MRCPsych
MA (Oxon)
Snr Lecturer (Guy's, King's St. Thomas'
& Institute of Psychiatry) and Honorary
Consultant Psychiatrist in Challenging
Behaviour and Intensive Care Psychiatry
(Oxleas NHS Trust)

Christian Betteridge RMN
Senior Staff Nurse
Greyfriars Psychiatric Intensive Care
Unit, Severn NHS Trust,
Gloucester, UK

Debbie Coleman RMN
Snr Nurse Manager
Bracton Centre
Bexley Hospital
Bexley
Kent, UK

Roland Dix RMN
Consultant Nurse in Intensive Care
Greyfriars Psychiatric Intensive Care
Unit, Severn NHS Trust
Gloucester, UK

Brenda Flood MSc Dip NZ OT SROT
Inpatient Therapy Development
Manager
Cornwall Healthcare NHS Trust
Cornwall, UK

Phil Garnham RMN Dip in
Counselling, MA in Counselling and
Psychotherapy
Snr Charge Nurse & Course Director
Diploma in Forensic Mental Health Care
Guy's, King's and St Thomas' Medical
School
Bracton Centre
Bexley Hospital
Bexley
Kent, UK

Marc Goldstein
BA (WITS) BA Hons (Applied
Psychology)(WITS) MA (Clinical
Psychology) (PRET)
Senior Clinical Psychologist (SA)
Specialist Clinical Psychologist in Adult
Mental Health
Goodmayes Hospital
Essex, UK

Harvey Gordon MRCPsych
Consultant Psychiatrist
Broadmoor Special Hospital
Crowthorne
Berks, UK

Caroline L Holmes MRCPsych
Specialist Registrar in Psychiatry
Addenbrooke's Hospital
Cambridge, UK

Sarah Hooton BScOT SROT
Snr Occupational Therapist
Bridging the Gap Challenging
Behaviour Service
Brook Lane Medical Centre
London, UK

Maurice Lipsedge FRCPsych FRCP
FFOM (Hons)
Consultant Psychiatrist and Senior
Lecturer
Keat's House
Guy's Hospital
London, UK

Brian Malcolm McKenzie
MA Clin Psychol (Natal), Dip For
Psychotherapy (UCL)
Clinical Forensic Psychologist
Bracton Centre
Bexley Hospital
Bexley, Kent

Tom Morahan RMN
Snr Nurse
Bracton Centre
Bexley Hospital
Bexley
Kent, UK

Chike I Okocha MRCPsych
Consultant Psychiatrist
Cygnet, Beckton PICU and
Community Mental Health Centre
Eltham
London, UK

Carol Paton BSc Dip Clin Pharm
MRPharmS
Chief Pharmacist
Bexley Hospital
Oxleas NHS Trust
Bexley, Kent UK

Stephen M Pereira MD MRCPsych
DPM MSc
Consultant Psychiatrist and
Honorary Snr Lecturer in Psychiatry
Guy's, King's and St Thomas' School of
Medicine
Pathways PICU
Goodmayes Hospital
Essex, UK

Lyn Sarah Pilowsky MRCPsych PhD
Senior Lecturer and Honorary
Consultant South London and Maudsley
NHS Trust
Maudsley Hospital
London, UK

Mark Polczyk-Przybyla PhD RMN
Forensic Charge Nurse
Bracton Centre
Bexley Hospital
Bexley
Kent, UK

Andrew W Procter FRCPsych
Consultant Psychiatrist
Oxford Ward PICU
Manchester Royal Infirmary
Manchester, UK

Helen Simmons MRCPsych
Specialist Registrar in Psychiatry South
London and Maudsley NHS Trust
Maudsley Hospital
London, UK

FOREWORD

I am very pleased to be able to write this foreword and to commend this book to all clinicians in psychiatric intensive care, low secure and general mental health settings. This book comes at an extremely valuable time in the life of this newest of psychiatric specialities. The Butler report of 1975 was clearly instrumental in the construction of regional and interim secure services for the offending patient in the United Kingdom, but made no provision for the highly disturbed or acutely distressed patient who was not in the judicial system.

Prior to the establishment of a network of psychiatric intensive care units (PICUs) in some countries care for these patients was usually spread around acute hospital wards that would occasionally lock their doors. This was often an unsafe and unsatisfactory situation. Over the past twenty years, hospitals have increasingly recognised the need for a specialist environment that provides security and high intensity nursing, medical and other multi-disciplinary input for our most seriously ill patients. Prior to the establishment of this network, it was always a conundrum in psychiatry that our most severely ill patients often encountered barriers to care due to lack of the 'right' facility – something that would be unthinkable in other areas of medicine.

Most major Mental Health Hospital Trusts now have PICUs and the establishment of the National Association of Psychiatric Intensive Care Units (NAPICU) marks the birth of an entirely new speciality in psychiatry. This book is therefore a landmark in the psychiatric literature, being the first definitive and authoritive text on the subject and an excellent one at that. The book covers all aspects of the speciality from techniques for rapid traquilisation through to physical, risk and management issues, as well as interfaces with forensic services. The book lays down important benchmarks of care and management in a current environment, which is subject to a great deal of regional variability. The three editors have been instrumental in the establishment of the National Association and the running of vanguard PICUs and they have done an excellent job in assembling a panel of authors who all work at the 'cutting edge' of intensive care and who all have extensive 'hands-on' experience. As the efficiency of community care increases, it is important to recognise that intensive care represents a vital core service for those who fall through this net and also for those who experience acute disturbances at first onset of psychosis. With a core service there must also be core knowledge. Such specialists will always be small in number compared to the general psychiatrists working mainly in a community setting and this book represents the first benchmark for this knowledge.

I am sure the book will grow in popularity and content as the speciality increases its sophistication and evidence base.

Robert Kerwin
Professor of Clinical Neuropharmacology and
Honorary Consultant in Intensive Care Psychiatry
Institute of Psychiatry
London SE5

August, 2000

PREFACE

'Why do we need a book about psychiatric intensive care?' 'What *IS* psychiatric intensive care?', 'Is there any difference between intensive care and general psychiatry?' 'Where is the distinction between forensic psychiatry and psychiatric intensive care?, 'What special skills do PICU staff require?' Our first attempt to address some of these questions came at the first national conference on psychiatric intensive care, held in Bexleyheath, England, in 1996. The enthusiasm of the delegates and their thirst for knowledge and networking has led to the publication of this book.

We, as editors, have attempted to cover as many elements of psychiatric intensive care provision as is possible within one book. We are, however, aware of certain deficiencies. Where there is an evidence-base, we have attempted to use it. Where there is not, we have used personal experience and the experience of others to guide us. We believe that psychiatric intensive care is at the heart of psychiatry and its good practice requires a full multidisciplinary team, strong leadership and effective managerial support. We have, therefore, included a wide variety of chapters, all written by professionals who have extensive expertise in this area of care. We have included examples of sample policies, which can be used as a guide, but these obviously need to be adapted and scrutinised for use locally. The editors would welcome any comments and suggestions on this work.

The first section addresses treatment issues. Effective treatment requires input from a wide variety of professionals. We have included contributions on the role of medication, psychological treatments, therapeutic activities, and more controversially, the use of both restraint and seclusion. The development and definition of psychiatric intensive care and the management of the acutely disturbed patient and of the complex needs patient also warrant chapters in their own right.

The second section specifically addresses areas of risk and the interface with forensic services. Contributions from colleagues working in forensic services, we hope, will encourage the breaking down of unnecessary barriers between different services.

The third section addresses management issues such as how to set up and design a new psychiatric intensive care unit and how to manage such a unit effectively once it has been established.

We believe that this book will be of use to all disciplines working in, or interacting with, psychiatric intensive care units, and also to managers who have the responsibility for commissioning, providing and monitoring this high risk area of care. Although the emphasis is towards practice in the United Kingdom, the general principles should be relevant and applicable in any care setting where the disturbed psychiatric patient is managed.

We would like to thank all the contributors to the book; those who have assisted in the publishing, especially Geoff Nuttall, Nora Naughton, Kathleen Orr and Gavin Smith; our secretarial staff, Mrs Linda Wells, Mrs Lorraine Wright, Miss Michelle Gilham and Mrs Rosemary McCafferty for their considerable hard work; our patients and colleagues who have taught us much; and our families, especially Drs Naomi Beer and Preeti Pereira, for their support and patience through this project.

Dominic Beer
Stephen Pereira
Carol Paton

August, 2000

SECTION 1:
THERAPEUTIC
INTERVENTIONS

1

PSYCHIATRIC INTENSIVE CARE – DEVELOPMENT AND DEFINITION

M Dominic Beer, Stephen M Pereira, Carol Paton

HISTORICAL BACKGROUND

Throughout human history different cultures have had to manage their most behaviourally disturbed and mentally ill members. Turner (1996) has written that historically psychiatry has been judged by its management of the 'furiously mad'. Nearly three thousand years ago the King of Babylon was put to pasture (literally) after he started to behave like a wild animal (Book of Daniel). Two thousand years ago we read in the New Testament of a wild man wandering naked amidst the tombs, having broken the chains that bound him.

Seven hundred and fifty years ago the first 'asylum' for mental patients in England was formed at the Priory of St Mary of Bethlehem in London. 'Bethlem' became the national hospital for the disturbed mentally ill. The patient's parish of origin would pay for a stay of usually up to a year. Abuses however came to light, none better known than the case of William Norris in 1814, which prompted a parliamentary enquiry. The unfortunate man had been kept for seven years in a cell and restrained mechanically so that he could move no more than twelve inches.

Nineteenth-century psychiatrists like John Conolly then embraced 'non-restraint', but many hospitals remained locked. The Mental Treatment Act 1930 introduced the concept of patients being admitted informally and by 1938 such patients constituted 35% of the total (Jones 1993). The Royal Commission on the Law Relating to Mental Illness and Mental Deficiency (1954–57) stressed that patients should be treated informally where possible. The Mental Health Act 1959 confirmed this and laid down strict guidelines for involuntary patients.

In the late 1950s there was another important development in the care of the mentally ill. This was the introduction of chlorpromazine, the first pharmacological treatment for psychotic illness. The potent combination of effective antipsychotic drugs along with the introduction of patients' rights, led to the unlocking of many hospital wards. By the early 1960s, only a handful of wards in our own hospital (Bexley Hospital, Kent) were still formally locked. Two of these wards housed a stable population of chronically disturbed patients. There was another transient group of acutely disturbed patients who were admitted for brief periods until their behaviour became containable on an open ward. Thus, the Psychiatric Intensive Care Unit (PICU or locked ward) function had evolved as a pragmatic solution to the patient management problems encountered on the open wards.

SECURE PROVISION IN THE 1970s IN THE UK

By the early 1970s each health region was being encouraged to develop services in district general hospitals. These facilities could not adequately manage difficult patients. The latter joined the mentally abnormal offenders in asylums, prison or special hospitals. The Department of Health and Social Security set up a working party in 1971 to review the existing guidance on security in NHS psychiatric hospitals and make recommendations on the need for security. Consequently, the Glancy Report (Revised Report of the Working Party on Security in NHS Psychiatric Hospitals) was published (DHSS 1974). The Report noted the almost total lack of secure facilities and recommended 1000 places for England and Wales.

The problem of the mentally abnormal offender was addressed by the Butler Committee which was formed after the case of Graham Young who was convicted of murder whilst on conditional discharge from Broadmoor.

The terms of reference were:

- To consider the criminal law in relation to mental disorder or abnormality and to recommend whether any changes in the powers and procedures were necessary.

- To recommend whether any changes were required in the provision of facilities and treatment for this group of patients.

The Butler Report (HMSO 1975), and its interim version of 1974, advocated the development of forensic psychiatric services in the NHS and suggested a figure of 2000 secure beds. This was double the Glancy figure, which was based on the need for security among general psychiatric patients. It was proposed that regional secure units (RSUs) would be crucial in supporting the general psychiatric hospital as well as relieving overcrowding in Special Hospitals and providing a service to courts and prisons.

The RSUs were to be 50–150-bedded units closer to major centres of population than the Special Hospitals. A particular point was made regarding difficult long-stay patients – that the RSUs should not be allowed to become blocked with such patients. If they did then the problem which they were supposed to address would recur; but no clear alternative model of care was proposed for them. The Department of Health and Social Security very quickly made money available for 1000 beds to be provided in RSUs and in Interim Secure units (ISUs) whilst the former were being built.

These ISUs were usually converted psychiatric wards; most had a double door 'airlock' system to enter the unit and secure external exercise areas, as well as unbreakable glass and alarm systems.

Bluglass (1976) proposed that the admission criteria should include any acutely ill patient whose illness was accompanied by difficult and dangerous behaviour but should exclude wandering demented patients, the severely learning disabled and the difficult acute patients.

Thus, historically, the RSU network has been centrally planned and funded whereas locked beds for acutely ill, non-offender patients (Glancy) have not.

DEVELOPMENT OF PSYCHIATRIC INTENSIVE CARE UNITS WORLD-WIDE

The first publications which described locked PICUs came from the USA. Rachlin (1973) stated that 'an open-door policy cannot provide adequately for the treatment needs of all psychiatric patients'. He described the establishment of a 'locked intensive care unit' serving the Bronx area of New York, 'to treat several types of patients who did not respond on open wards' (p. 829). Half were referred because they were absconders. Crain and Jordan (1979) also reported on a psychiatric intensive care unit in the Bronx which admitted mainly violent patients 'who simply cannot be treated with an acceptable level of safety on a regular ward'. It also provided a more humane treatment setting 'for such individuals whose behaviour ordinarily would provoke angry, punitive responses from the environment' (p. 197).

Other psychiatric intensive care units were described elsewhere in the world. Goldney *et al* (1985) described a locked unit for actively severely ill patients in Adelaide, Australia. Warneke (1986) described a psychiatric intensive care unit for acutely ill patients in a general medical hospital in Edmonton, Canada. The patients were mainly suicidal and the unit was not locked) nor were the patients legally detained. Musisi (1989) described a six-bedded unit in a provincial Toronto psychiatric hospital.

In England the first designated psychiatric intensive care unit was opened in St James's Hospital, Portsmouth; Mounsey (1979) described the setting up a 12-bedded PICU in Salisbury. This was a lockable converted ward for disturbed patients referred from the rest of the psychiatric hospital.

In Scotland, Basson and Woodside (1981, p. 132) described the working of a mixed 'secure/intensive care/forensic' ward and stated that 'the pendulum has swung from "open door" hospitals back to a recognition for some security . . .'.

SECURE PROVISION IN THE UK IN THE 1980s AND 1990s

The RSU model has been developed throughout England and Wales but not in Scotland. Several deficiencies of the RSU model have been noted. Snowden (1990) wrote that 'there is a group of patients who are not so dangerous that they require special hospital security but who are chronically ill or poor medication responders and who require a degree of security. . . . Some of the more severely ill and disabled patients will not manage in the community and long-term care will not be available. . . . 'The mentally ill who cannot manage in the community may become mentally ill offenders by default, and even if they do not, general psychiatric services could well put pressure on forensic services to take patients that would have been considered appropriate for RSU admission in the past.'

In 1991 only 635 medium secure beds existed as compared with 1163 in 1986, according to the Reed Report; this review of Health and Social Services for mentally disordered offenders and others requiring similar services (DoH/Home Office 1992) proposed that 1500 beds were needed. It also proposed that 'access to local intensive care and locked wards should be available more widely' and that 'secure provision . . . should include provision . . . for those who require long-term treatment and/or care'.

The Reed Report again referred to the lack of service provision. 'Many offenders needing in-patient care can be accommodated in ordinary psychiatric provision. But although many offenders can be managed satisfactorily in "open" wards, there must be also better access to local intensive care and locked wards: see Annex J' (local services 5.16 Hospital Services, p. 19). The Report recognised 'the need for each Health District to ensure the availability of secure provision . . . [which] should include provision for intensive care'. The Reed Report (Department of Health and Home Office, 1992) referred to ICUs as low secure units.

Smith et al (1990) hypothesised that the role of the RSU was changing. They compared patients admitted to the Butler Clinic RSU in South West England in 1983 and 1989. In the 1983 population there were significantly more patients who had been aggressive towards staff and had histories of absconding. The 1989 population was much more likely to have been referred from the criminal justice system. The authors speculated that the RSU was originally dealing with a 'backlog' of local hospital patients for which there was no secure provision before the RSU opened.

A survey of RSU patient characteristics in 1994 confirmed that the RSU population had high levels of serious offending (McKenna 1996) and warned that: 'The ability of the RSU to respond quickly, effectively or flexibly to acute difficulties in the services referring potential admissions must in turn be compromised'.

In order to respond quickly, NHS Trusts have now used the low secure wards or psychiatric intensive care units to take up this demand for urgent forensic patients. Dix (1996) pointed out that this group does not necessarily present high levels of behavioural disturbance but requires a degree of security because of their charge or offence. James et al (1996) also referred to a group of patients that had offended but did not require security. The suggestion is that local services should be able to provide low security in order to facilitate diversion of offenders from the criminal justice system, and aid the rehabilitation of patients discharged from Special Hospitals. As Dix (1996) writes, however, 'A significant number of PICUs do not consider themselves as "forensic units" and are reluctant to accept patients who, as a result of legal restrictions, cannot be discharged from the PICU when clinically indicated'. Cripps et al (1995) describe a mixed PICU/forensic unit and discuss some of the advantages and disadvantages of this type of unit. Many would argue that the forensic role conflicts with the more dominant function of local low secure units, namely the modus operandi outlined by Faulk (1995): 'The usual pattern is for the wards to accept the patient briefly, to get them over an acute disturbance, before returning them to the original ward'.

A third role which has been adopted by PICUs is the care of the chronically disturbed patient. Coid (1991a) noted that the private sector was being used increasingly for such patients because of the lack of NHS facilities and he also (Coid 1991b) stated that 'the game of pass the parcel must stop' with reference to 'difficult to place patients'. The Mental Health Act Commission (1995) also reported on the lack of provision for patients who demonstrate longer-term behavioural problems.

The Chief Medical Officer (1996) stated that the number of medium secure beds was planned to be 2350 by the end of 1998 and that there was also a need for a greater diversity of secure beds, particularly those offering longer-term care at medium and low security levels.

PSYCHIATRIC INTENSIVE CARE UNITS IN THE UK IN THE 1990s

In the UK, PICUs have developed independently of the RSU network, and have provided a range of services in line with local circumstances and needs. This development is wholly appropriate. Units may variably describe themselves as PICUs, extra care wards, intensive care, high dependency, special care, challenging behaviour, locked wards or low secure units. None of these terms have a universally agreed definition.

Many PICUs operate in isolation not only from the main hospital wards, but also from other similar units. Zigmond (1995) commented upon his personal experiences of such facilities in his role as a Mental Health Act Commissioner and Second Opinion Appointed Doctor and described them as 'Physically apart from other inpatient facilities, containing the most seriously disturbed, invariably detained patients who were cared for by staff who rarely rotated around other settings and became brutalised and dehumanised by the constantly high levels of disturbance and violence they faced'.

Although there is very little objective data concerning the service that these units provide, three published surveys have attempted to describe the role that they fulfil. Each of these surveys had a slightly different focus.

Ford and Whiffin (1991) surveyed the 169 Health authorities in England and asked them 'about their units providing services to acutely ill clients who require close observation and frequent nursing observation' (p. 48). They identified 39 units in England which admitted in varying proportions those with acute or chronic problems such as aggression or self harm (in the setting of mental illness) and those with a forensic history.

Mitchell (1992) surveyed psychiatric hospitals in Scotland to determine the numbers and characteristics of their patients. He identified 13 PICUs in Scotland with a total of 219 beds (3% of total inpatient psychiatric beds). Two-thirds of patients were compulsorily detained, half were under 30 years of age; schizophrenia was the most common diagnosis and co-morbid substance abuse/personality disorder was present in 10% of the under 30s.

Beer *et al* (1997) identified 110 PICUs in the UK, 45 of which had been operational for less than 3 years. Eleven units were intensive care areas of 4–5 beds which formed part of acute admission wards, 18 units were mixed PICU/challenging behaviour or PICU/forensic. The remainder were dedicated PICUs. Bed occupancy rates were high: at the 100% level particularly in the larger dedicated units. There was a wide variation in the level of security provided, ranging from 11 units which were built to medium secure specifications or above through to the 22 units which did not have permanently locked doors. Operational policies also differed widely, with many staff feeling that they might as well not have, for example, an admissions policy, because it was frequently overridden in order to accommodate a difficult patient who could not be placed elsewhere. Units accepted patients from acute psychiatric wards, prisons, RSUs and special hospitals, and the community, in various combinations. Sixty-three units were willing to admit informal patients and this was irrespective of whether the door was permanently locked or not. The terminology used to describe the patient group who were admitted was confusing. There is no accepted cut off point between acute and chronic disturbance or between intensive care and challenging behaviour. The point at which a patient is described as 'forensic' is similarly blurred. Medical staffing was also highly variable. Only 30 units had a dedicated consultant psychiatrist with no other inpatient beds. An equal number of units could be accessed by a number of consultants, none of whom had overall responsibility for the daily functioning of the unit. Junior doctors posts were not exclusively filled by experienced Registrars; over half the units accepted rotational Senior House Officers, often with no supervision from a more experienced staff grade doctor or Senior Registrar. Multidisciplinary team working was less developed than in general adult psychiatry and written guidelines or policies covering high risk areas such as rapid tranquilisation, control and restraint and seclusion were often absent confirming the informal observations of Zigmond (1995). The implications of these findings have been further developed by Pereira *et al* (1999).

Psychiatric intensive care, as a specialty in its own right, is only beginning to have an identity. The National Association of Psychiatric and Low Secure Units (NAPICU) has been formed as an organisation which can provide guidance on PICU issues in the UK.

Aims of NAPICU

- To advance PICU/low secure service.

- To discuss and improve mechanisms for the delivery of PICU/low secure care.

- To encourage the support of staff working in PICU/low secure services.

- To audit the effectiveness of the service provided.

- To organise educational opportunities for staff.

Unlike the standard services provided by the RSUs, PICUs have developed independently of each other. They seek to provide a service to fulfil local needs. It is therefore impossible to be prescriptive regarding the exact role of any individual PICU, although certain criteria should be broadly filled. Patients should be too disturbed to be nursed on open wards (because of aggression, self-harming behaviour or absconding). There is, therefore, a need for increased nursing and multi-professional input and perimeter security. Admissions and discharges should be governed by symptoms and behaviour and not by the courts (Dix 1996).

DEFINITION OF PSYCHIATRIC INTENSIVE CARE

There is no commonly accepted definition of psychiatric intensive care.

However three features should ideally be present in an PICU. Two of them have parallels with the general medicine ICU; one is unique to psychiatry.

Firstly, there is the 'intensive' level of care delivered by professionals. This results in both quantitative and qualitative differences from general psychiatric care. The need for increased speed of response is a key element. In terms of nursing, the nurse:patient ratios will be higher than on general wards because of the increased need for monitoring patients exhibiting increased levels of aggression or self harm, and observing those on large amounts of medication, e.g. for side-effects. Medical staff will also need to be present more often than on general wards because of the need to assess patients rapidly and reach working diagnoses, to formulate and to monitor management plans and to prescribe and review medication. Qualitatively, nursing staff require special training in some areas of expertise such as the management of aggression. Medical staff will need training in the use of medication. The presence of a senior doctor (MRCPsych) on most days will be required to supervise trainees. This parallels the daily consultant ward round on a medical ICU. Because patients are often locked in and disturbed, they will need more in terms of occupational input and therapeutic activity. Social needs require social workers. Psychological, emotional and behavioural concerns will require a clinical psychologist. Medication issues require the active participation of pharmacists. In addition, all team members need to meet regularly together to discuss all patients.

Secondly, there is a need for more facilities than on a general psychiatric ward. There are more facilities on a medical ICU and these are often 'high-tech'. On a PICU resources and facilities will be both environmental and human: more space, a garden, a quiet area, a seclusion suite, snoezelen area, activity and games room are all possible requirements. Just as the patient on a medical ICU is deemed to be in need of special care, so the psychiatric patient often has multiple and complex needs which require extra resources. In human resource terms there will be a need for a multidisciplinary team to address these needs.

Thirdly, in contrast to a medical ICU, psychiatric intensive care generally entails a degree of security which is known as low secure (Department of Health and Home Office 1992). This may be a locked area on a ward, a lockable door, a locked setting, or even an electronically operated ward with air locks. PICUs may be permanently locked or just lockable, but they are not absolutely secure settings which can guarantee containment. Admissions from courts or prisons should not be considered if absconding carries serious risk to the public. Behaviours driven by symptoms of mental illness should govern admission, not a court's requirements for security. Such patients should generally be dealt with by the RSUs.

CONCLUSION

Psychiatric intensive care is at the cutting edge of clinical psychiatry. It is a developing specialty. Patients are often very unwell and behaviourally disturbed. This book seeks to address the principles and practice of meeting the needs of this group of patients.

REFERENCES

Basson JV, Woodside M. 1981 Assessment of a secure/intensive care/forensic ward. Acta Psychiat Scand 64: 132–141

Beer MD, Paton C, Pereira S. 1997 Hot beds of general psychiatry: a national survey of psychiatric intensive care units. Psychiatr Bull 21: 142–144

Bluglass R. 1976 The design of security units, the type of patient and behaviour patterns. Hosp Engineering pp. 5–7

CMO's update 1996 London Department of Health quoted. In: P. Snowden, Regional Secure Units and Forensic Services eds R Bluglass, P Bowden. Principles and Practice of Forensic Psychiatry London: Churchill Livingstone 1990, p. 1379

Coid JW. 1991a A survey of patients from five health districts receiving special care in the private sector. Psychiatr Bull 15: 257–262

Coid JW. 1991b Difficult to place patients. The game of pass the parcel must stop. Br Med J 32: 603–604

Crain PM, Jordan EG. 1979 The psychiatric intensive care unit – an in-hospital treatment of violent adult patients. Bull Am Acad Psychiatry Law V11(2): 190–198

Cripps J, Duffield G, James D. 1995 Bridging the gap in secure provision: evaluation of a new local combined locked forensic/intensive care unit. J Forensic Psychiatry 6: 77–91

Department of Health and Home Office. 1992 Review of Health and Social Services for Mentally Disordered Offenders and other Requiring Similar Services. (Reed Report). London: DoH/Home Office

Department of Health and Social Services. 1974 Revised Report for the Working Party on Security in NHS Psychiatric Hospitals (Glancy Report). London: DHSS

Dix R. 1996 An investigation into patients presenting a challenge to Gloucestershire's Mental Health Care Services. Gloucestershire Health Authority

Faulk M. 1995 Basic Forensic Psychiatry, 2nd edn. Oxford: Blackwell

Ford I, Whiffin M 1991 The role of the psychiatric ICU. Nursing Times 87(51): 47–49

Goldney R et al 1985 The psychiatric intensive care unit. Br J Psychiatry 146: 50–54

Home Office, Department of Health and Social Security. 1975 Committee on Mentally Abnormal Offenders (Butler Report). London: HMSO

James AJ, Smith J, Hoogkamer R, Laing J, Donovan M. 1996 Minimum and Medium security: the interface: use of Section 17 trial leave. Psychiatr Bull 20: 201–204

Jones K. 1993 Asylums and After. A Revised History of the Mental Health Services: From the Early 18th Century to the 1900s. London: Athlone Press

McKenna J. 1996 In-patient characteristics in a regional secure unit. Psychiatr Bull 20: 264–268

Mental Health Act. 1959, London: HMSO

Mental Health Act Commission. 1995 Sixth Biennial Report. London: HMSO

Mitchell GD. 1992 A survey of psychiatric intensive care units in Scotland. Health Bulletin 50(3): 228–232

Mounsey N. 1979 Psychiatric intensive care. Nursing Times 1811–1813

Musisi S, Wasylenski DA, Rapp MS. 1989 A psychiatric intensive care unit in a psychiatric hospital. Can J Psychiatry 34: 200–204

Pereira S, Beer MD, Paton C. 1999 Good practice issues in psychiatric intensive care settings. Findings from a national survey. Psychiatr Bull 23: 397–400

Rachlin S. 1973 On the need for a closed ward in an open hospital: the psychiatric intensive-care unit. Hosp Community Psychiat 24: 829–833

Smith J, Parker J, Donovan M. 1990 Is the role of regional secure units changing? Psychiatr Bull 14: 713–714

Snowden P. 1990 Regional secure units and forensic service in England and Wales. In: Blueglass R, Boeden P (eds) Principles and Practice of Forensic Psychiatry. London: Churchill Livingstone, pp. 1375–1386

Turner T. 1996 Commentary on 'Guidelines for the Management of Acutely Disturbed Patients'. Adv Psychiatric Treatment 2: 200–201

Warneke L. 1986 A psychiatric intensive care unit in a general hospital setting. Can J Psychiatry 31: 834–837

Zigmond A. 1995 Special care wards: are they special? Psychiatr Bull 19: 310–312

2

MANAGEMENT OF ACUTELY DISTURBED BEHAVIOUR

M Dominic Beer, Carol Paton, Stephen M Pereira

Historically, psychiatry has been judged by its management of the 'furiously mad' (Turner 1996). In the current climate where inquiries into the care of patients are becoming increasingly common, considerable care has to be taken because of the risk of untoward incidents with acutely disturbed patients. On the one hand there is the necessity to protect the patient, their family, carers and staff from the consequences of disturbed behaviour. On the other hand there is the risk that overzealous sedation with inappropriate medication regimens might lead to physical complications for the disturbed patient. Banerjee *et al* (1995), reviewing eight cases of sudden death in detained patients, concluded that 'the risk of sudden cardiotoxic collapse in response to neuroleptic medication given during a period of high physiological arousal should be widely publicised'.

There is some evidence to suggest that the level of violence in society is rising (College Research Unit 1998) and that this is reflected in the increasing number of assaults on hospital staff. PICU staff are frequently called upon to manage patients who are violent or potentially violent. It is vital that staff work together in an informed and supported environment to minimise the potential risks to themselves and others.

Acute behavioural disturbance requires urgent intervention. It usually manifests with mood, thought or behavioural signs and symptoms and can either be transient, episodic or long lasting. It can have either a medical or psychological aetiology and may reflect a person's limited capacity to cope with social, domestic or environmental stressors. The use of illicit substances or alcohol can accompany an episode of acute disturbance, or can be causative. The acute disturbance can involve: threatened or actual violence towards others, destruction of property, emotional upset, psychological distress, active self harming behaviour, verbal abuse, hallucinatory behaviour, disinhibition, disorientation or confused behaviour and extreme physical overactivity – 'running amok'. More than one patient may be involved and everyday objects such as chairs, table knives or broken cups may be used to threaten or cause damage to others or to property.

Acutely disturbed behaviour can sometimes be anticipated. Informing patients of their detention under the Mental Health Act, denial of requests to leave hospital or enforcing medication against a patient's will are all potentially provocative actions. Disturbance can also be unpredictable. A member of staff or another patient may say or do something that is misinterpreted by a paranoid patient who then lashes out. The underlying thought processes may not be obvious to others.

Disturbed behaviour is often transient and associated with the severity of the underlying psychiatric disorder. As the illness responds to treatment, so does the behaviour. Acute disturbance can also become chronic disturbance. Such patients are often called 'challenging behaviour' and may require longer admission and a wide range of pharmacological and psychological treatments. Some patients in this group have associated cognitive deficits (e.g. head injury) or severe problems with impulse control (e.g. borderline personality disorder).

The management of patients with acutely disturbed behaviour is a high-risk activity and it is essential that this risk is recognised and addressed throughout the management hierarchy of the hospital.

The following summarises the relevant issues in PICUs:

- PICU staff should be familiar with the procedures to be followed to facilitate the safe admission of an acutely disturbed patient.

- PICU staff should be trained in risk assessment and in the prediction, prevention and management of aggression.

- The PICU should have a written policy for the management of aggression. This should include advice on psychological and pharmacological interventions and when to involve the police.

- Ward policies on aggression from patients should be communicated to them as soon as is appropriate after admission.

- Incident forms should be completed after all aggressive incidents. These incident forms should be regularly reviewed and feedback provided to staff.

- Time and resources should be provided for formal debriefing after incidents. Specialist counselling may be required for victims of serious incidents.

- Sufficient appropriately staffed units to manage disturbed behaviour should be available across all levels of security.

PREPARING THE WARD FOR THE ARRIVAL OF AN ACUTELY BEHAVIOURALLY DISTURBED PATIENT

While many patients admitted to PICUs are already well known to the service, a significant proportion will be being admitted for the first time. A standard admissions procedure will help staff to feel more in control and reduce the variability in approaches that may be seen when less experienced staff or staff unfamiliar with the ward are on duty. Such a procedure could be written in bullet point format and displayed ideally in a prominent position in the nursing office. An example is shown below.

- Ideally, the patient should have been assessed prior to admission by PICU staff and a management plan should be in place.

- All PICU nursing staff should be alerted.

- If the patient is waiting in a police vehicle, he should remain there until the PICU is ready to receive him.

- If there is no dedicated 'reception suite', ensure that the unit is safe (e.g. lock the servery, TV room etc.).

- Remove all other patients from the reception area.

- Ensure staff are prepared, e.g. that a control and restraint team is ready if required. Decide which member of staff will be talking to the patient.

- Inform medical staff and discuss any immediate requirement in advance if possible, e.g. a medical examination if the patient is already sedated or a rapid assessment if the patient is still very disturbed and requires sedation.

Nursing observations

Ideally, prior to admission, PICU staff should have assessed the patient and a clear nursing plan should be in place.

For new admissions unknown to staff, the level of nursing observations should be negotiated between the admitting doctor and the most senior nurse on duty.

The levels of observations are:

Level 1   Nominal supervision.
              Awareness of whereabouts of patient at all times.

Level 2   Close attention.
              15-minute checks plus awareness of whereabouts.

Level 3   Constant care.
              Continual presence of nursing staff for observation, but privacy granted for bathing.

Level 4   Intensive observations.
              Continual presence of nursing staff and constant direct visual observation.

On admission, it is wise to be cautious. It is easier to reduce observation levels if the patient is more settled than anticipated than to deal with the consequences of inadequate observation.

The level of nursing supervision should be determined by the multidisciplinary team and reviewed at least once each nursing shift. Nurses trained in the appropriate techniques should carry out close observation. It should be recognised that special observation can exacerbate behavioural disturbance and unobtrusive monitoring can sometimes be used effectively. Episodes of continuous observation lasting less than 72 hours have been shown to help two-thirds of patients (Shugar and Rehaluk 1990).

A sample observation policy can be found on pp. 335–36.

Mental Health Act status

Ideally the PICU should have a policy in place which clearly defines the legal status of patients who may be admitted. This should be subject to local agreement.

Some PICUs may be happy to accept informal patients, some may process all Section 136 patients and some may accept prison transfers or even Section 41 patients.

Although the Mental Health Act aims to facilitate care and not to be obstructive, it is a fact of life that PICU regimes may compromise basic human rights (Pereira *et al* 1999) while informal status may compromise the ability of staff to provide optimal care.

If patients are resisting, aggressive and refusing treatment or threatening to leave the ward and their status is still informal then the Consultant/Senior Registrar should be called to instigate formal detention under Section 2 or 3 of the Mental Health Act.

If it is immediately necessary, for example, to prevent serious injury, intramuscular medication can be given under common law (under the doctrine of necessity). Careful consideration needs to be given to this and clear documentation kept, because professionals may be open to prosecution for assault by an informal patient. A doctor may use Section 5 (2) to detain a patient or a registered mental health nurse can use Section 5 (4). However medication cannot be given against the patient's will under Section 5 – unlike those under Sections 2, 3 or 4.

For the use of control and restraint and for the use of seclusion please see Chapters 7 and 8.

Ensuring a safe environment

- There should be good visibility in all areas of the unit.
- Alarms should be within easy reach at all times.
- Staff response to alarms should be consistent.
- Movable objects should be kept to a minimum. Those that exist should be of safe size and construction.
- Structured activities should be provided e.g. gym, garden, games.

ASSESSMENT OF THE ACUTELY DISTURBED PATIENT

Staff safety

Staff on PICUs should be aware of the basic rules to be followed to reduce the risk to themselves. They should also ensure that other staff who may visit the ward on a sessional basis are aware of the rules.

- When interviewing a patient who has potential for aggressive behaviour always inform colleagues of your intentions and location.

- Try to conduct joint medical and nursing assessments to protect interviewers and to reduce stimulation to the patient.

- Ensure that there are alarms close by at all times.

- Sit at an angle to the patient at a safe distance away and in close proximity to the exit.

- Avoid interviewing with the patient between you and the door.

- Call the police if necessary.

Research performed in psychiatric intensive care units (Walker and Seifert 1994) has shown that a disproportionately high number of violent incidents are perpetrated by a few patients (two patients were responsible for 15 of the 37 violent incidents). Mortimer (1995) also showed that a few patients caused many incidents. As more staff were trained in control and restraint, the number of incidents fell. It is often very difficult to predict accurately who these perpetrators will be but patients who score heavily from the factors in the tables below should be deemed as those most at risk of disturbed behaviour.

Important factors from the patient's history, which may indicate an increased risk of violence (Royal College of Psychiatrists 1995, College Research Unit 1998) include:

- Previous violence towards others or self.

- Young male patients.

- Previous forensic history.

- Substance misuse.

- Antisocial, explosive or impulsive personality traits.

- Poor compliance with treatment or services.

- Association with a subculture prone to violence.

- Evidence of social restlessness or rootlessness.

- Presence of precipitants, e.g. loss events.

- Access to any named potential victims identified in mental state.

The following characteristics have been identified as predicting the 'potential for immediate violence/aggression' (College Research Unit 1998):

Primary characteristics

- Previous history of aggression or violence, overtly aggressive acts, forensic history.

- Hostile, threatening verbalisation, boasting of prior abuse.

- Suspicious, paranoid ideation.

- Delusions of control or hallucinations with violent content.

- Poor impulse control.

- Non-verbal expression of hostile intent such as increased motor activity, pacing, invading others personal space, angry facial expression.

- Refusal to communicate.

- Poor concentration or unclear thought processes.

- Possession of a weapon.

Secondary characteristics

- Fear, anger, anxiety and pain.

- Inappropriate and unrealistic demands.

- Exacerbation of psychotic illness particularly the changes in life events, low self estccm, vulnerability to interpersonal stress.

- Inability to verbalise feelings.

- Previous substance abuse.

Related factors and considerations

- Hypomanic excitement.

- Confusional states.

- Psychiatric or psychological motivation for problematic behaviour.

- Goal structure for aggressive/problematic behaviour.

There are also some behavioural clues which have been identified as being predictors of imminent violence (Wykes and Mezey 1994). These are mainly intuitive and include: dishevelled appearance, smell of alcohol, signs of increased physiological arousal, pacing, gesticulating and violent gestures, increased muscle tension such as clenched fists and teeth, flared nostrils, escalating volume of speech, swearing, direct threats, labile affect, and appearing frightened, confused and disorientated.

Precipitants of violent incidents on wards

- Enforcement of ward rules.
- Denial of patient's requests.
- Confrontational or irritable manner of staff.

Staff factors related to incidents

- Staff stability.
- Staff training (young untrained more likely to be victims).
- Poor leadership.
- Inadequate staff resources.

Older, more experienced staff (Hodgkinson 1985, James *et al* 1990, Carmel and Hunter 1991) and those that have been trained in the prevention and management of violence (Carmel and Hunter 1990) are less likely to be physically assaulted. Agency staff (James *et al* 1990) are more likely to be assaulted, particularly when they are unfamiliar with ward routines (Katz and Kirkland 1990). Several studies support an association between aggression and overcrowding on wards (e.g. Palmstierna *et al* 1991).

Milieu factors

- Access to weapons.
- No fresh air.
- Lack of privacy.
- Environment that is too hot or too cold.
- Uncared for environment.
- Lots of hidden corners in building.
- Overcrowding.
- Unclear staff functions.
- Unpredictable routines and structure.
- Over stimulation.
- Authoritarian conditions.

(Katz and Kirkland 1990, Palmstierna *et al* 1991, College Research Unit 1998)

Medical causes

Some medical or neurological conditions may present with disturbed behaviour and treatment of the underlying problem is vital. Such problems need to be excluded when accepting an unknown patient into the PICU. The exact screening tests required in any individual patient would depend, of course, on the clinical presentation.

Examples of medical conditions, that can present in this way are:

- Head injury with vascular lesions, especially subdural haematoma.
- Delirium tremens.
- Intoxication with illicit drugs or alcohol.
- Overdose with prescribed drugs, e.g. anticholinergics.
- Meningitis.
- Encephalitis.
- Hypoglycaemia.
- Diminished cerebral oxygenation of any aetiology, e.g. vascular, metabolic or endocrine.
- Hypertensive encephalopathy.
- Wernicke's encephalopathy.
- Temporal lobe epilepsy.
- Neoplastic conditions.
- Dementia.

On admission, or ideally prior to admission, a comprehensive history should be obtained from as many sources as possible. This may include the patient, family, police, general practitioner, social worker, community psychiatric nurse and previous notes.

Mental State Examination

Mental state examination should cover the mental state factors known to be associated with violence. These are:

- Evidence of any 'threat/control override' symptoms especially persecutory delusions and delusions of passivity.
- Emotions related to violence especially irritability, anger, hostility and suspiciousness.

- Erotomania or morbid jealousy symptoms.
- Misidentfication phenomena.
- Command hallucinations.

The severity and nature of the patient's symptoms in the acute situation often limit history taking and detailed examination of the mental state. However, this should be carried out at the first available opportunity.

In the mental state examination, special attention should be paid to the level of conciousness, attention and concentration, memory, language abnormalities, mood and affect. Brief and quantifiable tests such as the mini mental state examination can be useful for monitoring the progress of such patients (Folstein *et al* 1975). Signs of acute organic brain syndrome (delirium) should be suspected until proven otherwise if the following are present:

- Disorientation (especially if worse at night).
- Clouding of conciousness.
- Abnormal vital signs.
- No previous psychiatric history (especially if over 40 years old).
- Visual hallucinations.

Other signs and symptoms would include: an acute onset (hours to days), a reversed sleep–wake cycle, labile mood, shifting delusions, disjointed thoughts, poor attention and impaired memory.

SUICIDE RISK

Some patients are admitted to PICUs because they pose a risk to themselves. The PICU does not offer significant advantages over open acute wards in the management of many suicidal patients. However, in those patients where absconding from the ward in order to self-harm is potentially problematic, then the locked door of the PICU confers additional protection. There are predictors of suicide specific to different diagnostic groups of patients:

Depression

- Male.
- Older.
- Single.
- Separated.

- Socially isolated.

- Previous deliberate self-harm/suicide attempt.

- Insomnia/hypersomnia.

- Self neglect.

- Memory impairment.

- Agitation.

- Guilt.

- Bleakness about the future.

- Severe depression.

Schizophrenia

- Male.

- Younger.

- Socially isolated.

- Unemployed.

- Previous deliberate self-harm/suicide attempt.

- Depressive episode.

- Severe and relapsing illness.

- Insight and fear of deterioration in mental state.

Alcohol problems

- Male.

- Age 40–60 years.

- Depression.

- Previous deliberate self-harm/suicide attempt.

- Bereavement.

- Poor physical health.

Management of acutely disturbed behaviour

Attempts should be made to prevent violence by using de-escalation techniques. The key points are (adapted from College Research Unit 1998):

- Stay a safe distance from the patient and within easy access to alarms and escape routes.

- Stay calm, avoid sudden movements and explain your intentions clearly and confidently.

- Engage the patient in conversation and try to reason.

- If reasoning fails, consider other interventions depending on circumstances.

Turner (1996) states that there is a 'key need for much better audit and research of acute treatment approaches' in the management of acutely disturbed behaviour. All PICUs should have a written policy for the management of such patients. An example of such a policy is shown in Figure 2.1.

Detailed discussion of pharmacological management can be found in Chapter 5. Time out, seclusion and control and restraint are discussed in detail in Chapters 7 and 8.

MANAGEMENT AFTER AN AGGRESSIVE INCIDENT/DEBRIEFING

After all aggressive incidents formal debriefing should be offered, focusing on practical and emotional issues at the time although there is some controversy about the effectiveness of debriefing (Rick *et al* 1998), victims need sympathy, support and reassurance. For professionals who are assaulted it is advisable for them to return to work as soon as possible to prevent 'the incubation of fear'. Usually the team working at the time of the incident is sufficient to deal with the debriefing. However, in the case of very serious incidents it may be useful to have an external person to ensure that sufficient counselling is provided, particularly to anyone who has sustained significant physical or emotional injury. At the time of a serious aggressive incident, immediate safety issues must take precedence over any investigation. The latter should attempt, as sensitively as possible, to compile detailed reports of the incident so as to understand its causes, context and consequences.

The following may act as an *aide-mémoire* for those who are either directly involved in an aggressive incident or who may be required to support colleagues (for further reading, see Wykes and Mezey 1994):

Dealing with the aftermath of an incident if you are the victim

- Acknowledge that you may experience some symptoms of stress and be aware that these may be delayed for several hours.

- Do not become helpless, be explicit about what you want or do not want in the way of support.

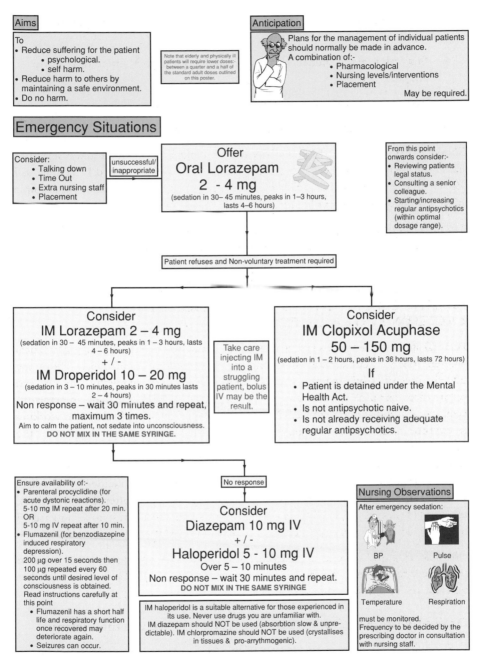

Aims

To
- Reduce suffering for the patient
  - psychological.
  - self harm.
- Reduce harm to others by maintaining a safe environment.
- Do no harm.

Note that elderly and physically ill patients will require lower doses:- between a quarter and a half of the standard adult doses outlined on this poster.

Anticipation

Plans for the management of individual patients should normally be made in advance. A combination of:-
- Pharmacological
- Nursing levels/interventions
- Placement

May be required.

Emergency Situations

Consider:
- Talking down
- Time Out
- Extra nursing staff
- Placement

unsuccessful/ inappropriate

Offer Oral Lorazepam 2 - 4 mg
(sedation in 30– 45 minutes, peaks in 1–3 hours, lasts 4–6 hours)

From this point onwards consider:-
- Reviewing patients legal status.
- Consulting a senior colleague.
- Starting/increasing regular antipsychotics (within optimal dosage range).

Patient refuses and Non-voluntary treatment required

Consider IM Lorazepam 2 – 4 mg
(sedation in 30 – 45 minutes, peaks in 1 – 3 hours, lasts 4 – 6 hours)
+ / -
IM Droperidol 10 – 20 mg
(sedation in 3 – 10 minutes, peaks in 30 minutes lasts 2 – 4 hours)
Non response – wait 30 minutes and repeat, maximum 3 times.
Aim to calm the patient, not sedate into unconsciousness.
DO NOT MIX IN THE SAME SYRINGE.

Take care injecting IM into a struggling patient, bolus IV may be the result.

Consider IM Clopixol Acuphase 50 – 150 mg
(sedation in 1 – 2 hours, peaks in 36 hours, lasts 72 hours)
If
- Patient is detained under the Mental Health Act.
- Is not antipsychotic naive.
- Is not already receiving adequate regular antipsychotics.

Ensure availability of:-
- Parenteral proclidine (for acute dystonic reactions). 5-10 mg IM repeat after 20 min. OR 5-10 mg IV repeat after 10 min.
- Flumazenil (for benzodiazepine induced respiratory depression). 200 µg over 15 seconds then 100 µg repeated every 60 seconds until desired level of consciousness is obtained. Read instructions carefully at this point
  - Flumazenil has a short half life and respiratory function once recovered may deteriorate again.
  - Seizures can occur.

No response

Consider Diazepam 10 mg IV
+ / -
Haloperidol 5 - 10 mg IV
Over 5 – 10 minutes
Non response – wait 30 minutes and repeat.
DO NOT MIX IN THE SAME SYRINGE

IM haloperidol is a suitable alternative for those experienced in its use. Never use drugs you are unfamiliar with. IM diazepam should NOT be used (absorbtion slow & unpredictable). IM chlorpromazine should NOT be used (crystallises in tissues & pro-arrythmogenic).

Nursing Observations

After emergency sedation:

BP   Pulse

Temperature   Respiration

must be monitored. Frequency to be decided by the prescribing doctor in consultation with nursing staff.

Figure 2.1 – Management of acutely disturbed patients (from Oxleas NHS Trust, with permission)

- Do not blame yourself. Try and learn from the experience.

- Try to return to work soon.

- Accept the necessary management investigations.

- Follow procedures carefully.

- Ensure that you get support, both formal and informal.

What colleagues and friends can do

- At the time, give the victim unconditional reassurance.

- Show that you are willing to talk at any time.

- Reassure the victim's family and ensure that the victim is not left alone after work. For example, offer a lift home.

- Help the victim to assimilate the experience and keep a sense of proportion, bearing in mind the nearly universal problem of unrealistic guilt.

- Do not treat victims as if they have an infectious disease (they do report being ignored).

What teams and ward managers can do

- Consider the need both for support and debriefing.

- Allow time to talk as a group.

- Consider what worked well/went wrong and how to prevent/deal with similar incidents in the future.

- Consider the feelings involved and make sure you have a chance to express them.

- Act on any suggestions which come out of the post-incident debriefing, given the tendency of organisations to experience denial after traumatic events.

Whether to charge a patient after an incident

This is often a very difficult decision and it may require considerable time and effort on the part of the clinical team to even persuade the local police service to interview the patient. It is essential that the multidisciplinary team have a view on whether to press charges and there will be issues for the victim if he or she is part of the clinical team. He or she will need the support of colleagues because there may be emotions such as guilt, which needs to be worked through. Factors that may influence the team's decision to press charges may include:

- The patient's mental state.
- The capacity of the patient to form intent.
- The degree of harm inflicted.
- The likely effect on the patient.
- Perceived need for more secure placement.

Advantages of charges being pressed include

- The possible therapeutic effect for the patient who may understand the concept and value of boundaries.
- The responsibility for managing difficult behaviour is shared with the Court/Criminal Justice System professionals.
- The patient may get a criminal record/hospital order/restriction order, which will alert others to possible danger in the future.
- Resources may be more forthcoming for the treatment of such a patient.
- Formal documentation of an incident is made.
- The patient has the opportunity to defend himself if he feels wrongly accused.
- It may increase the chance of compensation for the victim.

Further discussion of this subject is in Chapter 12. The Interface with Forensic Services.

'Trust-wide' issues regarding management of disturbed behaviour

- The PICU should have policies on the management of aggression.
- Staff should be trained in the management of aggression.
- Incident forms should be completed for all aggressive incidents.
- These incident forms should be regularly analysed and feedback provided to staff.
- Time and resources should be available for formal debriefing after incidents.
- Time and resources should be provided for specialist counselling of those victims of a serious incident.

- The MDT should be expected to confront and counsel patients who exhibit repeated episodes of disturbed behaviour.

- Ward policies on aggression designed for patients should be communicated to them as soon as appropriate after admission.

- Anger management groups should be provided for patients.

- Ensure that staff understand and have experience in risk assessment.

- Ensure that there is good cooperation between health and social services.

- Ensure that there is good record keeping and communication between community and in-patient facilities.

- Ensure that there are sufficient units to manage disturbed behaviour, e.g. intensive care units which are well staffed and arrange training of staff (ENB 956 Clinical Course) in the assessment and management of the acutely disturbed patient.

Leadership is essential. Basic skills in risk assessment and confidence in the management of disturbed behaviour are core skills that should be shared by all staff working in PICU.

CONCLUSION

This chapter has shown that there are many factors to the effective management of the acutely disturbed patient. It is essential that services are planned, resourced and supported to ensure the safety of the patients and staff in acute mental health services.

REFERENCES

Atakan Z. 1995 Violence on psychiatric in-patient units: what can be done? Psychiatric Bulletin 19: 593–596

Banerjee S, Bingley W, Murphy E. 1995 Deaths of Detained Patients: A Review of Reports to the Mental Health Act Commission. London: Mental Health Act Foundation

Carmel H, Hunter M. 1990 Compliance with training in managing assaultative behaviour and injuries from inpatient violence. Hospital & Community Psychiatry 41: 558–560

Carmel H, Hunter M. 1991 Psychiatrists injured by patient attack. Bulletin of the American Academy of Psychiatry and the Law 19: 309–316

College Research Unit. 1998 Management of imminent violence: Clinical Practice Guidelines to Support Mental Health Services. Occasional Paper 41, Royal College of Psychiatrists, London

Folstein MF, Folstein SE, McHugh PR. 1975 'Mini-Mental State': a practical method for grading the cognitive state of patients for the Clinician. J Psychiatr Res 12: 189

Hodgkinson P, McIvor L, Phillips M. 1985 Patient Assaults on Staff in a Psychiatric Hospital. A Two Year Retrospective Study. Medicine Science and the Law 28: 288–294

James DV, Fineberg NA, Shah AK, Priest RG. 1990 An increase in violence on an acute psychiatric ward: A study of associated factors. Br J Psych 156: 846–852

Katz P, Kirkland FR. 1990 Violence and social structure on mental hospital wards. Psychiatry, 53: 262–277

Macpherson R, Anstee B and Dix R. 1996 Guidelines for the management of acutely disturbed patients. Advances in Psychiatric Treatment 2: 194–199

Mortimer A. 1995 Reducing violence on a secure ward. Psychiatric Bulletin 19: 605–698

Noble P, Rodger S. 1989 Violence by psychiatric in-patients. Br J Psych 155: 384–390

Palmstierna T, Huitfeldt B, Wistedt B. 1991 The relationship of crowding and aggressive behaviour on a psychiatric intensive care unit. Hospital and Community Psychiatry 42: 1237–1240

Pereira S, Beer D, Paton C. 1999 Good practice issues in psychiatric intensive care units: findings from a national survey. Psychiatric Bulletin 23: 397–404

Powell G, Caan W, Crowe M. 1994 What events precede violent incidents in psychiatric hospitals? Br J Psych 165: 107–112

Rick J, Perryman S, Young K. 1998 Workplace Trauma and its management HSE books, London

Shugar G, Rehaluk R. 1990 Continuous observation for psychiatric inpatients: A critical evaluation. Compr Psychiatry 30: 48–55

The Royal College of Psychiatrists. 1993 Consensus Statement on the use of High-Dose Antipsychotic Medication. Council Report CR26: Royal College of Psychiatrists, London

The Royal College of Psychiatrists. 1995 Strategies for the Management of Disturbed and Violent Patients in Psychiatric Units. CR41. London: Royal College of Psychiatrists

The Royal College of Psychiatrists. 1997 The Association between Antipsychotic Drugs and Sudden Death. Report of the Working Group of the Royal College of Psychiatrists' Psychopharmacology Sub-Group, Council Report CR57. London: Royal College of Psychiatrists

Torpy D, Hall M. 1995 Violent incidents in a secure unit. Journal of Forensic Psychiatry 4: 517–544

Turner T. 1996 Commentary on 'Guidelines for the Management of Acutely Disturbed Patients'. Advances in Psychiatric Treatment 2: 200–201

Walker Z, Seifert R. 1994 Violent incidents in a Psychiatric Intensive Care Unit. Br J Psych 164: 826–828

Whittington R, Wykes T. 1994 An observational study of associations between nurse behaviour and violence in psychiatric hospitals. Journal of Psychiatric and Mental Health Nursing 1: 85–92

Whittington R, Wykes T. 1996 Aversive stimulation by staff and violence by psychiatric patients. Br J Clinical Psychology 35: 11–20

Wykes T, Mezey G. 1994 Counselling for victims of violence in violence and health care professionals. In: T. Wykes (ed) London: Chapman & Hall

3

DE-ESCALATION TECHNIQUES

Roland Dix

The past 15 years have seen a dramatic increase in attempts to investigate the nature of in-patient aggression (Whittington 1994). With aggressive behaviour being better understood, attention has turned more recently towards prediction and early intervention to reduce the incidents of physical assault (Cheung *et al* 1997). The process of de-escalating aggression is being recognised as an important skill for health care professionals (Leadbetter and Paterson 1995). Stevenson (1991) defined de-escalation as a 'complex, interactive process in which a patient is redirected towards a calmer personal space'. Becoming competent at de-escalation is in itself a sophisticated activity requiring much more than just a theoretical understanding of aggression. It cannot be considered in purely academic terms. The practitioner must undertake a developmental process, resulting in highly evolved self awareness enabling the skills of de-escalation to become instinctive.

The psychiatric intensive care unit (PICU) has an unavoidable role in setting limits to disturbed behaviour and thus is an excellent location for development and practice of de-escalation. Boettcher (1983), Kaplan and Wheeler (1983), McHugh and West (1995) and Turnbull *et al* (1990), for example, have proposed models of de-escalation. These models have much to offer the PICU although they do not specifically address the PICU patient. Experience in the PICU suggests three basic components for effective face-to-face de-escalation. They are: assessment of the immediate situation, communication skills designed to facilitate co-operation and tactics aimed at problem solving. This chapter will bring together all these components and to demonstrate their practical value within the context of the PICU. The model for de-escalation offered here is in daily use in a PICU and has shown good efficacy.

COMPONENT 1. ASSESSMENT OF THE AGGRESSIVE INCIDENT

Many studies have considered in-patient violence in terms of a behavioural expression of underlying psychopathology (Betempts *et al* 1993). Correlations between aggression with symptom profiles, diagnosis and other demographic details have been suggested (Davis 1991). An understanding of these factors is useful to the practitioner of de-escalation, but it does not provide the most practical theoretical framework. Situational analysis is a much more useful basis from which to consider de-escalation. To support this line of reasoning Cheung *et al* (1997) concluded that 69.9% of inpatient assaults (n=332) were precipitated by interaction with staff. There is also good evidence that issues such as administering medication, prevention of absconding and limit setting, all common in the PICU, are often the start of aggressive escalation (Blair 1991, Bensley *et al* 1995).

Frude (1989) suggested a model for the situational analysis of an aggressive incident. The model describes a progression of five factors through which aggression can result. This is illustrated in Figure 3.1.

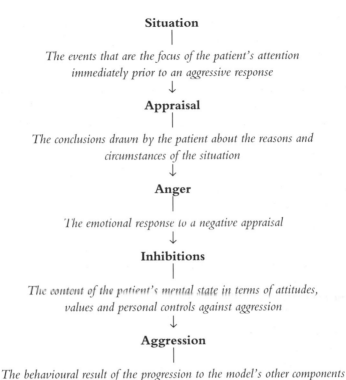

Situation

|

The events that are the focus of the patient's attention
immediately prior to an aggressive response

↓

Appraisal

|

The conclusions drawn by the patient about the reasons and
circumstances of the situation

↓

Anger

|

The emotional response to a negative appraisal

↓

Inhibitions

|

The content of the patient's mental state in terms of attitudes,
values and personal controls against aggression

↓

Aggression

|

The behavioural result of the progression to the model's other components

Figure 3.1 – Situational analysis of an aggressive incident

Within the context of the PICU, a common example of the model's application is as follows:

Situation

A detained patient requests to leave the PICU unescorted to go to the local shop. The clinical assessment and conditions of Section 17 of the Mental Health Act require a nurse escort. This is communicated to the patient.

Appraisal

The patient appraises this as punitive action by the staff in which his freedom is being restricted without therapeutic reason.

Anger

Frustration results from an inability to control this situation. The emotional result is a feeling of anger.

Inhibitions

The patient is suffering with mild manic symptoms resulting in a degree of grandiosity. He has a poor tolerance to his needs not being immediately met.

Aggression

He is verbally abusive to the staff member and kicks the unit entrance several times.

The above is an example of the model's application to a common PICU event. It can also be applied to many other situations that occur in the PICU, e.g. offering unwanted medication, etc. When interacting with the potentially aggressive patient, the practitioner of de-escalation should attempt to make a rapid assessment of the incident's components. During handovers and at other times when aggressive incidents are discussed, the incident in the example could have been simply described as 'the patient became aggressive because he could not go to the shop'. The application of Frude's model allows this situation to be more thoroughly interrogated resulting in a superior level of description. Through a comprehensive understanding of the incident, intervention may be applied at each point, attempting to derail the journey from event to aggression. This may be achieved by the use of specific communication skills in combination with de-escalation tactics.

COMPONENT 2. COMMUNICATION

It is not possible to set out a list of communication skills the cold application of which will de-escalate an aggressive patient. The communication skills set out here are merely tools that are to be used by the practitioner and moulded by their individual style and personality. The content of communication with an aggressive patient needs to appear genuine and sincere and not just a regurgitation of artificial techniques. A successful de-escalation will be firmly based within the principles of the therapeutic relationship.

Non-verbal communication principles

- Position your body so that you are communicating at an angle that is not confronting.

- Be aware of your body posture. Avoid postures that may appear authoritarian or defensive, e.g. folded arms or hands on hips.

- Attempt to communicate at the same height as the patient, i.e. standing or sitting. Being sat down during de-escalation is sometimes useful in appearing non-threatening. However, this may place the staff member at increased risk if physical assault actually occurs.

- Be aware of your facial expression, ensuring that it reflects what you are saying verbally.

- Comfortable proximity between individuals during communication may be approximately 1 metre. This may need to be increased at least 3-fold in response to escalating verbal aggression (Lanza 1988). As the intensity of the aggressive responses diminishes then the distance can be reduced accordingly.

- Avoid the temptation to use a reassuring touch early in the de-escalation process. As the situation calms, look for non-verbal and verbal cues suggesting permission to touch.

- Be aware of the use of eye contact. Maintain eye contact in the same way as if you were communicating with a non-aggressive person. Avoid intimidating stares. Good use of eye contact will communicate genuineness and confidence.

Verbal communication principles

- Use a calm, warm and clear tone of voice as a general principle. Voice tone may be altered as appropriate to reflect energy in the conversation (see Mood matching below).

- If a rapport is not already present, personalise yourself as quickly as possible, e.g. appropriate self disclosure. This will help to increase inhibitions against assault.

- In the early phase of de-escalation, ask for specific acts, avoiding long, complicated statements, e.g. 'Let's sit down and discuss what you need'.

- Avoid personal confrontation by remaining focused on the issues at hand, ignoring personally directed attack.

- In the early phase of de-escalation avoid being selective with your attention to the issues the patient is verbalising. Deal with what appears to be the main problem, even if this is uncomfortable.

- Avoid 'passing the buck'. Show yourself to be someone in a position to problem solve. Even if this means after initial de-escalation others are needed to resolve the issue.

- Avoid using jargon.

- Highlight the impact of the patient's behaviour, showing they are being listened to, e.g. 'You are scaring people with your shouting'. Statements of this kind can help to demonstrate that the patient is making an impact and thus diminish the need for further escalation.

- Reinforce your position as a helper rather than a restricter.

- Keep the communication fluid and attentive to the content of the problem. Mood matching is useful in achieving this. This is where the energy in the discussion is temporarily matched by the staff member, e.g. by facial expression or raising the energy in your voice (for further explanation see Davis 1989)

- There are limits to what can be achieved verbally. Remain astute to the progress made towards de-escalation. It may not be possible to return the patient to a state of complete calm. If the expressed aggression has significantly reduced, then be prepared to disengage rather than risk re-escalation. Avoid the need to have the last word.

COMPONENT 3. DE-ESCALATION AND NEGOTIATION: THE TACTICS

To suggest that the activity of de-escalation involves the use of tactics may be inappropriately interpreted as a lack of genuineness. However, many aggressive responses have areas of commonality; thus it is useful to hold a set of general de-escalating tactics that may be modified to suit the situation.

The win–lose equation

Many of the situations that may lead to aggression involve a perceived conflict of interests between the patient and staff member. A drama is often enacted where one part is left with a feeling of loss and frustration. This general issue has been tackled by management theorists and has been described by Le Poole (1987) as the win–lose equation. In essence a win or lose scenario is created. It is the objective of the de-escalator to as far as it is possible, negotiate a win–win situation. Figure 3.2 illustrates that basic situation.

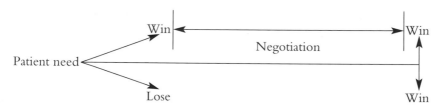

Figure 3.2 – The win–lose/win–win equation

A common situation in which a PICU patient may enter into the win or lose scenario is negotiating with a patient to accept unwanted medication. If the patient is given the medication against his will, then he feels he has lost and the staff have won, and aggression may result. Through the process of negotiation, a win–win is sought. One method of achieving this is, during the process of negotiation, offer the patient choices over which he has control. In the case of the unwanted medication, an example would be to offer the patient time to consider the benefits of medication, and then to return to you with his decision. This is usually employed in the latter stages of de-escalation. The overall tactic is to create a feeling of empowerment (real or perceived) for the patient. Experience of using this tactic shows that in many cases the patient will return with a statement like 'OK I will take it this time, but I want to speak to the doctor again before I take any more'.

Debunking

This is the process of debunking the patient's need to make his point by the use of aggression. This may be achieved by unconditionally accepting the content of the patient's grievance (Maier 1996). For example, a patient makes that statement, 'I am bloody sick of being locked up here, just let me go home'. A debunking response may be, 'I don't blame you, I would feel frustrated too, let's sit down and discuss what is needed for you to go home'. The general principle here is to shift the patient's focus from confrontation to discussion. This tactic is particularly usefully in the early stages of de-escalation as a means of grabbing the patient's attention and confidence.

Aligning goals

A frequent precipitant to aggressive escalation is a perceived state of affairs where the patient feels he has completely different goals to the staff. Examples of this include preventing a patient from leaving, the need to take medication and limit setting with disturbed behaviour. It is very easy to reinforce this perception by maintaining a linear focus on the issue of confrontation. If we look at the wider issues there may be far more common ground than there first appears. For example, the patient wishing to leave may feel in confrontation with the staff who are preventing him from doing so. During the de-escalation the staff may align these goals by saying, 'I want you to go home too, success for us is when you have no need for hospital, we are working towards this from the day you are admitted'.

Transactional analysis

The use of Berne's (1964) Transactional Analysis (TA) can be a useful strategy for de-escalating aggression (Farrell and Grey 1992). This involves a detailed understanding of three different contexts within which interaction takes place. These are defined by Berne as 'ego states' and during social intercourse they are in the form of either the Parental, Adult or Child context. During the course of de-escalation the basic idea is to ensure that the ego state within which the de-escalator is interacting is complementary to the patient's ego state. TA is a large area of study in itself and courses in its use are recommended.

CONCLUSION

The model of de-escalation offered here comprises three separate but interdependent components: Assessment, Communication and Tactics (ACT). The ACT model should be considered as cyclic, requiring the de-escalator to remain fluid during de-escalation. During the course of de-escalation, it is necessary continually to revisit each component and to ensure they remain complementary to each other. This is illustrated in Figure 3.3.

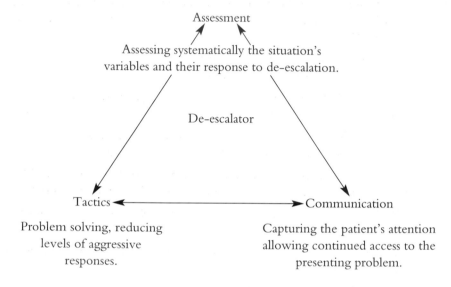

Figure 3.3 – The ACT model

Under each of the headings, tools have been suggested which experience has shown to be effective in the PICU setting. The list is by no means exhaustive, and each practitioner can modify the suggested tools to suit their own individual styles. In this chapter de-escalation has focused on the content of situations, rather than the psychopathology of the patient. There is good evidence that many aggressive responses are indeed precipitated by situations rather than driven by purely psychiatric symptoms (Poyner and Warne 1986, Whittington and Patterson 1996, McDougall 1997). In many situations, psychotic and other psychiatric phenomena no doubt play a part in the aggressive responses of patients. However, in many cases these can be considered as one of many variables that need to be incorporated into the ACT model of de-escalation.

Training in the management of aggression has demonstrated its value in significantly reducing the incidents of physical assault (Infantino and Musingo 1985). In the PICU however, it may have to be accepted that while de-escalation training will reduce the number of violent incidents, physical assaults and the ultimate use of restraint as a last resort may be unavoidable (Parkes 1996).

REFERENCES

Bensley L, Nelson N, Kaufman J, Silverstein B, Shield J. 1995 Patient and staff views of factors influencing assaults on psychiatric hospital employees. Issues in Mental Health Nursing, no. 16 pp. 433–446

Berne E. 1964 Games people play: The Psychology of Human Relationships. Harmondsworth. Penguin

Betempts E, Somoza E, Buncher C. 1993 Hospital characteristics, diagnoses, and staff reasons associated with the use of seclusion and restraint. Hospital and Community psychiatry. 44: 367–361.

Blair D. 1991 Assaultive behaviour: does provocation begin in the front office? J Psychosocial Nursing Mental Health Services, 29: 21–26

Boettcher E. 1983 Preventing violent behaviour: an integrated theoretical model for nursing. Perspectives in Psychiatric Care 21: 54–58

Cheung P, Schweitzer I, Tuckwell V, Crowley K. 1997 A prospective study of assaults on staff by psychiatric in patients. Med Sci Law 37(1); 46–52

Davis W. 1989 The prevention of assault on professional helpers. In: Clinical Approaches of Violence, eds: Howells K, Hollin C. Chichester: Wiley, 311–328

Davis S. 1991 Violence by psychiatric inpatients: a review. Hospital and Community Psychiatry, 42(6): 585–589

Farrell G, Gray C. 1992 Aggression: A Nurse's Guide to Therapeutic Management. London: Scutari Press

Frude N. 1989 The physical abuse of children. In: Clinical Approaches to Violence, eds: Howells K, Hollin C. Chichester: Wiley, 155–181

Infantino J, Musingo S. 1985 Assaults and injuries among staff with and without training in aggression control techniques. Hospital and Community Psychiatry 36(12): 1312–1314

Kaplan S, Wheeler E. 1983 Survival skills for working with potentially violent clients. J Contemp Social Work 339–346

Leadbetter D, Paterson B. 1995 De-escalating aggressive behaviour. In: Management of Violence and Aggression in Health Care eds Kidd B, Atark C. London: Gaskell, 49–84

Lanza M. 1988 Factors relevant to patient assault. Issues in Mental Health Nursing 9: 259–270

Le Poole S. 1987 Never Take No for An Answer: A Guide to Successful Negotiation, London: Kogan Page

Maier G. 1996 Managing threatening behaviour. The role of talk down and talk up. J Psychosocial Nursing 34(6): 25–30

McDougall T. 1997 Coercive interventions: the notion of the 'last resort'. Psychiatric Care 4: 19–21

McHugh I, West M. 1995 Handle with care. Nursing Times, 91(6): 62–63

Parkes J. 1996 Control and restraint training: a study of its effectiveness in a medium secure unit. J Forensic Psychiatry, 7(3): 525 534

Poyner B, Warne C. 1986 Violence to Staff: A Basis for Assessment and Intervention. London: HMSO

Stevenson S. 1991 Heading off violence with verbal de-escalation. J Psychosocial Nursing Mental Health Services 36: 6–10

Turnball J, Aiken I, Black L, Patterson B. 1990 Turn it around. Short-term management for aggression and anger. J Psychosocial Nursing 28(6): 7–10

Whittington R. 1994 Violence in psychiatric hospitals. In: Violence and Health Care Professionals, ed Wykes T. Chapman & Hall: London, 23–43

Whittington R, Patterson P. 1996 Verbal and non-verbal behaviour immediately prior to aggression by mentally disordered people: enhancing assessment of risk. J Psychiatric Mental Health Nursing 3: 47–54

4

RAPID TRANQUILISATION

Caroline L Holmes, Helen Simmons, Lyn S Pilowsky

INTRODUCTION

Violence is a continuing problem in both inpatient and outpatient psychiatry. Past authors have concluded that violence is no more likely in the psychiatric population than the general population, but there is an increasing consensus that people with psychotic illnesses are more likely to exhibit violence in the community (Mullen 1988, Monahan 1992, Mulvey 1994, Swanson et al 1996).

Violence in the psychiatric setting may be acute, as seen in a severely disturbed patient with paranoid schizophrenia or mania, or ongoing, as seen in-patients who are chronically psychotic or those with personality disorders. In the UK, the acutely violent patient should ideally be treated in a Psychiatric Intensive Care Unit (PICU) until more settled. In the context of acute violence on the ward, the primary concern is to ensure the safety of patients and staff and any intervention should be the minimum required to calm the patient. However, in many cases medication is needed.

Rapid tranquilisation (RT) is defined as 'the use of psychotropic medication to control agitated, threatening or destructive psychotic behaviour' (Ellison et al 1989). It should not be confused with rapid neuroleptisation (RN) that entails giving high loading doses of neuroleptics to achieve an early remission. There is no evidence that RN offers any therapeutic advantages over the use of standard doses while side-effects are significantly greater. It has been suggested that the confusion between RN and RT, concerns about excessive doses and side-effects of antipsychotic medication have, in part, led to the introduction of different classes of drugs for RT (Dubin 1988), i.e. benzodiazepines.

Several reviews of RT have been published (Dubin 1988, Sheard 1988, Ellison et al 1989, Goldberg et al 1989) and some studies looked at actual practice in clinical settings. Goldney et al (1986) looked at the use of high-dose neuroleptics in the PICU but did not look specifically at RT.

Work on RT is now focusing on auditing the use of RT in clinical settings (Pilowsky et al 1992) and psychiatric inpatient units are becoming more aware of the need for a defined policy for RT. Researchers have also noted that patients requiring RT tend to fall into two groups: those who require repeated injections due to persistent refusal of oral medication and resulting aggressive behaviour and those who require only one or two injections early on in their treatment (Pilowsky et al 1992).

A hospital policy for RT should include a discussion of the indications for its use, namely, that the patient is acutely disturbed and at high risk of harming himself or others in the very near future, and that non-pharmacological interventions have been considered (these will be discussed later). According to the Royal College of Psychiatrists' paper on the Management of Imminent Violence (Royal College of Psychiatrists 1998), training for RT should involve assessment and monitoring of the risks associated with the procedure. These include the cardiorespiratory effects, knowledge of the need to prescribe within therapeutic limits and the need to titrate dose to effect. Training should also include working and training as a team using cardiopulmonary resuscitation techniques as well as being familiar with the use of flumazenil. Ideally, violence should be anticipated and the use of alternative management strategies optimised. This will minimise the need for RT.

HOW TO USE RT

Staff should be aware of the procedures for RT before difficulties arise (Royal College of Psychiatrists 1998). The first step is to assess the situation with the multidisciplinary team. Safety is of paramount importance. Ensuring the patient, staff and other patients on the ward are safe allows further assessment to take place and may involve the need for physical restraint. Staff should be called in to help if need be. There should be enough staff available so that a staff member is free to review with the doctor, events leading up to the use of restraint, and to prepare medication. Ideally, there should be five nurses restraining, one person for each limb and one person to give orders and hold the head (Jacobs 1983). The doctor is present to manage the situation and to diagnose underlying conditions leading to disturbed behaviour, not to get involved in the restraining procedure itself. If there are not enough staff available, then either the patient should be allowed to leave and then the police called, or immediate assistance from the police should be requested.

Voluntary application of restraint may be possible, e.g. by explaining to the patient that it is necessary to restrain him for his own protection and to prevent others getting hurt. The patient should be held gently but firmly, on his back with one arm above his head and one arm by his side. He should be reassured, all procedures being explained during restraint, and should be able to respond to spoken messages throughout the period of sedation (Royal College of Psychiatrists 1998). Restraints should be checked to ensure good circulation to the limbs (Jacobs 1983). Staff should continue to observe the patient to see if he is continuing to struggle against restraint or whether the nurses have been able to relax their hold without the use of medication.

A review of case notes is necessary to check for contraindications to medication or any organic complications that may be contributing to the present situation. However, although establishing a differential diagnosis is extremely important, it should not delay intervention in a dangerous situation. If the patient does have an organic condition, further violence will worsen their physical health. In situations leading up to restraint, non-verbal signals may be necessary, e.g. to indicate when to restrain and these should be decided beforehand wherever possible.

If the patient is still aroused in spite of restraint, and staff members are unable to escort him to a safe environment without risk of injury to themselves or other patients, then RT is clearly necessary. Choice of drugs will depend on whether the patient has had neuroleptics previously and whether there is a history of severe extrapyramidal side-effects. The presence of complicating physical factors and the current physical and mental state of the patient will also be important. Clearly it will be impossible to examine a restrained patient adequately but, once the patient is calm, his physical state should be reviewed.

During and just before the administration of medication, vital signs should be measured including blood pressure, pulse and respiratory rate. Ideally, a pulse oximeter should be used to measure oxygen saturation. This is a non-invasive method for measuring oxygen saturation in arterial blood via a transmitter and detector placed on either side of a peripheral tissue such as a digit or earlobe. The tissue here is thin enough to allow visible red and infrared light transmission and it is the ratio between these two detected signals which is used to calculate oxygen saturation, oxygenated blood absorbing different amounts of light than deoxygenated (Jones 1995). Readings may be affected by tight clothing or tight restraint, which may affect blood flow. Nail varnish can interfere with digit readings and smokers can have raised carboxyhaemoglobin levels for up to 4 hours after smoking, resulting in false readings (Sims 1996). At the start of RT, the oximeter is attached usually to a digit and the machine switched on. A baseline oxygen saturation is recorded. While treatment is given, the monitor shows continuously the oxygen saturation in the blood and should be observed closely. Blood pressure, pulse and respiratory rate should be recorded every 5 minutes (Taylor *et al* 1996). If a pulse oximeter is not available, respiratory rate should be monitored more closely.

Facilities for mechanical ventilation and cardiac resuscitation should be readily available as should the benzodiazepine antagonist flumazenil. If the patient's oxygen saturation starts to drop then the attachment of the oximeter should be checked and the patient closely observed for falling respiratory rate, rising pulse and cyanosis. A sudden drop in saturation is an immediate indication to stop tranquilisation, as is a fall in systolic blood pressure to less than 80, or diastolic to less than 60 mmHg. If the respiratory rate drops below 6–8 breaths per minute then 200 mcg of flumazenil should be given IV. It should be emphasised that the above are recommendations based on clinical practice and are suggestions only. Pilowsky recommends the use of small bolus doses of medication titrated to the effect on the target symptoms, e.g. overt aggression, in order to minimise the risks of the procedure (Pilowsky *et al* 1992).

CHOICE OF MEDICATION

Dubin in his review of RT suggested that the choice of drugs for RT should be in part dictated by the diagnosis of the underlying cause of the disturbed behaviour (Dubin 1988). He advised that schizophrenic patients should be given primarily neuroleptics possibly with the addition of a benzodiazepine to lower the dose of the antipsychotic required, but that manic patients should be given mainly benzodiazepines and neuroleptics should only be used if these fail to control the situation. Patients with a history of substance abuse should receive benzodiazepines if the degree of agitation and violence is mild to moderate, but neuroleptics should be used in severe violence.

However, more recent opinion is that RT primarily controls behaviour (Ellison *et al* 1989, Swanson *et al* 1996) and hence there is no reason why benzodiazepines should not be used preferentially to achieve behavioural control, even if the patient has schizophrenia. A few studies have supported the use of benzodiazepines alone for RT (Bick and Hannah 1986, Modell 1986, Salzman 1988, Salzman *et al* 1991).

Benzodiazepines

Benzodiazepines were introduced as an alternative to neuroleptics for controlling acutely disturbed behaviour, as it was becoming clear that the use of neuroleptics in a dose necessary for sedation can result in severe extrapyramidal side-effects and postural hypotension.

Benzodiazepines, classically lorazepam IM or diazepam IV are the drugs of choice in cases where organic factors have caused the disturbed behaviour, e.g. acute confusional states secondary to alcohol/drug withdrawal, infection, cerebral upset and epilepsy. They are widely used in conjunction with neuroleptics in RT to reduce the antipsychotic requirement.

Benzodiazepines should be administered very slowly and hence are better given IV to allow for titration of the dose. Generally, diazepam 10 mg IV (as Diazemuls) or lorazepam 2 mg IM is used. Diazepam should never be given IM due to its prolonged and erratic absorption. The IV route is safe and effective (Lerner *et al* 1979), and should be achieved via a large vein to minimise the risk of painful extravasation into the tissues and thrombophlebitis.

Lorazepam has a short half-life with no active metabolites and is safer in liver impairment than diazepam, which has a longer half-life and has active metabolites, hence tending to accumulate with frequent administration. Clonazepam is used as maintenance treatment in epilepsy, but has also been found to be helpful in the treatment of agitation and arousal not responding to other treatment. Clonazepam also has a long half-life of (19–60 hours compared with 8–24 for lorazepam and 14–70 for diazepam). From recent studies it appears that benzodiazepines, particularly clonazepam, are more useful than previously thought for the management of drug-induced agitation, for mania in combination with lithium and when used alone in mania without psychotic symptoms (Freinhar and Alvarez 1985).

IM lorazepam has been used alone in the management of the violent patient, even when psychosis is present, and found to be at least as effective as neuroleptics in controlling violent behaviour (Pilowsky *et al* 1992). Arana *et al* (1986) looked at 14 psychotic patients treated with lorazepam alone and compared their progress with patients treated with lorazepam and haloperidol. They concluded that lorazepam is a useful treatment in the first 48 hours, but that the initial improvement in psychotic symptoms is temporary and does not improve with increasing doses. Modell (1986) also found that lorazepam alone has limited use in maintaining improvement. However, Salzman *et al* (1991) compared IM lorazepam with IM haloperidol and concluded that 2 mg of lorazepam may be better in RT than 5 mg of haloperidol. Midazolam, a rapid acting benzodiazepine has been used in doses of 1–3 mg IM in RT. It has a low incidence of side-effects and its intramuscular absorption is predictable (Mendoza *et al* 1987).

Neuroleptics

Traditionally, sedative drugs such as chlorpromazine have been used for agitated patients but Kane's review of the treatment of schizophrenia points out that there is no evidence to show they are more effective in controlling aggressive behaviour than non-sedating drugs (Kane 1977). There are also many difficulties with their parenteral use in that IV administration is not always possible, due to problems titrating the dose and because of the numerous side-effects of sedating neuroleptics such as phenothiazines, some potentially fatal.

Haloperidol and droperidol are used most commonly in RT and are the drugs of choice for two reasons. Not only has their use in RT been best evaluated, but also they have a very good safety record. In fact, haloperidol has been used to treat critically ill, confused patients on medical and surgical wards (Adams 1988). The cardiorespiratory safety of haloperidol has been established, even in the coronary care unit (Tesar *et al* 1985).

Haloperidol can be given IV or IM; IV administration is more rapid and between 5 and 10 mg is given initially, and may be repeated after 10 minutes (IV) or 30 minutes (IM) if it has had no effect. Droperidol can also be given IM or IV (5–10 mg) although unlike haloperidol there is little difference in the onset of action between IM and IV administration, taking approximately 5–20 minutes in both cases. Droperidol is shorter acting than haloperidol and so is particularly useful in patients who have been prescribed large doses of neuroleptics prior to the incident, where there is a risk of accumulation. In addition, in a double blind study of 27 acutely agitated patients, 81% of patients treated with haloperidol required a second injection compared with only 36% given droperidol (Resnick and Burton 1984).

Minimum doses of neuroleptics should be used and this is facilitated by concomitant use of benzodiazepines. The combination of haloperidol and diazepam has been particularly recommended due to its synergistic effect (Dubin 1988), although droperidol and lorazepam are also highly effective. Small bolus doses should be given and there should be at least a 10-minute wait between IV boluses or a 30-minute wait if the IM route has been used. If there is concern about the possibility of EPS, either because the patient has a history of EPS or the patient is neuroleptic naïve, then IM procyclidine (5–10 mg) should also be given.

Combined therapy with both neuroleptics and benzodiazepines is becoming increasingly common. There is no evidence of a higher incidence of adverse effects with this approach, and it may have therapeutic advantages. Kerr and Taylor (1997) have suggested two points in favour of a combination of benzodiazepines and neuroleptics. Firstly, the use of benzodiazepines allows a lower dose of the more toxic neuroleptic to be used and secondly, through their anticonvulsant effect, benzodiazepines may offset the lowering of the seizure threshold caused by neuroleptics. It has been shown in one survey that, when the combination is used, a second administration of medication is less likely and serious adverse effects are rare (Pilowsky et al 1992).

Other drugs

Clopixol acuphase (zuclopenthixol acetate) has been purported to be useful in RT and has the advantage that its effect lasts for 2–3 days, thus avoiding repeated injections and further confrontations with a disturbed individual. It is an intermediate acting neuroleptic, lasting 72 hours (peak 24–36 hours). Dosage is between 50 and 150 mg. However, it can take up to 3 hours to have an effect and the few controlled clinical studies available have given equivocal results (Coutinho et al 1997). Bourdouxhe et al (1987) compared 20 patients given acuphase to 13 patients given IM haloperidol, but found no difference with respect to effectiveness and side-effects between both groups. Baastrup et al (1993) compared acuphase with oral and IM haloperidol and conventional zuclopenthixol. They noted increased rigidity and hypokinesia in the first 24 hours in the haloperidol group, but otherwise no differences between the treatments. However, they observed that acuphase had an equal rapidity of action to the other treatments. Chouinard et al (1994) also found acuphase as effective as IM haloperidol, but observed an increase in dyskinesia in the acuphase group.

These studies confirm acuphase as an effective alternative to conventional IM medication. However, there is little evidence to suggest that it has fewer side-effects and the drug seems to have been evaluated in acute psychotic relapse, but not in the control of acute behavioural disturbance. A common problem with studies in this area is that many are conducted in 'acutely disturbed and disruptive individuals' without a clear definition of what constitutes such behaviour (Royal College of Psychiatrists 1998).

Acuphase is not generally recommended for use in RT because its onset and length of action cannot always be predicted. For this reason it should never be given to a highly aroused, struggling patient because of potential adverse effects on the myocardium (see below). In addition, because the drug may have an onset of action between 20 minutes and 3 hours after administration, it limits the safe use of further medication.

Both loxapine and thiothixene have been evaluated in RT. Tuason (1986) found 25 mg loxapine IM to be at least as effective as haloperidol 5 mg IM in the initial treatment of aggressive patients with schizophrenia and there was no difference between the two with regard to side-effects. 25 mg of IM Loxapine was compared to haloperidol 5 mg IM and has also been compared to 10 mg IM thiothixene (Dubin and Weiss 1986). Both were found to be comparable in terms of efficacy and side-effect profile, but response to IM loxapine was faster. Molindone has also been used in RT. Thiothixene, IM loxapine and molindone are not available in the UK.

Chlorpromazine has been used extensively in the past to control agitated and aggressive patients due to its sedative properties. Cunnane's (1994) review of consultant psychiatrists looked at their suggestions for medication, having been given the clinical vignette of a young schizophrenic patient in his first admission. The most frequent suggestion was chlorpromazine 100 mg IM (above BNF limits) repeated 1–6 hourly. This is no longer recommended. Man and Chen compared IM chlorpromazine with IM haloperidol and concluded that the incidence of hypotension with chlorpromazine was higher than reported and suggested using a test dose of 10 mg to test sensitivity, although suggesting that overall haloperidol was the safer drug to use in RT (Man and Chen 1973).

In rare, exceptional cases, sodium amytal and paraldehyde have been used but their use is no longer recommended.

AFTER RT

Unless the patient remains highly sedated, oral medication should be resumed. If oral medication is refused, then the patient can be managed on a droperidol or haloperidol oral/IM regime where, if oral dose is refused, the equivalent dose is given IM. For example, 10 mg of droperidol orally is equivalent to 7.5 mg IM; 10 mg of haloperidol orally is equivalent to 5 mg IM. Clinicians appear to have poor knowledge of equivalent doses and tend to overestimate the dose (Mullen et al 1994).

Clopixol acuphase can also be used following RT, although it should never be administered to a neuroleptic naïve patient. It is important to determine the patient's underlying diagnosis and also their legal status before giving an antipsychotic that could last up to 72 hours. The efficacy of lithium as an acute antimanic agent should not be forgotten in the aftermath of RT.

DANGERS OF RAPID TRANQUILISATION

As with any pharmacological intervention, RT is not without its hazards, and the clinician must assess the risk–benefit ratio of treatment. It is important not to underestimate the risks of inadequate tranquilisation, which in the violent patient can lead to harm to self and others. Other factors to consider include the patient's current treatment regimen and possible drug interactions, their age and physical state, and the proposed route of administration. RT, if administered with care and if there is good aftercare, is generally very safe, particularly when balanced against the risks of not medicating the patient.

To reduce risks inherent in the procedure, the patient should be securely restrained. Injecting a struggling patient can lead to inadvertent intra-arterial injection, nerve damage, and a higher than expected rate of absorption of the drug from the injection site due to increased bioavailability from IM or IV use (up to five times) and due to increased blood flow to the muscles IM use (Thompson 1994). Highly aroused patients are also more sensitive to adrenergic and noradrenergic effects on the myocardium. Even restraint alone is not without risks, and it has been suggested that restraint in the prone position with tying of the ankles and hands leads to splinting of the respiratory apparatus. This can result in respiratory muscle fatigue and death due to positional asphyxia (Bell *et al* 1992). Following administration of medication, close monitoring including measurement of saturation with pulse oximetry gives early indication of hypoxaemia secondary to oversedation (Charlton 1995).

Complications of RT include minor or local complications, and major systemic complications. In Pilowsky's survey of 102 incidents of rapid tranquilisation, 70% of patients had no or only minor local complications with 30% reporting minor bruising, pain or extravasation. Cardiovascular or respiratory complications were seen in four cases, with only one of these being serious (Pilowsky *et al* 1992). It was felt that the complications that did occur were related primarily to idiosyncratic drug reactions, predictable side-effects and interactions, and overmedication, of which the majority could have been prevented by adequate training in RT.

Goldberg has also reviewed fully the other side-effects of rapid tranquilisation which include local complications (bruising, pain or extravasation in up to 30% of patients), respiratory complications in 2%, cardiovascular complications in 3% (again particularly with phenothiazines) and seizures due to lowering of the seizure threshold (Goldberg *et al* 1989).

If we first consider the use of antipsychotics in RT, chlorpromazine is no longer recommended for parenteral administration as intravenous administration is not licensed and IM injection is painful. Parenteral chlorpromazine can also cause profound hypotension, particularly dangerous in the elderly and those with coronary artery disease and has been associated with prolonged unconsciousness (Quenstedt *et al* 1992). Together with other phenothiazines, chlorpromazine has a quinidine-like effect on the myocardium and cardiac conduction system. Prolongation of the QT interval is responsible for the rare appearance of torsade de pointes (Wilson and Weiler 1984). Although droperidol and haloperidol have been found to be relatively safe to use in RT, problems of sudden cardiac death and neuroleptic malignant syndrome have been reported (Konikoff *et al* 1984, Huyse and Stack van Schijndel 1988), emphasising the need for good after-care of the patient, to ensure prompt intervention when necessary.

Finally, antipsychotics should not be used in a suspected case of PCP psychosis as they may precipitate anticholinergic psychoses.

Benzodiazepines are a recommended choice for RT in psychiatric emergencies due to their low toxicity, with diazepam and lorazepam being the two most frequently employed. However, withdrawal seizures can occur and benzodiazepines are associated with confusion, nausea, vomiting and oversedation, particularly in the elderly. In Modell's study of the use of lorazepam for behavioural control in 75 agitated patients, 50% of patients developed ataxia, and 25% experienced nausea and vomiting (Modell 1986). Benzodiazapines should only be used in the acute phase, and not for long-term management as there is a high risk of dependence. In the practice of RT, the most serious complication of benzodiazepine use is respiratory depression due to sedation. All benzodiazepines are contraindicated in patients with pulmonary disease, as they depress hypoxic respiratory drive. As previously noted, respiratory depression can be reversed by the use of the benzodiazepine antagonist flumazenil. Flumazenil is not an easy drug to use and clear instructions should be easily accessible. For example, the half-life of flumazenil is short compared to the benzodiazepines used in RT and repeated doses may be required. Flumazenil may also precipitate withdrawal seizures in those with significant prior exposure to benzodiazepines.

Other drugs previously used in psychiatric emergencies are no longer recommended. These include the barbiturates, which are associated with dependence, tolerance, hazardous drug interactions, profound hypotension and irreversible respiratory depression. Paraldehyde may be used where all other methods have failed, but it is painful when given intramuscularly and may cause profound respiratory depression. Its use is also associated with sterile abscesses and nerve damage. Paraldehyde should not be administered via plastic syringes. It should never be administered intravenously in the psychiatric setting.

CURRENT USE OF RT

Several studies have looked at the use of RT in everyday practice. Surveys of trainees (Ellison *et al* 1989, Mannion *et al* 1997) and of consultants and senior registrars (Cunnane 1994, Simpson and Anderson 1996) have revealed worrying discrepancies. Generally, although most senior psychiatrists advised sensible drug regimes. Of them 10% advised the use of clopixol acuphase in a neuroleptic naive patient (Simpson and Anderson 1996), a practice not advised by the Royal College of Psychiatrists Consensus Statement (Thompson 1994). Only 15% of psychiatrists reported that their units had protocols for RT and only 48% reported that their juniors had received training in the use of RT.

Nearly 50% of psychiatrists felt that the BNF was unhelpful in providing advice about RT and that maximum doses stated in the BNF were not relevant to RT (Simpson and Anderson 1996). Mannion *et al* (1997) found that 39% of trainees surveyed used doses within the high range and 24.4% prescribed more than one neuroleptic. The study also suggested that trainees tended to prescribe the same dose whether given orally or intramuscularly and had little knowledge of dose equivalents. Simpson and Anderson (1996) point out that the BNF does not report RT as an indication for the use of benzodiazepines. Moreover, it does not indicate clearly the best drugs to use in RT. Although the BNF cites tranquilisation as an indication for haloperidol and droperidol, it does not give a consensus view and does not specify which drugs are *not* suitable for RT.

A recent study has looked at patient satisfaction in a Psychiatric Intensive Care Unit and found there was no significant association between patient dissatisfaction and experiencing side-effects of medication and receiving RT. However, patients who received RT at least once during their stay had significantly higher total side-effects than those who did not. In the group who received RT, patients who had a number of different antipsychotics experienced more side-effects than those who had mono-therapy, and those who had clopixol acuphase had fewer side-effects than those given haloperidol (Hyde *et al* 1998).

ALTERNATIVES TO RT

Although psychotropic medication in the form of RT remains the mainstay of treatment for the aggressive patient, it should always be used in conjunction with psychological and behavioural techniques. Some patients may be amenable to psychological and behavioural strategies alone, although this has not been examined in a controlled manner. McLaren *et al* (1990) have shown that even after other strategies have been used, up to 20% of patients in a locked ward setting still need enforced medication. However, a broad psychotherapeutic approach should still be encouraged.

Psychological and behavioural approaches to the aggressive patient include: decelerative/de-escalation techniques (Corrigan *et al* 1993) (also known as talking-down), time-out from reinforcement, and seclusion and restraint. Basic techniques can be found in any textbook of nursing skills with a fuller discussion in Kidd and Stark (1995). Even if these skills do not prevent the administration of RT, they can help to preserve the therapeutic relationship and the safety of all involved.

De-escalation, also described as 'defusing' or 'talking down', has been defined as a set of verbal and non-verbal responses which, if used selectively and appropriately, reduce the level of a person's hostility by reducing anger and the predisposition to assaultative behaviour (Leadbetter and Paterson 1995). It assumes a proactive approach to manage anger or aggression before a violent incident occurs. Unfortunately, there is not a standard method and little systematic research on the content of the current approaches.

In addition to de-escalation techniques, behavioural interventions may also be useful with the aggressive client (Corrigan *et al* 1993). These include self-controlled time-out, a technique based on operant principles. Patients undergo short-term removal for a few minutes from overstimulating situations, the emphasis being on their control over the process. A similar method involves the use of a low stimulus environment, where staff support and counsel patients for a 15-minute period in a specifically allocated quiet area. The successful use of such an area within a psychiatric intensive care unit has been described in the literature (Hyde and Harrower-Wilson 1994). Continuous observation may be another useful method for managing patients representing an acute risk. A continuous observation protocol provides several elements that may be important in reducing violent episodes including reduced stimulation, protection, intensive observation and an opportunity for therapeutic contact. It is also less restrictive than seclusion or restraints. Shugar and Rehaluk (1990) evaluated a continuous observation protocol and found brief episodes of observations for less than 72 hours to be effective and practical. Clinical review should take place if more than 72 hours of observation are required.

Physical restraint has also been advocated as a therapeutic procedure, with several authors discussing clinical guidelines for its use (Bursten 1975, Rose and DiGiacomo 1978). Restraint may be applied by mechanical means (e.g. by leather straps) as described by Jacobs (1983). In the UK, physical restraint is most often seen in the form of 'control and restraint' (C&R), a term referring to a set of intervention skills involving wrist locks used by a team of trained staff to facilitate control of an assaultative patient. These techniques have been endorsed by professional nursing bodies in accordance with the Mental Health Act Code of Practice, which advises the use of 'the minimum necessary restraint to deal with the harm that needs to be pre-vented' (Department of Health and Welsh Office 1993). Thus, C&R is not perceived as a therapeutic procedure, although clinical experience suggests that it can sometimes act as one. The most important criterion for its use is that it must be performed by staff who are fully trained to apply it in a safe, rapid and effective manner.

The most restrictive of alternatives to RT is the use of seclusion, a topic fully discussed elsewhere in this book. It should not be confused with time-out, which occurs with the patient's agreement and understanding as part of their care plan. Instead, seclusion is often an emergency measure used to contain or deal with a situation on a short-term basis. It differs from restraint in that all social contact and interaction is removed. The Mental Health Act Code of Practice defines seclusion as 'supervised confinement of a patient alone in a room which may be locked for the protection of others from significant harm' (Department of Health and Welsh Office 1993). The Code of Practice also gives guidelines for its use suggesting that this should be as infrequently as possible, for the smallest possible duration and only when alternative methods have failed. It does not advise use for those with a risk of self harm or suicide. Surveys show that seclusion is used for a wide variety of conditions and behaviours (Mattson and Sacks 1978, Plutchik et al 1978, Russell et al 1986). It may also serve to contain staff anxiety as well as patient disturbance (Russell et al 1986). However, there is little evidence to suggest that seclusion results in any long-term changes in behaviour, and the Code of Practice is careful to state that its use may be damaging to staff–patient relationships (Soliday 1985) and to the patient's mental state (Plutchik et al 1978, Binder and McCoy 1985, Wadeson and Carpenter 1976).

ECT may be another alternative to RT in the management of the acutely aggressive patient, particularly when the patient is only responding slowly to pharmacological methods. It is known to be an effective treatment of the positive symptoms of schizophrenia (Taylor and Fleminger 1980), although its principal benefit appears to be in speeding up the response to antipsychotics (Taylor 1993). ECT is also effective in mania. However, it cannot act as a replacement for RT in the emergency situation.

LEGAL CONSIDERATIONS

The use of RT clearly involves infringement of an individual's civil liberties and hence the giving of medication to someone against their will is a decision not to be taken lightly. One has to consider the protection of patients' rights against the safety of others. An important issue is the patient's right to refuse treatment, debated in Rogers v. Commissioner in the USA (Gutheil 1985). The opinion of the court was that a committed mental patient is considered competent and has the right to refuse treatment until declared incompetent by a judge. If the patient is incompetent, then the judge decides the patient's most likely choice regarding medication, if the patient had been competent. The court stated that the only instance where antipsychotic drugs can be given without consent is in an emergency to prevent 'immediate, substantial and irreversible deterioration of a serious mental illness'. In all other situations, then the psychiatrist has to take the patient to court before compulsory treatment can be given.

Gutheil (1985) criticised the court's view of antipsychotic medication as 'extraordinary treatment' and also pointed out that the court's ruling assumed and could create an adversarial relationship between patient and doctor. In addition, the ruling would result in unnecessary delay in a patient's treatment and a longer stay in hospital. Other concerns were that the restriction of involuntary medication to severe behavioural emergencies would actually put others at risk because it would not allow medical staff to give treatment to avoid such incidents (Gutheil 1985, Moldin 1985). The suggestion by the courts that violence is predictable in certain patients and hence consent for medication should be obtained when a patient is 'competent and calm' is clearly impractical. In reality, violence is often unpredictable. Furthermore, if a patient is 'competent and calm', then they are likely to be well and hence the possibility of violence is a remote event. When violence occurs some time later, how valid is the consent given weeks or months previously? Such a discussion regarding emergency medication is liable to be detrimental to the therapeutic relationship.

Fortunately in the UK, such legal restraints have not been introduced and reasonable clinical judgement is accepted. Certain constraints do have to be kept in mind. Occasionally, RT may have to be given to a patient who is informal, hence treatment is given under common law. In this case, it is inadvisable to give longer-acting neuroleptics such as clopixol acuphase or depot medication. Generally, a section of the Mental Health Act should be instituted as soon as possible. The same applies to a patient on Section 5(2) since this section is a holding order only. Close relatives should be informed about the giving of forced medication at the appropriate time and told why it was necessary.

Lord Donaldson clarified the indications for medical treatment under common law. Firstly, the doctor needs to assess the capacity to give informed consent; if the patient is unable to give consent, then the duty of the doctor is to treat the patient in his best interests, e.g. to save life. The doctor is deemed to have acted in the best interests of the patient if he acts in accordance with current practice by a responsible body of medical opinion.

The following statements cover RT under common law:

- That it is permissible to give treatment to a non-consenting capable patient who is suffering from 'a mental disorder which is leading to behaviour that is an immediate serious danger to himself or to other people' (Department of Health and Welsh Office 1993).

- 'Any patient whose mental disorder leads to such behaviour is unlikely to possess the high level of mental capacity that is required' (Jones 1996).

Clearly the ability to give informed consent presents a problem for the assessing doctor.

A disturbed aggressive patient will not be able to co-operate in the assessment of competence, but could be assumed to be incompetent as above. But arguably, even if aroused and actively psychotic, the patient may be capable of giving consent.

Clearly, in RT, assessment of capacity presents a problem, although even if a patient is capable of giving consent, medication can be given if he is mentally ill and presenting a danger to others.

Clearly, rapid tranquilisation is a procedure that should not be carried out without consideration of alternatives. But as long as strict guidelines are followed with respect to patient's rights, choice of medication and physical monitoring, then it remains a safe, acceptable procedure for controlling disturbed, potentially dangerous behaviour in mental illness.

All PICUs should have RT guidelines and all staff should be familiar with their content. An example can be found in Chapter 2.

REFERENCES

Adams F. 1988 Emergency intravenous sedation of the delirious, medically ill patient. J Clin Psychiatr, December 49(12) (suppl): 22–27

Arana GW, Ornsteen ML, Kanter FF, Friedman HL, Greenblatt DJ, Shader SI. 1986 The use of benzodiazepines for psychotic disorders: A literature review and preliminary clinical findings. Psychopharmacol Bull 22(1): 77–87

Baastrup PC, Alhfors UG, Bjerkenstedt L, et al. 1993 A controlled Nordic multicentre study of zuclopenthixol acetate in oil solution, haloperidol and zuclopenthixol in the treatment of acute psychosis. Acta Psychiatr Scand 87: 48–58

Bell MD, Rao VJ, Weitli C, Rodriguez RN. 1992 Positional asphyxia in adults: 30 cases. Am J Forensic Med Pathol 13: 101–107

Bick PA, Hannah AL. 1986 Intramuscular lorazepam to restrain violent patients. Lancet, 25 January: 206

Binder RL, McCoy SM. 1985 Patients attitudes towards placement in seclusion. J Nerv Ment Dis 173: 273–286

Bourdouxhe S, Mirel J, Denys W, Bobon D. 1987 L'acetate de zuclopenthixol et l'haloperidol dans la psychose aigue. Acta Psychiat Belg 87: 236–244

Bursten B. 1975 Using mechanical restraints on acutely disturbed psychiatric patients. Hosp Comm Psych 30: 48–55

Charlton JE. 1995 Monitoring and supplemental oxygen during endoscopy. Br Med J 310: 886–888

Chouinard G, Safadi G, Beauclair L. 1994 A double-blind controlled study of intramuscular zuclopenthixol acetate and liquid oral haloperidol in the treatment of schizophrenic patients with acute exacerbation. J Psychpharmacol 14(6): 126–129

Corrigan PW, Yodufsky SC, Silver JM. 1993 Pharmacological and behavioural treatments for aggressive psychiatric inpatients. Hosp Comm Psych 44: 125–133

Coutinho E, Fenton M, Campbell C, David A. 1997 Details of studies of zuclopenthixol are needed (letter). Br Med J 4 October 315: 884

Cunnane JG. 1994 Drug management of disturbed behaviour by psychiatrists. Psychiatric Bulletin 18: 138–139

De la Fuenta JR, Rosenbaum AH, Martin HR. 1980 Lorazepam-related withdrawal seizures. Mayo Clin Proc 55: 190–192

Department of Health. April 1999 Draft outline proposals by the Scoping Study Committee. Review of the Mental Health Act 1983.

Department of Health and Welsh Office. 1993 Code of Practice – Mental Health Act 1983. London: HMSO

Dubin WR, Weiss KJ. 1986 Rapid tranquilization: a comparison of thiothixene with loxapine. J Clin Psychiatr, 47(6): 294–297

Dubin WR. 1988 Rapid tranquilization: antipsychotics or benzodiazepines? J Clin Psychiatr 49(12) (suppl): 5–11

Ellison J, Hughes D, White K. 1989 An emergency psychiatry update. Hospital and Community Psychiatry 40(3): 250–260

Freinhar JP, Alvarez WH. 1985 Use of clonazepam in two cases of acute mania. J Clin Psychiatr 46(1), 29–30

Goldberg RJ, Dubin WR, Fogel BS. 1989 Review. Behavioural emergencies, assessment of psychopharmacologic management. Clin Neuropharmacol 12(4): 233–248

Goldney RD, Spence ND, Bowes JA. 1986 The safe use of high-dose neuroleptics in a psychiatric intensive care unit. Austra New Zeal J Psychiatry 20: 370–375

Gutheil TG. 1985 Rogers v. Commissioner. Denouement of an important right-to-refuse-treatment case. Am J Psychiatr 142(2)

Huyse F, Strack Van Schijndel R. 1988 Haloperidol and cardiac arrest. Lancet ii: 568–569

Hyde CE, Harrower-Wilson C, Morris J. 1998 Violence, dissatisfaction and rapid tranquilisation in psychiatric intensive care. Psychiatric Bulletin 22: 477–480

Hyde CE, Harrower-Wilson C. 1994 Psychiatric intensive care: principles and problems. Hospital Update, May 287–295

Jacobs D. 1983 Evaluation and management of the violent patient in emergency settings. Psychiatr Clin N Am June 6(2): 259–269

Jones R 1996 (ed). Mental Health Act Manual, 5th edn. Sweet & Maxwell, London

Jones SE. 1995 Getting the balance right. Professional Nurse: 368–373

Kane JM. 1977 Treatment of schizophrenia. Schizophrenia Bulletin 13(1): 133–156

Kerr IB, Taylor D. 1997 Acute disturbed or violent behaviour: principles of treatment. J Psychopharm 11(3): 271–277

Kidd B, Stark C (eds). 1995 Management of Violence and Aggression in Health Care. London: Gaskell

Konikoff F, Kuritzky A, Jerushalmi Y et al. 1984 Neuroleptic Malignant Syndrome induced by a single injection of haloperidol (letter) Br Med J 289: 1228–1229

Leadbetter D, Paterson B. 1995 De-escalating aggressive behaviour. In: Kidd B, Stark C (eds) Management of Violence and Aggression in Health Care. London: Gaskell, 49–84

Lerner Y, Lwow E, Levitin A, Belmaker R H. 1979 Acute high-dose parenteral haloperidol treatment of psychosis. Am J Psychiatr 136: 1061–1064

Man PL, Chen CH. 1973 Rapid tranquilization of acutely psychotic patients with intramuscular haloperidol and chlorpromazine. Psychsomatics 14: 59–63

Mannion L, Sloan D, Connolly L. 1997 Rapid tranquilisation: are we getting it right? Psychiatric Bulletin 21(7): 411–413

Mattson MR, Sacks MH. 1978 Seclusion: uses and complications. Am J Psychiatry 135: 1210–1213

McLaren S, Browne FWA, Taylor PJ. 1990 A study of psychotropic medication given as required in a regional secure unit. Br J Psychiatr 156: 732–735

Mendoza R, Djenderedjian A H, Adams J, Ananth J. 1987 Midazolam in acute psychotic patients with hyperarousal. J Clin Psychiatr 48(7): 291–292

Modell JG. 1986 Further experience and observations with lorazepam in the management of behavioural agitation. J Clin Psychopharm 6(6): 385–387

Muldin SO. 1985 The Effect of Rogers on forensic, emergency psychiatry. Am J Psychiatr 142 (12): 1521–1522

Monahan J. 1992 Mental disorder and violent behaviour. Am Psychologist April: 511–521

Mullen P. 1988 Violence and mental disorder. Br J Hosp Med 40: 460–463

Mullen R, Caan AW, Smith S. 1994 Perception of equivalent doses of neuroleptic drugs. Psychiatric Bulletin 18(6): 335–337

Mulvey EP. 1994 Assessing the evidence of a link between mental illness and violence. Hospital and Community Psychiatry 45(7): 663–668

Pilowsky LS, Ring H, Shine PJ, Battersby M, Lader M. 1992. Rapid tranquilisation. A survey of emergency prescribing in a general psychiatric hospital. Br J Psych 160: 831–834

Plutchik R, Karasu TB, Conte HR, Siegal B, Jerret I. 1978 Toward a rationale for the seclusion process. J Nerv Ment Dis 166(8): 571–579

Quenstedt M, Ramsey R, Bernadette M. 1992 Rapid tranquilisation. Br J Psych 161: 573

Resnick MD, Burton BT. 1984 Droperidol vs haloperidol in the initial management of acutely agitated patients. J Clin Psychiatr 45(7): 298–299

Rosen H, DiGiacomo JN. 1978 The role of physical restraint in the treatment of psychiatric illness. J Clin Psychiatr 39: 228–232

Royal College of Psychiatrists. 1998 Management of Imminent Violence. Clinical Practice Guidelines to Support Mental Health Services. OP41 March

Russell D, Hodgkinson P, Hillis T. 1986 Time out: are disturbed patients secluded for purely clinical reasons? Nursing Times, 26 February: 47–49

Salzman C, Soloman D, Miyawaki E et al. 1991 Parenteral lorazepam versus parenteral haloperidol for the control of psychotic disruptive behaviour. J Clin Psychiatr, 52(4): 177–180

Salzman C. 1988 Use of benzodiazepines to control disruptive behaviour inpatients. J Clin Psychiatr 49(12) (suppl): 13–15

Sheard MH. 1988 Review: clinical pharmacology of aggressive behaviour. Clin Pharmacol 11: 483–492

Shugar G, Rehaluk R. 1990 Continuous observation in-patients: a critical evaluation. Comp Psych 30: 48–55

Simpson D, Anderson I. 1996 Rapid tranquilisation: a questionnaire survey of practice. Psychiatric Bulletin 20(3): 149–152

Sims J. 1996 Making sense of pulse oximetry and oxygen dissociation curve. Nursing Times 92(1): 34–35

Soliday SM. 1985 A comparison of patient and staff attitudes towards seclusion. J Nerv Ment Dis 173: 273–286

Swanson JW, Borum R, Swatrz MS, Monahan J. 1996 Psychotic symptoms and disorders and the risk of violent behaviour in the community. Criminal Behaviour and Mental Health 6: 309–329

Taylor D, Kerwin R, Duncan D. 1996 The Bethlem and Maudsley NHS Trust Prescribing Guidelines 3rd edn. July

Taylor P, Fleminger JJ. 1980 ECT and schizophrenia. Lancet 1380–1382

Taylor PJ. 1993 Mental illness and violence. In: Taylor PJ (ed) Violence in Society. London: Royal College of Physicians

Tesar GE, Murray GB, Cassem NH. 1985 Use of high-dose intravenous haloperidol in the treatment of agitated cardiac patients. J Clin Psychopharm 5(6): 344–347

Thompson C. 1994 Consensus statement: The use of high-dose antipsychotic medication. Br J Psychiatr 164: 448–458

Tuason VB. 1986 A comparison of parenteral loxapine and haloperidol in hostile and aggressive acutely schizophrenic patients. J Clin Psychiatr 47(3): 126–129

Wadeson H, Carpenter WT. 1976 Impact of the seclusion room experience. J Nerv Ment Dis 163: 318–328

Wilson WH, Weiler SJ. 1984 Case report of phenothiazine induced torsade de points. Am J Psychol 141: 1265–1266

5

PHARMACOLOGICAL THERAPY

Chike I Okocha

GENERAL PRINCIPLES

In the past few decades, drugs have become the cornerstone of treatment for mental disorders. With the refinement of diagnostic categories and the development of newer drugs it has become important to have guidelines underpinning such treatments.

These guidelines are largely based on assumptions such as the existence of:

- clear-cut diagnostic categories;
- effective drug treatments; and
- disorders that are either life-long or represent life-long vulnerabilities.

A further important assumption is that exacerbations and recurrences are unfavourable for patients, their families, and society.

In intensive care psychiatry, treatment goals are generally short-term although, where appropriate, long-term goals can also be set. These goals are to reduce symptoms as rapidly as possible; build an alliance for long-term management; educate the patient and their families about the illness, its treatment, and its course (treated and untreated); and lay the groundwork for a return to premorbid levels of functioning.

Effective strategies for achieving these goals include:

- the use of medication in adequate doses for adequate durations before abandoning a drug trial;
- avoiding polypharmacy where possible;
- optimising long-term drug treatment regimes; and
- combining drug treatment with psychological treatment strategies, and providing systematic psycho-education for patients and their families.

Although the ideal duration of treatment for mental disorders remains debatable, it is generally accepted that almost all acute treatments should continue for at least 6 months, and with disorders like schizophrenia it may take 18 months, until symptom remission. Furthermore it is recommended that a discrete 6-month period of remission passes before tapering of therapeutic medication commences.

In the longer-term, the primary goals of treatment are to aid return to pre-morbid levels of functioning and prevent relapse, as this results in symptom exacerbation as well as impairment in social and vocational functioning. In patients where the benefits of continuing long-term medication outweigh the risks, it is important to aim for the minimal effective dose while continuously monitoring side-effects and life circumstances. It is also beneficial to maintain contact with families and carers to maximise compliance and reduce the burden of living with someone with a chronic psychiatric illness.

USE OF ANTIPSYCHOTICS

The term 'antipsychotic' was originally coined to describe drugs that had the capacity to alter neuronal activity, but the term is now used almost exclusively to describe drugs with antipsychotic potency. The modern era of the use of such drugs started in the 1950s with the introduction of chlorpromazine. Since that serendipitous discovery a number of other drugs have also been discovered. More recently, however, drugs with more clearly defined receptor sites of action and, as a consequence, better adverse effect profiles have been manufactured.

Although the biochemical effects of antipsychotics are known in some detail, the relationship between these effects and therapeutic properties is often unclear. Their use is largely, therefore, empirical rather than wholly evidence based. They are not generally curative but accelerate recovery and prevent or postpone relapse in the course of major illnesses.

In using antipsychotics, it is important to remember that their pharmacokinetic properties determine their bioavailability. Orally administered drugs are influenced by factors such as, gastric motility and emptying and first pass metabolism in the liver. For example, only 30–60% of orally administered chlorpromazine reaches the general circulation compared to parenteral administration. Other factors influencing bioavailability are frequency of administration, lipophilicity, and protein binding. The breakdown of drugs can be influenced by genetic factors, as is the case with the oxidative metabolism of risperidone which is subject to genetic polymorphism, or the drug itself, as with chlorpromazine which induces its own metabolism.

Antipsychotic drugs have a number of uses, which can broadly be grouped as follows:

- Calming of disturbed patients ('tranquilisation') with a range of diagnoses, such as schizophrenia, mania, and organic mental disorders.

- Treatment of acute symptoms of psychotic illnesses.

- Provision of maintenance treatment.

- Treatment of symptoms of anxiety.

These indications are described individually below.

Tranquilisation

This refers to the practice of rapidly loading medication to decrease behavioural agitation when other non-drug strategies have failed. Patients with psychosis do sometimes become acutely disturbed for a variety of reasons, including their abnormal experiences, and may endanger themselves or others at such times. This practice does not in any way refer to an attempt to rapidly 'treat' the underlying cause of psychosis, e.g., schizophrenia.

Antipsychotics alone, or in combination with, benzodiazepines are typically administered parenterally to patients for their calming effects (Chapter 4). The choice of antipsychotics and benzodiazepines vary and depend to a large extent on local policy. Butyrophenones, such as haloperidol and droperidol, are now commonly used alone or in combination with diazepam or lorazepam. The use of chlorpromazine has been limited because of its potential to cause postural hypotension. In patients with an established history of antipsychotic treatment, zuclopenthixol acetate with or without a benzodiazepine, should be considered. This short acting depot lasts for up to 72 hours and may reduce the need for repeated confrontation with reluctant or struggling patients.

Acute psychosis

Psychosis is characterised by loss of touch with reality which may manifest as hallucinations, delusions, bizarre behaviour, and disorders of thought. Its underlying causes include detectable brain disease, such as may result from a head injury, dementia, psychoactive substance abuse, and psychiatric disorders such as schizophrenia, affective disorder, and various other brief disorders.

The use of antipsychotic drugs in the treatment of acute psychosis aims to alleviate psychotic symptoms and shorten the acute episode of illness. Several 'typical' and 'atypical' antipsychotics are now available. The antipsychotic potency of the typical antipsychotics were thought to depend entirely on dopamine-2 (D_2) receptor blockade in the mesolimbic and cortical areas of the brain. Similar blockade of basal ganglia dopamine receptors in excess of about 75% results in extrapyramidal symptoms especially parkinsonism. The newer 'atypicals', however, do not have such a high affinity for D_2 receptors but appear to have affinity for other receptor types, particularly serotonin receptors. They all share a high 5-HT_{2A}: striatal D_2 receptor blockade ratio (Kapur and Remington 1996).

Irrespective of mode of action, there is no convincing evidence that any one drug or class of drugs, except clozapine, is more effective than the other. Despite this equal efficacy across classes of drugs, patients do not respond equally to all classes. Side-effects, which differ from drug to drug or class to class, seem to be the main determinant for choice of drug. Equally important is a previous history of response to a particular antipsychotic. Therapeutic response with lessening of symptoms is observed in up to 3–4 weeks following the onset of treatment.

Maintenance treatment in psychosis

The use of antipsychotics in the maintenance treatment of psychosis is aimed at the prevention of relapse or worsening of psychotic symptoms and disability. About 80% of untreated patients with schizophrenia relapse. Maintenance treatment is, therefore, indicated but it raises issues about antipsychotic dosage and the length of time patients should be exposed to antipsychotics to minimise the risk of long-term side-effects, especially tardive dyskinesia.

Two commonly adopted strategies are:

- the intermittent or targeted approach where antipsychotics are withdrawn and then reintroduced at the first symptomatic signs of psychosis; and

- the fixed low dose approach where treatment is continuous with a low dose of medication in combination with close follow-up (Kane and Marder 1993; Schooler 1991).

Both strategies have their critics and are not thought to be very successful at preventing relapse (Kane and Marder 1993; Schooler 1991). Studies on patients with schizophrenia have shown that 75% of patients who switched to placebo after a year of being symptom-free relapsed within 6–24 months. This is in contrast to a relapse rate of 23% in patients receiving continuous antipsychotic medication (Hegarty et al 1994). The strategy used will depend largely on the patient's history but close collaboration with the patient over medication strategies and doses may enhance their engagement.

The advantages and disadvantages of oral medication are well rehearsed as are those for depot antipsychotics. It is argued that the use of low-dose depot medication, as opposed to oral medication, may have additional benefits in terms of relapse prevention (Davis et al 1994). The use of atypical antipsychotics for long-term maintenance has not yet been fully validated but there are no reasons to suggest that they are not effective. Drug treatment must be combined with appropriate psycho-socio-educational strategies to achieve maximum benefits (Bellack and Mueser 1993; Mortimer 1997).

Alleviation of symptoms of anxiety

Some antipsychotics, in much smaller doses than are used in psychoses, are useful as sedatives particularly in patients who are likely to become dependent on benzodiazepines (Okocha 1996). Thioridazine (Melleril), in doses of 10–25 mg, is particularly favoured in this regard but small doses of flupenthixol hydrochloride (Fluanxol), in doses of up to 3 mg a day, and chlorpromazine are also effective. Although these drugs do not pose the same problem of dependence as benzodiazepines, they can cause acute side-effects such as akathisia and dystonia and in the longer-term, dyskinesias. The benefits of using them should therefore be weighed against these risks.

Adverse effects of antipsychotics

As there are no significant differences between antipsychotics in terms of efficacy, the choice of drug in clinical practice depends to a large extent on the anticipated side-effect profile of the drug. Other factors of importance are patient characteristics, diagnosis, and the clinician's knowledge of available drugs. Considering the prevalence of side-effects in patients prescribed antipsychotics, it is important that these are discussed. Side-effects, particularly akathisia, weight gain, sexual dysfunction and the unpleasant feeling of dysphoria tend to reduce compliance.

Typical antipsychotics consist of drugs in a number of chemical groups:

- The phenothiazines which are grouped on the basis of the side-chain, e.g. aliphatic (chlorpromazine), piperidene (thioridazine), and piperazine (fluphenazine, trifluoperazine).

- The thioxanthenes, e.g. flupenthixol and thiothixene.

- The butyrophenones, e.g. droperidol and haloperidol.

- The diphenylbutylpiperidenes, e.g. fluspirilene and pimozide.

These drugs cause a range of side-effects: those that are predictable from the pharmacology of the drugs and those resulting from an allergic or idiosyncratic response. Dopamine blocking effects underlie some adverse effects and blockade of other receptors most of the others.

Extrapyramidal syndromes

These consist of a range of reactions which are mostly well defined although occasionally atypical. They occur at different times during treatment: some early, others later.

Acute dystonia develops within 1–2 days of exposure to antipsychotics or on increasing the dose. Approximately 10% of patients are affected. With depot formulations, it may take three days to develop. It usually affects young males and may involve the tongue, lip and jaw although the trunk and limbs can also be affected. Treatment is by parenteral anticholinergic medication.

Akathisia is a subjective sense of restlessness accompanied by ceaseless movements of the hands or feet with repeated standing or pacing. It occurs in 20–25% of patients taking antipsychotic drugs. To the inexperienced, it can be mistaken for increasing agitation. Akathisia has been associated with aggression, both towards others and self directed. Benzodiazepines, cyproheptadine or a beta-adrenoceptor blocker such as propanolol, may provide relief. Anticholinergic drugs are not particularly beneficial.

Parkinsonism is perhaps the most common extrapyramidal side-effect and ranges from bradykinesia in its mildest form, to akinesia with rigidity, festinant gait, crouched posture, coarse tremor, hypersalivation, and seborrhoea. It is more common in women and the elderly and can be confused with apathy, depression, or dementia. Its onset is usually in the first month of treatment and it tends to lessen with time, after dose reduction or anticholinergic drug administration. The common practice of concomitant administration of an anticholinergic drug with a antipsychotic, in the absence of this side-effect, is not advisable as they worsen the anticholinergic side-effects of the antipsychotic such as dry mouth and constipation, and are liable to abuse for their euphoriant effects.

Tardive dystonia and dyskinesia are long-term extrapyramidal side-effects of antipsychotic use. Tardive dystonia is relatively rare, with a prevalence of about 2%, and typically presents as a craniofacial syndrome in younger patients. Tardive dyskinesia, however, is more common with a prevalence of 15–25% or more, and starts months or years following antipsychotic medication although non–drug related cases in the elderly have been reported. Relevant risk factors for its development are female sex, affective disorder, organic brain disease, parkinsonian side-effects during acute treatment, alcohol abuse, negative symptoms of schizophrenia, and increasing age. It usually presents as choreoathetoid movements of the mouth and face but the trunk and limbs can also be affected. It's precise aetiology is unclear and theories abound. It is thought that using the smallest possible dose of antipsychotics and treating for short periods if practicable, are likely to minimise the risk of developing tardive dyskinesia. The treatment of tardive dyskinesia is difficult and strategies that have been tried include dose reduction, benzodiazepines such as clonazepam as muscle relaxants, tetrabenazine (a dopamine-depleting agent), vitamin E (a free radical scavenger) and lithium. The evidence base underpinning most of these strategies is weak. In severe cases, switching to clozapine should be considered. It is wise to examine for abnormal movements before prescribing antipsychotic drugs and to review patients every 6 months. If necessary, consideration should be given to the use of the Abnormal Involuntary Movement Scale (AIMS).

Neuroleptic malignant syndrome

This is perhaps the most dangerous neuromuscular adverse effect from antipsychotics. In moderate to severe cases, the incidence in antipsychotic treated patients is in the range of 0.2–1%, although milder cases are often unrecognised. Symptoms often develop early in treatment or are associated with rapid upward dosage titration.

The key clinical features are :

- hyperthermia;

- muscle rigidity;

- varying degrees of unconsciousness;

- labile hypertension;

- sweating;

- tachycardia; and

- elevated creatinine phosphokinase (CPK).

The hyperthermia is thought to be mediated by dopaminergic systems in the striatum and hypothalamus and is fatal in 20% or so of patients. More serious cases can result in death from shock, renal failure (with myoglobinuria), respiratory failure, or disseminated intravascular coagulation. The treatment of this condition is by cooling, rehydration, and specific drug treatments to counter muscle stiffness and promote dopamine activity. Dopamine agonists such as bromocriptine and amantadine and the antispasticity drug, dantrolene, are useful specific treatments although the precise regimen for use in this condition remains to be established.

Other side-effects of antipsychotics

These are:

- Anticholinergic effects, e.g. blurred vision, dry mouth, constipation, and difficulty with micturition.

- Sedation which varies between drugs.

- Postural hypotension, reflex tachycardia, and delayed ejaculation result from α_1-adrenergic antagonism.

- Weight gain which may result in poor compliance.

- Endocrine effects such as an increase in prolactin level due to dopaminergic blockade may cause galactorrhoea (and amenorrhoea), and loss of libido in men.

- Neuropsychological effects include impairment of co-ordination, attention, and memory, and the emergence of secondary negative symptoms or the antipsychotic induced deficit syndrome which is sometimes indistinguishable from depression. This can cause patients' compliance to falter.

- Granulocytopenia and other blood dyscrasias.

- Cardiac irregularities, and lowering of epileptic fit threshold are other less common side-effects.

USE OF 'HIGH-DOSE' ANTIPSYCHOTICS

High-dose antipsychotic treatment can be defined as the use of a dose in excess of the upper limit recommended by the *British National Formulary* (BNF) or the product data sheet produced by the manufacturers of the antipsychotic (Thompson 1994). There remains some uncertainty about whether low- or high-dose antipsychotics is the most appropriate treatment for psychosis (McEvoy *et al* 1991). Studies with high-doses have shown little evidence of superior effectiveness in the treatment of psychosis: with a similar proportion of patients responding to high and standard doses (Kane and Marder 1993; McCreadie and MacDonald 1977; McCreadie *et al* 1979). It is thought, however, that about 10–20% of schizophrenic patients may require higher than recommended doses of medication but there is no effective way of identifying this subgroup (Little *et al* 1989).

Indiscriminate use of higher than necessary doses of antipsychotics, which will have initial sedative benefits, may produce more potentially bothersome side-effects of dystonia, extrapyramidal syndrome, and general dysphoria that correlate with poor compliance and therefore, poor long-term outcome (Barnes and Bridges 1980; King *et al* 1995). Other serious adverse effects include cardiac arrhythmias (Fowler *et al* 1976; Committee on the safety of Medicines, 1990), and sudden death (Mehtonen *et al* 1991; Jusic and Lader 1994).

The Royal College of Psychiatrists' consensus statement on the use of high-dose antipsychotic medication (Thompson, 1994) notes that there are three main circumstances in which high-doses are commonly used and advises alternatives to the use of such high-doses.

These circumstances are:

- psychiatric emergencies;

- acute treatment; and

- long-term treatment.

In the latter, high-dose use seems to be largely driven by treatment resistance, polypharmacy, where two or more drugs are prescribed concurrently, and limited resources in in-patient units.

The Research Unit of the Royal College of Psychiatrists in a recent audit of the use of antipsychotics in the United Kingdom (of which the author was the organising psychiatrist member – unpublished data) found that of a total of 3132 patients receiving antipsychotics on the audit date, 47% were receiving more than one antipsychotic drug concurrently (polypharmacy). Approximately 20% were receiving antipsychotic medication in doses exceeding the BNF upper limit (high-dose). In 6% of these patients the high-dose prescription was due solely to a single antipsychotic and in the remaining 14% it was due to polypharmacy. The audit showed that the three common reasons, which were not mutually exclusive, advanced for multiple prescribing (polpharmacy) were:

- a single antipsychotic drug failed to control the patient's symptoms (76% of cases);

- two or more drugs were needed to treat an acute exacerbation (38%); and

- the patient was being switched from one antipsychotic drug to another (27%).

As these reasons were not mutually exclusive, it follows in some patients that two or more of these reasons were present.

Although the use of high-doses is to be discouraged, they may be necessary in some patients (Hirsch and Barnes, 1994). In such cases, high-doses should be used with caution and under specialist guidance. The Royal College of Psychiatrists has set out guidelines and suggestions for such prescribing. These guidelines are considered good practice and should minimise the risk of litigation. They include the need to:

- seek consent from the patient;

- discuss the treatment with a specialist colleague; and

- undertake investigations before initiating treatment and review these as appropriate, and check vital signs regularly.

Dose increases should be slow and regular reviews of the treatment must be instituted so that the dose can be reduced to an acceptable level as soon as possible (Thompson 1994, Hirsch and Barnes 1994).

ATYPICAL ANTIPSYCHOTICS

There is no consensus view about the definition of an atypical antipsychotic (Meltzer 1991). This group of drugs have become important over the last decade, although the prototype, clozapine, was first synthesised in 1959.

Atypical antipsychotics have been described as:

- producing antipsychotic action at doses that do not cause significant acute or subacute extrapyramidal side-effects (EPSE), such as parkinsonism and akathisia. Using this definition, it follows that substituted benzamides like remoxipride and sulpiride are atypicals;

- being associated with a reduced risk of tardive dyskinesia;

- having low dopamine receptor occupancy in clinically effective doses;

- having a high $5HT_2:D_2$ affinity;

- failing to increase serum prolactin levels (except substituted benzamides, zotepine and risperidone); and

- having improved efficacy in negative symptoms and treatment refractory patients. Only clozapine has proven efficacy in refractory illness.

With the exception of clozapine, which remains the most efficacious treatment in otherwise refractory patients, there are no clear clinical differences between the atypicals. Clozapine is effective in at least 30% of schizophrenic patients who had failed to respond to at least two trials of antipsychotic drugs of different classes (treatment-resistant) when given for 6 weeks (Kane *et al* 1988). After 1 year, up to 60% respond.

The following is a brief account of atypical antipsychotics, based on chemical grouping and *in vitro* receptor binding profile, and covers relevant prescribing information, side-effects, and precautions.

Clozapine is a dibenzapine tricyclic and is chemically related to loxapine. It has a spectrum of action across a range of receptor types: D_1, $5HT_2$, $5HT_6$, $5HT_7$, adrenergic α-1 and α-2, H_1 and Ach. It has a low D_2 receptor occupancy of 30–60%. Clozapine is licensed for the treatment of people with schizophrenia who are intolerant of conventional antipsychotics due to adverse effects or who fail to respond to them. Clozapine should be started at a low dose and ideally be used as monotherapy. The dose should be increased gradually and ideally administered in two divided doses because the half-life is 12–16 hours. The maximum daily dose is 900 mg. Response to clozapine in antipsychotic-resistant patients may not be evident until after 6 months or longer have elapsed (Meltzer, 1992). Blood levels may be useful in optimising therapy if no response occurs. A good response is more likely when the level is above 350 ng/ml (Taylor and Duncan 1995; Cooper 1996; Perry *et al* 1998).

Clozapine causes agranulocytosis in up to 1% of patients, a rate higher than that found with standard antipsychotics (about 1:2,000). The great majority of these cases occur in the first to fifth months (Atkin *et al*, 1996). Regular blood monitoring through the Clozaril Patient Monitoring Service aims to reduce this risk. Weekly blood counts are required in the first 18 weeks of treatment, followed by two weekly counts until 1 year and then monthly checks thereafter.

Clozapine causes sedation, sialorrhoea, and postural hypotension. It can cause epilepsy (Wilson and Claussen 1994) especially in doses of over 600 mg a day where the risk is approximately 5% (Devinsky, 1991). It has been proposed that patients on such doses should be routinely commenced on the anti-convulsant drug, sodium valproate.

Some patients who may benefit from clozapine treatment refuse to co-operate with blood tests, oral medication or both. It is important to fully explore reasons for refusal and work with the patient to encourage adherence to treatment. Full discussion of this issue is in Pereira *et al* (1999).

Risperidone is a benzisoxazole derivative and like clozapine is a potent antagonist of $5HT_{2A}$, $5HT_7$, α-1 and 2 adrenergic, and histamine H_1 receptors. It does, however, have a higher D_2 receptor affinity but its potency as an antagonist at D_1 receptors is low. Because it produces hyperprolactinaemia, EPSEs at higher doses (Marder and

Meibach 1994), and a somewhat inconsistent benefit in negative symptoms, some have disputed its place as an atypical (Cardoni 1995).

Risperidone is metabolised in the liver to an active metabolite, 9-hydroxyrisperidone which has a half-life of 17–22 hours. In doses of 4–8 mg/day, it appears to be at least equivalent and possibly superior to haloperidol, 10–20/day, in decreasing positive and negative symptoms (Castelao et al 1989; Claus et al 1992; Chouinard et al 1993, Marder and Meibach, 1994). Common adverse effects of risperidone are insomnia, anxiety, agitation, sedation, dizziness, rhinitis, hypotension, weight gain, and menstrual disturbances. It has been reported to cause Neuroleptic Malignant Syndrome and careful observation is therefore advised (Sharma et al 1995). Unlike clozapine, no special monitoring is required with risperidone.

Olanzapine is a thienobenzodiazepine similar in structure to clozapine. It has a high affinity for several of the 5HT receptor subtypes, α-1 adrenoreceptors, histaminergic, and muscarinic receptors. It has a weak affinity for D_2 receptors compared to typical antipsychotics but more than clozapine (Reus 1997).

Olanzapine is well absorbed after oral administration and reaches peak blood levels in 5–8 hours. It is metabolised to inactive metabolites by the liver mostly via CPY1A2. In a number of studies, it was at least as effective as haloperidol, in a range of doses (5–20 mg), and caused a similar frequency of EPSE to placebo (Beasley et al 1996a,b; Beasley et al 1997; Tollefson et al 1997). Serum level measurements are now readily available and may be necessary in patients for whom there may be a problem with compliance.

Apart from use in pregnant or breast-feeding women and patients with narrow-angle glaucoma there are no contra-indications to the use of olanzapine. Common side-effects are drowsiness and weight gain which can be significant. Others are anticholinergic effects like dry mouth and constipation, dizziness, peripheral oedema, and postural hypotension. Asymptomatic elevation of liver enzymes has been reported (Beasley et al 1996b) and it may therefore be necessary to perform a baseline liver function test and re-check this after treatment with olanzapine has started.

Quetiapine has a broad receptor binding profile with low to moderate affinity for D_1, D_2, $5HT_{1A}$ and $5HT_{2A}$ receptors; moderate affinity for α-1 and -2 adrenoceptors; and high affinity for histamine-1 receptors. A number of double-blind randomised trials have shown it to be as effective as conventional antipsychotics in the treatment of schizophrenia (Hirsch et al, 1996; Markowitz et al, 1999). Trials have shown that the incidence of EPSE in patients taking quetiapine was similar to those taking placebo across the full dosage range (150–750 mg). The most frequent side-effects reported from short-term controlled trials included sedation (17.5%), dizziness (10%), and constipation (9%). Quetiapine does not raise serum prolactin levels. It is contra-indicated in breast feeding mothers. Quetiapine has been associated with the development of cataracts in laboratory animals and there have been a small number of reports in humans (causality has not yet been determined).

Treatment is usually initiated with 25 mg twice a day and increased over several days to the usual range of 300–450 mg a day in two divided doses. A starter pack is available in the UK to make the dose titration easier.

Substituted benzamides, e.g. sulpiride, amisulpiride, and remoxipride. This group of drugs are classified as atypicals because of their selectivity for limbic or cortical dopamine receptors rather than striatal dopamine receptors. They therefore have a considerably reduced potential for EPS but do, however, raise serum prolactin.

Sulpiride is a very well established drug in the UK, having been around for about a decade. It is specific for dopamine D_2, D_3, and D_4 receptors. Maximum dosages differ for patients depending on whether they present with positive or negative symptoms. Positive symptom patients should be treated with doses of up to 2.4 g a day and negative symptom patients 800 mg a day.

Amisulpiride also has a high affinity for D_2 and D_3 receptors predominantly at limbic sites. It is commonly prescribed in France and seems to be effective against negative symptoms when used in low doses such as 100 mg a day (Boyer *et al* 1995, Loo *et al* 1997), although no more effective than low dose haloperidol. EPSE and raised prolactin are dose-dependent.

Remoxipride, which is selective for D_2 receptors, is available in North America. In the UK it is available on a named patient basis only with the need for specific monitoring because of reports of aplastic anaemia and pancytopenia (Markowitz *et al* 1999). Its clinically effective dose lies between 150 and 600 mg a day. It does not appear to have any significant impact on the negative symptoms of schizophrenia (Vartiainen *et al* 1993).

Zotepine is also available in the UK. It has a complex pharmacology. Zotepine causes hyperprolactinaemia, EPSEs at higher doses and precipitates epilepsy.

Ziprasidone is a potent D_2 and $5HT_2$ receptor antagonist. It is still undergoing clinical trials and is said to have an effect on co-morbid anxiety and depression (Tandon 1977) is devoid of weight gain. It causes somnolence in 20% of patients.

TREATMENT RESISTANCE

There is no firm agreement about the definition of treatment resistance. It is, however, accepted by most to mean a lack of satisfactory clinical improvement despite the use of at least two antipsychotics from different chemical classes prescribed at an adequate dose for an adequate duration (Brenner *et al* 1990). A much stricter criteria, proposed by Kane (1992), requires the patient to have had several treatment trials for over 6 weeks with different antipsychotics in doses of over 500 mg chlorpromazine equivalents per day. Daniel and Whitcomb (1998) argue for a multi-axial classification of treatment resistance that focuses attention on specific target problems in the belief that this may be more helpful in directing treatment. They suggest the following target problems: misdiagnosis or co-morbidity; positive symptoms, negative symptoms, and agitation; treatment intolerance due to side-effects; and poor compliance.

About a third of patients with schizophrenia do not respond to conventional or classical antipsychotics. This non-response, by which is meant the continuation of symptoms with considerable functional disability and or behavioural disturbance (Brenner et al, 1990), is commoner in patients with negative symptoms, aggressive behaviour, cognitive impairment, and co-morbid mood symptoms.

Strategies for the management of treatment resistance include ensuring compliance and increasing insight into dose response relationships, dosage adjustment, change of antipsychotics, and augmentation with other drugs or treatment methods (Daniel and Whitcomb, 1998).

Compliance issues

It is important to ensure that patients are compliant with their medication as poor compliance contributes significantly to poor response and prognosis (Kemp et al, 1996). It appears to be perpetuated by lack of insight, psychosis, and intolerable side-effects. Two other important factors are a complicated drug regimen and poor follow-up. It may be necessary to measure the plasma level of some drugs to check compliance and, where applicable, therapeutic levels. A review of the patient's diagnosis, drug regimen, and follow-up programme may be required.

High dose antipsychotics

The use of high-doses of conventional or typical antipsychotics is discussed above. This is arguably the most common treatment approach for the treatment-resistant patient (Hirsch and Barnes, 1994). There have been a number of anecdotal and controlled reports supporting such an approach although not all studies favour high-doses (Ital et al 1970; Rifkin et al 1971; Quitkin et al 1975). The use of high-doses must be guided by the patient's response and should be reviewed on a regular basis. In the absence of clinical improvement, a medication review is needed.

Atypical antipsychotics

Atypical antipsychotics are worth trying particularly clozapine which is licensed in treatment-resistant illness. A number of open design studies suggest that risperidone in modest doses of 4–8 mg/day is effective in treatment-resistant patients. However, studies that have compared risperidone to clozapine have reported inconsistent findings: some reported similar efficacy others significantly less (Bersani et al 1990; Chouinard et al 1994; Cavallero et al 1995; Sharif 1998).

Clozapine is an established treatment for this group of patients. About 30% of patients improve after 6 weeks of treatment and up to 60% improve after 1 year. It has been suggested that a clozapine plasma level of over 350 ng/ml distinguishes responders from non-responders (Perry et al 1991; Hasegawa et al 1993; Lieberman et al 1994; Potkin and Bera 1994). There is no evidence for a therapeutic window and some patients respond at plasma levels below 350 ng/ml. It may, however, be prudent to exceed the recommended maximum daily dose of 900 mg if the plasma level of clozapine is less than 350 ng/ml and the patient is free of major side-effects (Hasegawa et al 1993). Closer monitoring will, of course, be required.

The usefulness of combination treatments is being researched in patients who do not respond to clozapine. Of particular interest are combinations of clozapine with ECT or risperidone. No robust data is currently available in favour of either combination. The primary literature must always be consulted before using such combinations as additional side-effects have been reported.

Adjunctive treatments

Adjunctive treatments have been in use in treatment resistant patients for some time. Most of these strategies were in use before the availability of drugs such as clozapine, for the treatment of this recalcitrant population. They are, however, useful in a number of patients.

Antidepressants

Research into the aetiology and treatment of postpsychotic depression, negative symptoms, and antipsychotic-induced akinesia indicates that a small group of patients respond to adjunctive tricyclic antidepressants (Siris et al 1991; Meltzer 1992). Newer SSRIs are also beneficial (Geoff et al 1990). It is suggested that the $5HT_{1A}$ agonist, buspirone, may also be beneficial (Brody et al 1990). However, further research is needed to establish the role of buspirone in the treatment of these patients. In practice antidepressants are recommended if significant symptoms of depression exist.

Lithium

Lithium has been used for over two decades for the effective treatment of patients with manic–depressive psychosis. A number of studies have reported a reduction in symptoms in patients who have been given lithium in addition to conventional antipsychotics (Small et al 1975; Carman et al 1981). Patients with significant affective symptoms or those diagnosed as suffering from schizoaffective disorder seem to particularly benefit (Biederman *et al* 1979; Hirschowitz *et al* 1980). The combination of lithium with high-doses of haloperidol should be avoided as neurotoxicity may result (Cohen and Cohen 1974).

Propranolol

Some studies have examined the usefulness of propranolol in addition to antipsychotics in treatment resistant-schizophrenia. Some report improvement (Yorkston *et al* 1977; Lindstrom and Persson 1980) whereas others do not (Myers *et al* 1981). Dosages in these studies are large and range from 400 to 2,000 mg a day. It is however, difficult to predict which patients will respond or indeed what dose of propranolol to use. Furthermore, propranolol increases the plasma levels of antipsychotics and may therefore lead to considerably more side-effects (Peet *et al* 1980).

Carbamazepine

Carbamazepine in combination with antipsychotics may be beneficial to some patients with schizophrenia, particularly those with EEG abnormalities, history of violence or aggression, or manic symptoms (Hakola and Laulumaa 1982; Klein *et al* 1984; Luchins 1984). The risk of lowering antipsychotic plasma levels, probably through induction of hepatic enzymes, should be borne in mind as this may require an increase in the dose of the antipsychotic. Carbamazepine should not be combined with clozapine as it may increase the risk of bone marrow depression.

ECT

The use of ECT in schizophrenia has been a long-established practice although available evidence indicates that it is not as effective as medication (Salzman 1980). In treatment resistant patients, it may improve symptoms in about 5–10% of cases but, the response is usually short-lived and maintenance treatments may be required. Response is better in patients with a long history of illness, significant affective symptoms, or catatonia (Meltzer 1992).

Others

Benzodiazepines are other agents proposed in the treatment resistant patient. Benzodiazepines have not resulted in consistent improvement and can produce violent behaviours in some patients (Karson *et al* 1982). Advocates suggest modest improvement (Wolkowitz *et al* 1992). Their use should, however, be limited to the anxious patient who has not responded to other management strategies. The risk of abuse and dependence should always be borne in mind.

ANXIOLYTICS AND OTHER MEDICATIONS

Anxiety is a commonly used word which is defined as 'uneasiness of the mind and concern about imminent danger' (*The Concise Oxford Dictionary*, 1995). It is common in the day to day life of virtually everyone. Anxiety disorder, however, implies excessive, severe, and prolonged anxiety, which compromises normal functioning. The prevalence of moderate to severe anxiety in the general population ranges from 2.5 to 6.5% depending on definition and gender (Weissman and Merikangas 1986; Kessler *et al* 1994). This pathological anxiety, which occurs in a range of clinical states, often requires treatment.

Range of anxiety disorders

Although most psychiatric disorders such as schizophrenia and organic brain syndromes, may be associated with pathological anxiety requiring treatment, only the group of disorders that share the subjective, physiological, and behavioural features of anxiety are grouped under the term 'anxiety disorders'. The 10th edition of the International Classification of Diseases (ICD10) groups these disorders under 'neurotic, stress-related, and somatoform disorders' (F40-F48). They include:

- Phobic anxiety disorders such as agoraphobia, social and specific phobias.

- Panic disorder.

- Generalised anxiety disorder (GAD).

- Obsessive-compulsive disorder (OCD).

- Post-traumatic stress disorder (PTSD).

- Adjustment disorder with anxiety (and depression).

Management

The treatment of anxiety disorders depends on the type and severity of the disorder as well as other associated factors, which will be evident from the assessment of the patient. Non-pathological anxiety and panic attacks, rather than panic disorder, which are attributable to an identifiable stress, can effectively be treated with reassurance about symptoms, counselling, and relaxation techniques.

Patients with anxiety disorders typically require both psychological treatment, aimed at addressing any underlying problems, and drug treatment for the relief of symptoms. For a significant number of these patients, drug treatment may be indicated initially before the patient can participate effectively in psychological treatment, especially, when depression is present (Okocha 1996a).

Drug treatments

Available drugs for the treatment of anxiety disorders include: benzodiazepine and non-benzodiazepine anxiolytics, antidepressants, beta-blockers and antipsychotic drugs.

Benzodiazepines

These drugs, which are very effective anxiolytics, were for many years the mainstay of treatment but the risk of dependence has now greatly limited their use (Okocha 1996b). They do, however, still have a role in the management of some patients. The benefits of treatment must be weighed against the risk of dependence in individual cases. Patients with incapacitating generalised anxiety disorder, panic disorder or post-traumatic stress disorder may benefit from an initial course of a benzodiazepine e.g., diazepam, 6 mg in divided doses, or lorazepam, 1–4 mg a day, to control their symptoms until longer-term drug treatment and psychological therapy become effective.

The triazolo-benzodiazepine, Alprazolam, which has a different chemical structure to typical benzodiazepines like diazepam, is effective in the treatment of generalised anxiety (and panic) disorder. However, it is also associated with dependence, which may be worse than with typical benzodiazepines. Furthermore, it is not available for prescription on the NHS.

Whenever possible, intermittent use of benzodiazepines, rather than regular use, must be encouraged and the risk of dependence discussed with patients before and during use.

Buspirone hydrochloride

This drug, unlike the benzodiazepines, which act on the GABA-chloride complex, acts via 5HT receptors. It is indicated in the short-term management of anxiety disorders and appears to have moderate efficacy in this regard. Unlike benzodiazepines, however, buspirone has a slow onset of action but does not appear to impair psychomotor function or cause dependency problems. Nausea, dizziness, headache, and fatigue, can be bothersome for patients, such that up to 10% default from treatment. Patients who have previously been treated with benzodiazepines respond poorly to buspirone and may suffer more side-effects.

Antidepressants

The use of antidepressants in the treatment of anxiety disorders is well established. Antidepressants are effective even in the absence of depression and this has led to the suggestion that the two conditions may share a common underlying biological cause.

The three main groups of antidepressants that are used in the treatment of anxiety disorders are:

- Tricyclic antidepressants (TCAs).

- Selective serotonin reuptake inhibitors (SSRIs).

- Monoamine oxidase inhibitors (MAOIs).

As with the treatment of depression, there is no consensus among specialists on whether a TCA or an SSRI should be used first line in the treatment of anxiety disorders. Some drugs in each of these groups are, however, licensed for the treatment of particular disorders or have shown significantly more efficacy. Once good effect has been achieved, antidepressant treatment should be continued for about 6–8 months and then tapered to minimise the likelihood of symptom recurrence on withdrawal.

Tricyclic antidepressants

These drugs act by blocking the neuronal uptake of catecholamines and serotonin thus increasing the effective concentrations of these monoamines at central receptor sites (monoamine re-uptake inhibition). Their effectiveness varies in different conditions. For example, clomipramine, which inhibits reuptake of serotonin and to some degree noradrenaline through its metabolite methylclomipramine, is reputed to be effective in obsessive-compulsive disorder. Tricyclics with weak serotonergic activity, such as imipramine, appear to be ineffective in OCD. Both clomipramine and imipramine are, however, effective in panic disorder, although the doses must be increased gradually as their side-effects can be bothersome. The common side-effects are dry mouth, blurred vision, constipation, sedation, weight gain, sexual dysfunction, and urinary retention. They are also dangerous when taken in overdose and are slow in onset of action; taking up to 3 weeks to produce an effect.

Selective serotonin reuptake inhibitors (SSRIs)

With the evidence that serotonin may be implicated in the pathogenesis of anxiety, has come an increased interest in these drugs. They do not bind to any specific neuroreceptors but selectively block serotonin re-uptake through inhibition of the re-uptake 'carrier'. This inhibition results in an increase of serotonin in the synapse. It is thought that the lack of clinical efficacy for at least two weeks or so is due to the stimulation of pre-synaptic autoreceptors resulting in a reduction in serotonergic turnover in the synaptic cleft. Eventual desensitisation of the pre-synaptic autoreceptors results in increased serotonin release and enhancement of serotonergic transmission. This process takes about 2 weeks to occur. Although other explanations have been put forward for the delay in onset of action, this is perhaps the most favoured, as the reduction in serotonergic turnover from stimulation of the auto-receptors is thought to be responsible for the exacerbation of anxiety that occurs soon after these drugs are started.

These drugs are preferred to TCAs because of their relative safety in overdose although some deaths have recently been attributed to citalopram (Ostrom *et al* 1996).

Their common side-effects are nausea, headache, agitation, and sexual dysfunction. Advising patients of these and starting treatment at a low dose will minimise these problems. A benzodiazepine can be added for a short period.

All SSRIs have been used in the treatment of various anxiety disorders. However, they are not all licensed for the treatment of these disorders.

Monoamine oxidase inhibitors

These drugs inhibit the intracellular enzyme monoamine oxidase (MAO) thereby increasing the concentration of noradrenaline, dopamine, and serotonin. MAOIs such as phenelzine, have been found to alleviate generalised anxiety, panic and phobic disorders. Phenelzine is, however, not licensed for the treatment of panic disorder. Their use is limited by dietary restrictions and dangerous interactions with a range of other drugs like pethidine and cold remedies. They also have troublesome side-effects like weight gain, oedema, postural hypotension, sexual dysfunction, and urinary retention. The reversible and selective MAOI, moclobemide, has fewer side-effects and minimal dietary restrictions but has not been used extensively in the treatment of these disorders.

Beta-blockers

Propranolol, has long been used to treat anxiety, particularly where autonomic symptoms such as palpitations, tremor and gastro-intestinal upset are prominent. Patients with performance anxiety may also respond well. Propranolol does not, however, have any effect on the subjective or behavioural manifestations of anxiety such as, impaired concentration and avoidance. Its effectiveness in relieving a patient's anxiety disorder depends, to some extent, on the significance of the bodily symptoms in the maintenance of the disorder.

Mood stabilisers

Mood stabilisers are drugs that lower and maintain mood at euthymic levels in patients with mania or hypomania. They also sustain euthymic mood in patients with unipolar depression when combined with an appropriate antidepressant. These drugs, which are particularly useful in the treatment of patients with bipolar-affective disorder, include: lithium, carbamazepine, and sodium valproate.

Lithium

Lithium is an alkali earth element, similar to sodium and potassium. It is an established treatment in patients with bipolar-affective disorder. Its precise mode of action is uncertain but it is known to reduce the neurotransmitter-induced activation of adenylate cyclase at certain post-synaptic receptors. Adenylate cyclase is required for the formation of cyclic adenosine monophosphate (cAMP), which mediates changes in most neurotransmitter target cells. This inhibition of adenylate cyclase also occurs in other organs, such as the thyroid gland and the kidneys. In the thyroid, it results in hypothyroidism due to poor response of the gland to thyroid stimulating hormone. In the kidneys, nephrogenic diabetes insipidus with the typical symptom of polyuria occurs as a result of poor response to antidiuretic hormone.

Lithium is effective in acute mania although recent studies have indicated that 30–60% of patients do not respond well (Kukopulos *et al* 1980; Small *et al* 1988; 1991). Poor response is commoner in patients with mixed mania i.e., presence of manic symptoms with dysphoria, and rapid or continuous cycling patients (Faedda *et al* 1991; Bauer *et al* 1994). Clinical improvement with lithium is relatively slow, with an initial response generally occurring 1–2 weeks after commencing treatment. Initial improvement may not occur for up to 4 weeks in some patients. Antipsychotic medication is often required during this lag period due to the aggressive and disruptive behaviour of the acutely manic patient. The combination of lithium with high-doses of haloperidol should be avoided because of the risk of neurotoxicity (Cohen and Cohen 1974).

Lithium has also been shown to markedly reduce the risk of recurrence of manic and depressive episodes in patients with bipolar-affective disorder (Baastrup *et al* 1970; Coppen *et al* 1971; Fieve *et al* 1976). Its protective effect against subsequent episodes appears however, to be lower for depressive episodes than for manic episodes (Dunner and Fieve 1974). Maintenance lithium appears to be most effective in patients with an uncomplicated manic episode, good functioning between episodes, and a family history of bipolar illness (Goodwin and Jamison 1990). As with acute treatment, mixed mania and rapid cycling mania respond poorly to maintenance treatment with lithium. Other predictors of poor response are severe or chronic depression, mood incongruent psychotic symptoms, significant substance abuse, and personality disorder.

Before commencing lithium, thyroid and kidney function should be tested. Hypothyroidism due to lithium is common and occurs in up to 20% of women (Linstedt *et al* 1977). Lithium should be discontinued or thyroxine treatment commenced. The effects on the kidneys are two-fold: nephrogenic diabetes insipidus, which is largely reversible, and persistent impairment of concentrating ability, which occurs in 10% of cases. Reversible ECG changes due to the displacement of potassium in the myocardium have been described. These look like those of hypokalaemia, with T-wave flattening and inversion or widening of the QRS.

A suitable starting dose of lithium carbonate is 400 mg daily. Plasma levels need to be monitored 12 hours after the last dose and at weekly intervals initially. Plasma levels of between 0.4 and 1.0 mmol/l should be aimed for. Levels above 1.5 mmol/l lead to lithium toxicity.

Patients on lithium may complain of side-effects such as:

• Nausea.

- Metallic taste in the mouth.

- Excessive thirst and polyuria.

- Tremor.

- Weight gain.

These side-effects are worse with higher plasma levels. Lithium interacts with a number of non-steroidal anti-inflammatory drugs, which are known to delay its clearance. Lithium should be avoided in pregnant women especially in the first trimester: it is known to increase cardiovascular anomalies (Kallen and Tandberg 1983). In such patients, antipsychotics should be used if manic symptoms occur following discontinuation of lithium.

Symptoms of lithium toxicity are:

- Coarsening tremor.

- Nausea.

- Vomiting and dizziness.

- Ataxia.

- Dysarthria.

- Drowsiness.

- Confusion.

- Epileptic fits.

- Coma.

Carbamazepine

Carbamazepine has been established as being effective in both the acute and prophylactic treatment of mania, mixed states, rapid cycling bipolar illness, and other lithium non-responsive patients (Ballenger and Post 1980). There is evidence that it is superior to placebo and as effective as lithium and antipsychotics in the treatment of acute mania (Klein *et al* 1984; Post *et al* 1987, 1989; Small *et al* 1991). The addition of lithium to the regimen of poor responders appears to lead to clinical improvement (Kramlinger and Post 1989). Carbamazepine does, however, produce a less robust response in acute bipolar depression than it does in mania (Ballenger and Post 1980; Post *et al* 1986).

For prophylactic and maintenance treatments, carbamazepine is superior to placebo and at least as effective as lithium although there is evidence that patients on carbamazepine relapsed earlier than those on lithium (Ballenger and Post 1980; Okuma *et al* 1983; Placidi *et al* 1986; Watkins *et al* 1987).

It has a number of side-effects like, drowsiness, ataxia, and diplopia, which develop when the plasma concentrations are too high. Others are erythematous rash, water retention, hepatitis, and leucopenia or other blood dyscrasias. Carbamazepine induces liver enzymes and may therefore accelerate the metabolism of other drugs like contraceptive pills, antidepressants, and antipsychotics.

Valproate

Valproate, which is commonly available as sodium valproate, has been shown in well-designed studies to be effective for the treatment of manic patients (Emrich *et al* 1985; Pope *et al* 1991; Freeman *et al* 1992). It is superior to placebo (Emrich *et al* 1985), and as effective as lithium in acute mania (Pope *et al* 1991). Freeman *et al* (1992), found that valproate and lithium were both effective in improving manic symptoms, although lithium was slightly more effective overall. Furthermore, they found valproate to be superior to lithium in the management of acute episodes of mania accompanied by co-existing depression, i.e., mixed states or dysphoric mania. Double-blind controlled studies examining the use of valproate for prophylaxis or maintenance treatment of mania are rare. However, open studies show that it is as effective as lithium or carbamazepine (Puzynski and Klosiewicz 1984; Emrich *et al* 1985; Hayes 1989; Pope *et al* 1991).

The common adverse effects of valproate are gastro-intestinal disturbance, potentiation of the effects of sedative drugs, and obesity. Thrombocytopenia, tremor, and impairment of liver function tests occur occasionally.

ELECTROCONVULSIVE THERAPY (ECT)

Meduna first introduced convulsive therapy for schizophrenia using camphor in 1934 but electrical induction of convulsions was not introduced until 1938. At the time, it was thought that schizophrenia and epilepsy never co-existed (Abrams 1992). Convulsive treatments were used widely in the 1940s and 1950s to the extent of being the standard against which new drugs were compared. Interest in ECT died down as new and effective drugs became available, and public concern about its frequency of use increased. It is now used in limited circumstances (American Psychiatric Association Task Force on ECT 1990) and remains a very effective treatment. Real ECT has been shown to be more effective than sham ECT (Freeman *et al* 1978; Johnstone *et al* 1980; West 1981; Brandon *et al* 1984; Gregory *et al* 1985).

Changes in the use and practice of ECT over the past decades have increased its safety and efficacy. Modified ECT is achieved with the use of short-acting anaesthetics and muscle relaxants. These considerably reduce the frequency of bone fractures and the unpleasant awareness of paralysis of the respiratory muscles during treatments with muscle relaxants only. Modern ECT is given as brief pulse stimulation from a constant-current machine with a stimulus setting that can be altered to take into account the individuals' seizure threshold. The aim of treatment is thus to produce a seizure that will lead to amelioration of symptoms whilst minimising adverse cognitive side-effects.

Unilateral ECT, where the two treatment electrodes are placed over the non-dominant hemisphere, produces minimal adverse cognitive effects compared with the more traditional bilateral treatment. The main adverse effect of ECT is post-treatment confusion and variable degrees of anterograde and retrograde amnesia. Patients treated with unilateral ECT suffer these side-effects less (Squire et al 1986). There does, however, appear to be significant differences in clinical efficacy between the two methods of ECT treatment, with bilateral treatments being more effective (Gregory et al 1985). Evidence shows that the dose of electricity must be increased several fold in unilateral treatments to achieve the same clinical efficacy as bilateral treatment (Sackeim et al 1993).

Although the frequency and number of treatments vary, ECT is commonly administered two or three times a week in courses that range from 4–12 treatments (Weiner 1994). More treatments have been proposed in patients with schizophrenia (Salzman 1980). In some patients, maintenance or continuation treatments are given 2 weekly or monthly for 6 months or more to prevent relapse and maintain improvement (Weiner 1994; Karliner 1994).

Indications

By far the commonest reason for the use of ECT is major depression, particularly if it is life threatening or resistant to treatment (Fink 1994). Other uses are, mania especially manic delirium, and catatonic schizophrenia. In developing countries where ECT is an available and inexpensive treatment, schizophrenia continues to be an important indication for the use of ECT (Salzman 1980). The elderly also represent a high percentage of ECT recipients, presumably because ECT has a better safety profile compared to some pharmacological alternatives and because rates of life threatening depression are probably higher in the elderly. Further, medication resistance and intolerance are commoner in the elderly (Sackeim et al 1990). ECT can be life-saving in cases of neuroleptic malignant syndrome and can be used across all ages. In pregnancy and certain physical illnesses, it may be considered safer than antidepressant medication (Royal College of Psychiatrists, 1995).

Mode of action

The exact mode of action of ECT is yet to be determined (Fink 1990). Previous theories have focused largely on psychological factors such as, induction of fear, punishment, memory loss for underlying cause of depressive symptoms, and euphoria akin to that seen in some types of brain damage, and have all been discarded. There is, to date, no evidence that ECT produces any kind of brain damage as shown by the absence of quantitative or qualitative changes using imaging techniques (Devanand *et al* 1994).

Animal and human studies, using a range of techniques, show that ECT causes a variety of neurophysiological changes in the brain. These changes include an increase in cerebral blood flow, oxygen consumption, and glucose metabolism; short-lasting reversible inhibition of protein synthesis which is thought to play a role in the cognitive effects through loss of neuronal plasticity necessary for consolidation of memory, and transient disruption of the blood–brain barrier leading to permeability of larger molecules (Davis and Squire 1984; Sackeim 1994).

Therapeutic benefit from ECT is thought to be associated with enhanced function of the serotonergic, dopaminergic, and noradrenergic pathways. There is also an associated increase in gamma aminobutyric acid concentration in specific brain regions and like most antidepressants, ECT results in increased density of the GABA-B receptor. Cholinergic activity is, however, reduced and this is thought to be partly responsible for the amnestic effects of ECT (Nutt and Glue 1993; Mann and Kapur 1994).

Adverse effects and dangers

The mortality rate associated with ECT is comparable with that of general anaesthesia in minor surgery and is estimated to be about one death per 10,000 patients treated (Abrams 1992; Royal College of Psychiatrists 1995). ECT related complications are more likely in the elderly, particularly the oldest age groups, those with other medical conditions, particularly cardiac illnesses, and those receiving medication for medical illnesses.

Patients with any of the following medical conditions are believed to be at considerably higher risk of mortality from ECT:

- Space-occupying cerebral lesions or other conditions that increase intracranial pressure.

- Recent myocardial infarction associated with unstable cardiac function.

- Recent intracerebral haemorrhage.

- Unstable vascular aneurysm or malformation.

- Retinal detachment.

- Phaeochromocytoma.

Although there are no absolute contra-indications to the use of ECT, except perhaps raised intracranial pressure, patients with any of the above are best not treated with ECT until the medical condition has stabilised.

Ethical and legal issues

The responsibility for appropriate use of ECT and adoption of guidelines for obtaining informed consent remains that of the psychiatrist. Every patient must give a written and valid informed consent before treatment can commence. In life-saving circumstances, one or possibly two treatments can be given under common-law but a second opinion, under the Mental Health Act 1983, must be sought for subsequent treatments, if consent is unobtainable. In patients under 16 years, the Royal College of Psychiatrists recommends that the opinion of a Child and Adolescent psychiatrist be sought in addition to the consent of the child and their parents (Royal College of Psychiatrists 1995).

Antilibidinal drugs

Antilibidinal drugs are of some use in patients who commit sexual offences, in whom they complement psychological and social treatments. Sexual offences refer to a breach of acceptable sexual behaviour. Sexual disorders, which largely fall into dysfunctions such as anorgasmia, and problems related to orientation and body image difficulties, do not necessarily result in offences. Paraphilias are perhaps the most likely disorders to lead to offending behaviour. Depending on the findings during assessment, antilibidinal drugs may be required. Their use, however, is often involuntary in that patients are forced to receive them by the law as an alternative to imprisonment or an aid to early release from prison or secure hospital.

By far the most commonly used drug is cyproterone acetate, a steroidal antihandrogen which has a direct blocking effect at the cellular level but also with additional anti-androgen properties, blocking gonadotropin secretion. It reduces sexual interest, drive, arousal, and deviant fantasies (Bradford 1983; Cooper 1986). It may take 2–3 weeks to work. Anti-androgens are available in tablet or depot injection forms. It is necessary to explain anticipated effects and side-effects before prescribing antilibidinal drugs. Written consent is desirable, where applicable and regular liver function tests are required.

The butyrophenone, benperidol is also widely believed to be effective for the control of deviant sexual behaviour (Tennent et al 1974). This effect is probably due to hyperprolactinaemia and is unlikely to be different from the sexual dysfunction commonly reported with all antipsychotic drugs.

CONCLUSION

Almost all patients admitted to PICUs receive pharmacological interventions and for many, medication is the major treatment intervention. Staff should be aware of the uses and side-effects of commonly used drugs and be able to access information to assist in planning drug strategies for those patients with more refractory illness.

REFERENCES

Abrams R. 1992 Electroconvulsive Therapy. New York: Oxford University Press

American Psychiatric Association. 1990 The Practice of ECT: Recommendations for Treatment, Training, and Privileging. Washington, DC: American Psychiatric Press

Atkin K, Kendall F, Gould D. 1996 Neutropenia and aggranulocytosis in patients receiving clozapine in the UK and Ireland. Br J Psych: 169: 483–488

Baastrup PC, Paulsen JC, Schou M, Thomsen K, Amidsen A. 1970 Prophylactic lithium: double-blind discontinuation in manic-depressive and recurrent depressive disorders. Lancet ii: 326–330

Ballenger JC, Post RM. 1980 Carbamazepine in manic-depressive illness: a new treatment. Am J Psych 137: 782–790

Barnes TRE and Bridges PK. 1980 Disturbed behaviour induced with high-dose antipsychotic drugs. BMJ 281: 274–275

Bauer MS, Calabrese JR, Dunner DL. 1994 Multisite data vs analysis: validity of rapid cycling as a course modifier for bipolar disorder in DSM-IV. Am J Psych 151: 506–515

Bellack AS and Mueser KT. 1993 Psychosocial treatment for schizophrenia. Schiz Bull 19: 317–336

Beasley Jr CM, Tollefson G, Tran P. 1996a Olanzapine versus placebo and haloperidol. Acute phase results of the North American double-blind olazapine trial. Neuropsychopharm 14: 11–1123

Beasley Jr CM, Sanger T, Satterlee W. 1996b Olanzapine versus placebo: results of a double-blind, fixed-dose olanzapine trial. Psychopharm 124: 159–167

Beasley Jr CM, Hamilton SH, Crawford AM. 1997 Olanzapine versus haloperidol: acute phase results of the international double-blind olanzapine trial. European Neuropsychopharm 7: 125–137

Biederman J, Lerner Y, Belmaker RH. 1979 Combination of lithium carbonate and haloperidol in schizoaffective disorder: a controlled study. Arch Gen Psychiatry 36: 327–333

Bersani G, Bressa GM, Meco G. 1990 Combined 5HT2 and Dopamine D2 antagonism in schizophrenia: clinical, extrapyramidal and human neuroendocrine response in a preliminary study with risperidone. Hum Psychopharm 5: 225–231

Boyer P, Lecrucibier Y, Puech AJ. 1995 Treatment of negative symptoms of schizophrenia with Amisulpiride. Br J Psych 166: 68–72

Brandon S, Cowley P, McDonald C, Neville P. 1984 Electroconvulsive therapy: Results in depressive illness from the Leicestershire trial. BMJ 288: 22–25

Brenner HD, Dencker SJ, Goldstein M. 1990 Defining treatment refractoriness in schizophrenia. Schiz Bull 16: 551–561

Brody D, Adler LA, Kim T. 1990 Effects of Buspirone in seven schizophrenic subjects. J Clin Psychopharm 10: 68–69

Cardoni AA. 1995 Risperidone: Review and assessment of its role in the treatment of schizophrenia. Ann Pharm 29: 610–618

Carman JS, Bigelow LB, Wyatt RJ. 1981 Lithium combined with neuroleptics in chronic schizophrenia and schizoaffective patients. J Clin Psychiatry 42: 124–128

Castelao JF, Ferrerira L, Gelders YG, Heylen SLE. 1989 The efficacy of the D_2 and $5HT_2$ antagonist risperidone in the treatment of chronic psychoses. An open dose finding study. Schiz Res 2: 411–415

Cavallero R, Colombo C, Smeraldi E. 1995 A pilot, open study on the treatment of refractory schizophrenia with risperidone and clozapine. Hum Psychopharm 10: 231–243

Chouinard G, Jones B, Remington G. 1993 A canadian multicenter placebo-controlled study of fixed doses of risperidone and haloperidol in the treatment of chronic schizophrenic patients. J Clin Psychopharm 13: 35–40

Chouinard G, Vainer JL, Belanger MC. 1994 Risperidone and clozapine in the treatment of drug-resistant schizophrenia and neuroleptic-induced supersensitivity psychosis. Prog Neuropsychopharm Biol Psy 18: 1129–1141

Claus A, Bollen J, de Cuyper H. 1992 Risperidone versus haloperidol in the treatment of chronic schizophrenic inpatient: a multi-centre double-blind comparative study. Acta Psych Scand 85: 295–305

Cohen NJ and Cohen NH. 1974 Lithium carbonate, haloperidol and irreversible brain damage. Journal of the American Medical Association 230: 1283–1287

Committee on the Safety of Medicine. 1990 Cardiotoxic effects of Pimozide. Current problems No. 29

Cooper T. 1996 Clozapine plasma level monitoring: current status. Psychiatr Q 67: 297–311

Coppen A, Noguera R, Bailey J. 1971 Prophylactic lithium in affective disorders: a controlled trial. Lancet ii: 326–330

Daniel and Whitcomb 1998 Treatment of the refractory schizophrenic patient. J Clin Psy 59 Suppl 1: 13–19

Davis H and Squire L 1984. Protein synthesis and memory. Psychological Bulletin 96: 518–559

Davis JM et al. 1994 Depot antipsychotic drugs: place in therapy. Drugs 47: 120–127

Devanand DP, Dwork AJ, Hutchinson ER, Bolwig TG, Sackeim HA. 1994. Does electroconvulsive therapy alter brain structure ? Am J Psych 151: 957–970

Devinsky O, Honigfield G, Patin J. 1991 Clozapin-related seizures. Neurol 41: 369–371

Dunner DL, Fieve RR. 1974 Clinical factors in lithium carbonate prophylaxis failure. Arch Gen Psych 30: 229–233

Emrich HM, Dose M, von Serssen D. 1985 The use of sodium valproate and oxycarbamazepine in patients with affective disorders. J Aff Disorders 8: 243–250

Faedda GL, Baldessarini RJ, Tohen M, Strakowski SM, Waternaux C. 1991 Episode sequence in bipolar disorder and response to lithium treatment. Am J Psych 148: 1237–1239

Fieve RR, Kumbaraci T, Dunner DL. 1976 Lithium prophylaxis of depression in bipolar I, bipolar II, and unipolar patients. Am J Psych 133: 925–930

Fink M.1990 How does ECT work? Neuropsychopharm 3: 77–82

Fink M. 1994 Indications for the use of ECT. Psychopharm Bull 30(3): 269–280

Fowler NO, McCall D, Chuan T. 1976 Electrocardiographic changes and cardiac arrhythmias in patients receiving psychotropic drugs. Am J Cardiol 37: 223–230

Freeman CPL, Basson JV, Creighton A. 1978 Double-blind controlled trial of electroconvulsive ttherapy(ECT) and simulated ECT in depressive illness. Lancet i: 738–740

Freeman TW, Clothier JL, Passaglia P, Lesem MD. 1992 A double blind comparison of VPA and LI in the treatment of acute mania. Am J Psych 149: 108–111

Geoff DG, Brotman AW, Waites M, McCormick S. 1990. Trial of fluoxetine added to neuroleptics for treatment resistant schizophrenic patients. Am J Psych 147: 492–494

Goodwin FK, Jamison KR. 1990 Manic-Depressive Illness. New York: Oxford University Press

Gregory S, Shawcross CR, Gill D. 1985 The Nottingham ECT study: a double blind comparison of bilateral, unilateral, and simulated ECT in depressive illness. Br J Psych 146: 520–524

Hakola HP, Laulumaa VA. 1982 Carbamazepine in treatment of violent schizophrenics. Lancet (Letter) ii: 1358

Hasegawa M, Gutierrez-Esteinou R, Way L, Meltzer HY. 1993 Relationship between clinical efficacy and clozapine plasma concentrations in schizophrenia: effect of smoking. J Clin Psychopharm 13: 383–390

Hayes SG. 1989 Longterm use of VPA in primary psychiatric disorders. J Clin Psych 50: 35–39

Hegarty JD et al. 1994 One hundred years of schizophrenia: a meta-analysis of the outcome literature. Am J Psych 151: 1409–1416

Hirsch SR and Barnes TRE. 1994 Clinical use of high-dose neuroleptics. Br J Psych 164: 94–96

Hirsch SR, Link CGG, Goldstein JM. 1996 ICI204,636: A new atypical antipsychotic drug. Br J Psych 168 (suppl. 29): 45–56

Hirschowitz J, Casper R, Garver DL 1980 Lithium response in good prognosis schizophrenia. Am J Psych 137(8): 916–920

Ital T, Keskiner A, Heinemann L. 1970 Treatment of resistant schizophrenics with extreme high dosage fluphenazine. Psychosomatics 11: 496–491

Johnstone EC, Deakin JFW, Lawler P, Frith CD. 1980 The Northwick Park electroconvulsive therapy trial. Lancet ii: 1317–1320

Jusic N, Lader M. 1994. Post-mortem antipsychotic drug concentrations and unexplained deaths. Br J Psych 165, 787–791

Kallen B, Tandberg A. 1983 Lithium and Pregnancy – a cohort study of manic-depressive women. Acta Psych Scand 62: 134–139

Kane J, Honigfield G, Singer J, Meltzer HY. 1988 The clozaril collaboration study group. Clozapine for the treatment-resistant schizophrenic: a double-blind comparison with chlorpromazine. Arch Gen Psych 45: 789–796

Kane JM. 1992 Clinical efficacy of clozapine in treatment refractory schizophrenia: an overview. Br J Psych (suppl. 17): 41–45

Kane JM, Marder SR.1993 Psychopharmacological treatment of schizophrenia. Schiz Bull 19: 287–302

Karliner W. 1994 Maintenance ECT. Convul Ther 10: 238–242

Karson CN, Weinberger DR, Bigelow L, Wyatt RJ. 1982 Clonazepam treatment of chronic schizophrenia: negative results in a double-blind, placebo-controlled trial. Am J Psych 139: 1627–1628

Kemp R, Hayward P, Applewhaite G, Everitt A, David A. 1996 Compliance therapy in psychotic patients: randomised controlled trial. BMJ 312: 345–349

Kessler RC. 1994 Lifetime and 12 month prevalence of DSMIIIR psychiatric disorders in the United States: results from the National Co-morbidity Survey. Arch Gen Psych 51: 8–20

King DJ, Burke M, Lucas RA. 1995 Antipsychotic drug-induced dysphoria. Br J Psych 167: 480–482

Klein E, Bental E, Lerer B, Belmaker RH. 1984 Carbamazepine and haloperidol v placebo and haloperidol in excited psychoses. Arch Gen Psych 41: 165–170

Kramlinger KG, Post RM. 1989 Adding lithium carbonate to carbamazepine: antimanic efficacy in treatment-resistant mania. Acta Psych Scand 79: 378–385

Kukopulos A, Reginaldi D, Laddomada P, Floric G. 1980 Course of the manic depressive cycle and changes caused by treatment. Pharmacopsych 13: 156–167

Lieberman JA, Kane JM. 1994 Predictors of response to clozapine. J Clin Psych 55(9): 126–128

Lindstedt G, Nilsson LA, Walinder J, Skott A, Ohman R. 1977 On the prevalence, diagnosis and management of lithium induced hypothyroidism in psychiatric patients. Br J Psych 130: 452–458

Lindstrom LH, Persson E. 1980 Propranolol in chronic schizophrenia controlled study in neuroleptic treated patients. Br J Psych 137: 126–130

Little KY, Gay TL, Vore M. 1989 Predictors of response to high-dose antipsychotics in chronic schizophrenics. Psych Res 30: 1–9

Loo H, Poirer-Littre MF, Theron M. 1997 Amisulpiride versus placebo in the medium term treatment of negative symptoms of schizophrenia. Br J Psych 170: 18–22

Luchins DL. 1984 Carbamazepine in violent non-epileptic schizophrenics. Psychopharm Bull 20(3): 569–571

Mann JJ, Kapur S. 1994 Elucidation of the biochemical basis of the antidepressant action of electroconvulsive therapy by human studies. Psychopharm Bull 30(3): 445–453

Marder SR, Meibach RC. 1994 Risperidone in the treatment of schizophrenia. Am J Psych 15: 825–835

Markowitz JS, Candace SB, Moore TR. 1999 Atypical antipsychotics: pharmacology, pharmacokinetics, and efficacy. Annals Pharmacother 33: 73–85

McCreadie RG, MacDonald IM. 1977. High-dose Haloperidol in chronic schizophrenia. Br J Psych 131: 310–316

McCreadie RG, Flanagan WL, McKnight J. 1979 High-dose flupenthixol decanoate in chronic schizophrenia. Br J Psych 135: 175–179

McEvoy JP, Hogarty GE, Steingard S. 1991 Optimal dose of neuroleptic in acute schizophrenia. A controlled study of the neuroleptic threshold and higher haloperidol dose. Arch Gen Psych 48: 739–745

Mehtonen OP, Aranko K, Malkonen L. 1991 A survey of sudden death associated with the use of antipsychotic or antidepressant drugs. Acta Psychiatrica Scand 84: 58–64

Meltzer HY. 1991 The mechanism of action of novel antipsychotic drugs. Schiz Bull 17: 263–287

Meltzer HY. 1992 Treatment of the neuroleptic, non-responsive schizophrenic patient. Schiz Bull 18: 515–542

Mental Health Act 1983. London: HMSO

Mortimer A. 1997 Treatment of the patient with long-term schizophrenia. Adv Psych treatment 3: 339–346

Myers DH, Campbell PL, Cooks NM. 1981 A trial of propranolol in chronic schizophrenia. Br J Psych 139: 118–121

Nutt DJ, Glue P. 1993 The neurobiology of ECT: animal studies. In: Coffey CE. (ed), The Clinical Science of Electroconvulsive Therapy. Washington DC: American Psychiatric Press. 213–234

Okocha CI. 1996a Managing anxiety disorders in general practice. *Hospital Update* November: 415–419

Okocha CI. 1995 Treating addiction to benzodiazepines. *Hospital Update* September: 396–401

Okuma T. 1983 Therapeutic and prophylactic effects of carbamazepine in bipolar disorders. Psych Clin North America 6: 147–174

Ostrom M *et al.* 1996 Fatal overdose with citalopram. Lancet 348: 339–340

Peet M, Middlemiss DN, Yates RA. 1980 Pharmacokinetic interaction between propronolol and chlorpromazine in schizophrenic patients. Lancet ii: 978

Pereira S, Beer D, Paton C. 1999 When all Else Fails: A locally devised structured decision process for enforcing clozapine therapy. Psychiatric Bulletin 23: 654–656

Perry PJ, Miller DD, Arndt SV, Cadoret RJ. 1991 Clozapine and norclozapine plasma concentrations and clinical response of treatment refractory schizophrenic patients. Am J Psych 148: 231–235

Perry PJ, Bever KA, Arndt S, Combs MD. 1998 Relationship between patient variables and plasma clozapine concentrations: a dosing nomogram. Biol Psych 44: 733–738

Placidi GF, Lenzi A, Lazzerini F, Cassano GB, Akiskal HS. 1986 The comparative efficacy and safety of carbamazepine versus lithium: a randomized, double-blind 3-year trial in 83 patients. J Clin Psych 47: 490–494

Post RM, Uhde TW, Roy-Byrne PP, Joffe RT. 1986. Antidepressant effects of carbamazepine. Am J Psych 143: 29–34

Post RM, Uhde TW, Roy-Byrne PP, Joffe RT. 1987 Correlates of anti-manic response to carbamazepine. Psych Res 21: 71–83

Post RM, Rubinow DR, Uhde TW. 1989 Dysphoric mania: clinical and biological correlates. Arch Gen Psych 46: 353–358

Potkin SG, Bera R. 1994 Plasma clozaril concentrations predict clinical response in treatment resistant schizophrenia. J Clin Psych 55(9): 133–136

Pope HG, McElroy SL, Keck P, Brown S. 1991. Valproate in the treatment of acute mania: a placebo controlled study. Arch Gen Psych 48: 62–68

Puzynski S, Klosiewicz L. 1984 Valproic acid amide in the treatment of affective and schizoaffective disorders. J Aff Dis 6: 115–121

Quitkin F, Rifkin A, Klein DF. 1975 Very high dosage versus standard dosage fluphenazine in schizophrenia: a double-blind study of non-chronic treatment refractory patients. Arch Gen Psych 32: 1276–1281

Rifkin A, Quitkin F, Carrillo C. 1971 Very high-dose fluphenazine for non-chronic treatment refractory patients. Arch Gen Psych 25: 398–403

Royal College of Psychiatrists. 1995 The ECT Handbook. Council Report CR 39. London: Royal College of Psychiatrists

Sackeim HA, Prudic J, Devanand DP, Decina P, Kerr B, Malitz S. 1990 The impact of medication resistance and continuation pharmacotherapy on relapse following response to electroconvulsive therapy in major depression. J Clin Psychopharm 10: 96–104

Sackeim HA. 1994 Central issues regarding the mechanisms of action of ECT: directions for future research. Psychopharmacology Bulletin 30(3): 281–312

Sackeim HA, Prudics, Devonod DP. 1994 Effects of stimulus intensity and electrode placement on the efficacy and cognitive effect of electroconvulsive therapy. N Engl J Med 328: 839–846

Salzman C. 1980 The use of ECT in the treatment of schizophrenia. Am J Psych 137: 1032–1041

Schooler JVR. 1991 Maintenance medication for schizophrenia: strategic for dose reduction. Schiz Bull 17: 311–324

Sharif Z. 1998 Treatment refractory schizophrenia: how should we proceed? Psych Quaterly 69(4): 263–281

Sharma R, Trappler B, Ng YK, Leeman CP. 1995 Risperidone induced neuroleptic malignant syndrome. Ann Pharmacother 30: 775–778

Siris S, Bermonzohn PC, Gonzalez A, Manson SE. 1991 Use of antidepressants for negative symptoms in a subset of schizophrenic patients. Psychopharmacol Bull 27: 331–335

Small JG, Klapper MH, Kellams JJ. 1988 Electroconvulsive treatment compared with lithium in management of manic states. Arch Gen Psych 45: 727

Small JG, Klapper MH, Milstein V. 1991 Carbamazepine compared with lithium in treatment of mania. Arch Gen Psych 48: 915–921

Squire LR. 1986 Memory functions as affected by electroconvulsive therapy. Ann New York Acad Sci 462: 307–314

Tandon R, Harrigan E, Zorn SH. 1997 Ziprasidone: a novel antipsychotic with unique pharmacological and therapeutic potential. J Serot Res 4: 159–177

Taylor D and Duncan D. 1995 The use of clozapine plasma levels in optimising therapy. Psychiatr Bull 19: 753–755

Tennent G, Bancroft J, Cass J. 1974 The control of deviant sexual behaviour by drugs: A double blind controlled study of benperidol, chlorpromazine, and placebo. Arch Sex Beh 3: 261–271

The Concise Oxford Dictionary 1995: 9th edition Oxford: Oxford University Press

Thompson C. 1994 The use of high-dose antipsychotic medication. Br J Psych 164: 448–458

Tollefson GD, Beasley Jr CM, Tran PV. 1997 Olanzapine versus haloperidol in the treatment of schizophrenia, schizoaffective, and schizophreniform disorders: results of an international collaborative trial. Am J Psych 154: 457–465

Vartiainen H, Leinonen E, Putkonen A, Lang S, Hagert U, Tolvanen U. 1993 A long-term study of remoxipride in chronic schizophrenic patients. Acta Psych Scand 87: 114–117

Watkins SE, Callender K, Thomas DR, Tidmarsh SF, Shaw DM. 1987 The effect of carbamazepine and lithium on remission from affective illness. Br J Psych 150: 180–182

Weiner RD. 1994 Treatment optimization with ECT. Psychopharm Bull 30(3): 313–320

Weissman MM, Merikangas KR. 1986. The epidemiology of anxiety and panic disorders. J Clin Psych 47 (suppl.): 11–17

West ED. 1981 Electric Convulsion therapy in depression: a double blind controlled trial. BMJ 282: 355–357

Wilson WH, Claussen AM. 1994 Seizures associated with clozapine treatment in a state hospital. J Clin Psych 55: 184–188

Wolkowitz OM, Tureksky N, Reus VI. 1992 Benzodiazepine augmentation of neuroleptics in treatment resistant schizophrenia. Psychopharmacology Bulletin 28: 291–295

Yorkston NJ, Zaki SA, Pitcher DR, Gruzelier JH, Hollander D, Sergeant HGS. 1977 Propronolol as an adjunct to the treatment of schizophrenics. Lancet ii: 575–578

6A

PSYCHOLOGICAL APPROACHES
TO THE ACUTE PATIENT

Marc Goldstein

INTRODUCTION

The aim of this chapter is to highlight some important features of psychological work within the context of acute psychiatric services. The specific focus is on psychological work within psychiatric intensive care settings. This offers an important opportunity to expand on the growing literature on multidisciplinary team activities within such contexts.

Psychiatric Intensive Care treatment offers a short-term multidisciplinary intensive treatment plan for patients admitted from a number of referring wards. An important feature of this treatment is the inclusion of psychological work. The role of the psychologist on such units may vary, and differences in treatment approaches may be expected.

A psychological perspective on patient admissions on PICU settings offers a valuable opportunity for mental health professions to investigate the holistic experience of ward culture and patient treatment on such wards. Such a holistic approach will be essential for the overall management of such patients admitted to acute psychiatric services, and is in line with preferred practice outlined in clinical governance. Clinical Governance has been defined as a 'Framework to ensure that all NHS organisations have proper processes for monitoring and improving clinical quality' (Kings Fund Briefing 1999). It is within the above contextual framework that some important functions the psychologist may offer will be highlighted.

The role of the psychologist within a PICU will include a number of functions:

- Providing a psychological assessment of patients:

  - Delineating the link between the patient's current admission and their life history

  - Forming a developmental history of the patient

  - Providing a description of the underlying personality structure of the patient

  - Providing an assessment of the patient's family and social dynamics.

- Providing psychotherapeutic input to patients.

- Providing staff support (supervision and training).

- Contributing to ward activities (ward rounds, staff groups).

- Research studies.

Box 6A.1

PROVIDING A PSYCHOLOGICAL ASSESSMENT OF THE PATIENT

Patients admitted on to acute psychiatric wards and PICU settings have a multitude of diagnoses and symptom presentations. The inability for such wards to have a homogeneous group of patients will result in patients with a number of different reasons for admission. A crucial aim of the psychologist in such a setting is to offer a psychological formulation of the patient's difficulties. The major impetus to such formulations is to offer the multidisciplinary team a glimpse into the patient's emotional world and the psychological triggers that may have contributed to the current episode and admission. Often, on acute ward admissions, the focus is narrowed to the symptom presentation and medication review, and the rich depth of emotional antecedents may be lost.

One of the key elements through which such psychological formulations are achieved, is the provision of a psychological assessment; the format may vary but the following points offer some preliminary outline of the assessment.

Attempting to delineate the link between the patient's current admission and life history

The significance of such links can help the team gain a broader and more detailed recognition of underlying psychological factors that have contributed to the current presentation. Such historical links may be overlooked when patients present with overriding symptom descriptions. A case example may help illustrate this point

Case history

An example is the case of a 30-year-old woman who presented to the psychiatric intensive care unit with symptoms of agitation and mood lability. The psychiatric history of the patient was extensive and included a family history of Bipolar Affective Disorder. The patient's life history was presented to the ward in short discharge summaries, but little was known of her developmental years. A psychological assessment gauged that the patient had lost her mother to suicide at the age of five years. She was cared for by her older sister who became a maternal figure. The patient functioned well until the time of her sister's marriage, shortly after which the patient had her first episode of depression. The patient described feeling like she had 'lost' a mother again. The psychological assessment gathered evidence of times in which the patient relapsed: a common theme seemed to be the patient's experience of loss or abandonment, and her regression to an earlier emotional state.

The above vignette gives recognition to the importance of an extensive developmental history for the team (Wallace 1983). An investigation into the patient's significant life events and developmental milestones can offer the psychologist the opportunity to formulate an outline for the ward of the patient's emotional life and personality structure. A detailed developmental history does not need to be exclusively for the psychologist, but can be used by all team members to expand on the holistic understanding of the patient. A detailed description of developmental history-taking, see Wallace (1983). However, some important pointers to consider when taking a developmental history are outlined below:

- A patient's life history is integral to the understanding of their subjective experience.

- A developmental approach recognises the significance of developmental milestones in the course of life maturity.

- Significant life courses include the stages of infancy, early childhood, middle childhood, adolescence and adulthood.

- The developmental history will attempt to track the patient's experiences through such a life course.

- Detailed recognition will be given to situations in which the patient has been adversely affected emotionally (emotional deprivation).

- The links between such adverse life experiences and later personality development will be traced.

- It must be recognised that, for so many psychiatric patients, their life history is a history of emotional deprivation, neglect, loss and abuse (Wallace 1983).

Box 6A.2 Some important features of a developmental perspective

Good and detailed history-taking will outline the relevant and significant life events that may be of importance to the overall understanding of the patient. An aspect of this may be to consider a model in which the current difficulties are seen as reactions to unresolved life events and difficulties, and not only always the result of a biochemical illness.

Providing a description of the patient's underlying personality structure

An important feature to investigate in the psychological assessment is the personality structure of the patient. The extent to which varying patient groups are found in the

PICU setting makes this an especially significant aspect of detection. The recognition of how the underlying personality structure of the patient makes him/her more vulnerable to admission will be outlined. An important aspect of this work is to differentiate those patients for whom their personality has been an integral and long-standing factor in their admissions from other patients for whom recovery from episodes of psychiatric illness leaves them reasonably intact. The ability to trace the patient's emotional functioning from developmental histories can help to distinguish these two groups.

The idea of personality structure has been investigated and outlined by a number of theorists and clinicians (e.g. Kernberg 1975). The outline of such models of personality is beyond the scope of this paper. The basic outline, however, is for the psychologist to give the ward a basic formulation of the patient's ego functioning. Ego functioning can be broadly defined as that area of the person's personality that is primarily involved in adapting to internal drives as well as external environmental demands (Kaplan *et al* 1994). Basic pointers that indicate weakened ego functioning (Kernberg 1975) include:

- Poor control of basic impulses (sexual and aggressive).

- Difficulties with tolerating frustration or emotional pressure.

- Maladaptive coping mechanisms (defences) in the event of stress and anxiety.

- Poor/diffuse emotional boundaries.

- Poor object-constancy. Constantly changing experiences of both self and others.

The impact of psychiatric illness can often result in weakened ego functioning, and the observation of the above-mentioned features. However, in some patients, such defects in ego functioning are an aspect of their underlying personality structure and are found even in the absence of psychiatric illness. It can be of use to the team treating the patient to have a clearer understanding of long-standing ego functioning of patients on the ward. This is particularly important in their management and treatment. Those patients for whom long-standing ego weakness remains an integral part of their personality structure have particular therapeutic needs that will be described later.

Providing an assessment of the patient's family and social dynamics

Providing a psychological profile of the patient should include addressing broader sociocultural issues which have an impact on patient admission and care. An important area is that of family dynamics. Much literature has been written on the role of the family in the lives of psychiatric patients; however, within the context of intensive care treatment, we can focus on some particular areas.

The experience of the admission to hospital for the patient's family

Admission on to a PICU is an emotional experience for both the patient and his/her close contacts. Coming to terms with the reality of a psychiatric illness is an important area for engagement treatment for the patient. This is equally an issue of concern for the patient's family and friends. The need for family members to have the opportunity to engage with staff members about this situation cannot be underestimated. The role of the psychologist on the ward would be to guide the team within this area of treatment.

For many family members, having to face an illness of a loved one is a difficult and painful process to bear (Mervis 1999). This applies to facing mental illness as much as to physical illness. The feelings associated with such a process can be complex and depend on the unique history of each family. However, overall, the experience can often be described as a grieving process in which loss can be a central dynamic (Mervis 1999). The team must be aware of the potential for the family to experience loss, or in certain cases to defend against feelings of loss, when the patient becomes ill or is admitted to the hospital. Understanding these feelings can assist the team to cope with the emerging dynamics and reactions experienced when dealing with families.

Case history

An example is the case of a 30-year-old patient admitted on to the unit. The ward soon began to receive phone calls from the mother who was angry and demanding. Letters of complaint often arrived about the quality of treatment care on the ward. Staff members felt defensive and angry in the mother's presence. A psychological formulation uncovered how the patient had had a steady decline in emotional functioning from early adulthood. Prior to the first admission, the patient had been a high achiever and very successful. The psychological formulation helped to shed light on how painful the process was for mother to watch her daughter steadily declining in mental health. The mother's anger helped her ward off feelings of underlying sadness and grief. Furthermore, the projection of 'poor care' on to the ward could have been linked to the mother's anxieties of not having offered sufficient emotional nourishment for her child

The above vignette offers an example of how important it is for the ward to be aware of the meaning for a family to face the psychiatric illness of the patient. The case, however, is also found on the ward where rather than loss being the overriding feeling, it is fear and avoidance. The experience of family and other close members facing a patient when in the grips of acute mental illness can have a lasting affect. Often, family members witness bizarre or violent behaviour, and are left with feelings that need to be worked through. Without an opportunity for the family to face these feelings, elements of acting-out by family members can otherwise occur, such as avoidance of the patient, with missed or short visits.

Family dynamics spilling over onto the ward

The importance of underlying family dynamics needs to be assessed, so as to be aware of such dynamics when they are lived out on the ward. Staff may gain insight into the functioning of the family through observation of various interactions as they unfold on the ward. For example, it is important for staff to assess the patient's mental state following interactions with family or friends. Another area in which this may be investigated is through family interactions in ward rounds.

Case history

An example is the case of a 37-year-old male with a diagnosis of paranoid schizophrenia. The patient spent most of his time isolated from the staff and fellow patients. He seemed suspicious and guarded. From the onset of his admission to the unit the patient refused to eat hospital food. A query about his paranoia was raised. However, it later unfolded that the patient would eat after cookery groups, and preferred his mother's cooking. The family continually brought in food to the ward, spoke for the patient in the ward rounds, and made decisions on his behalf. An examination of his home life indicated that the patient spent the majority of his time in his room, being brought meals by his mother and making minimal independent decisions. The team considered that there was evidence of an enmeshed family with poor boundaries, and it became apparent that this family dynamic was being replayed on the unit.

THE PROVISION OF PSYCHOTHERAPY TO PATIENTS

A core role of the psychologist on the intensive care unit is to be involved in the provision of psychotherapy to patients. The significance of psychotherapy within the spectrum of acute psychiatry is a debated area (Kaplan *et al* 1994). It is important for the team to have some idea of the variety of psychotherapeutic approaches that prevail, and what form of psychotherapy will be offered to the patient. Without an outline of this, many staff members remain doubtful of the effectiveness of therapy on such a setting (Clinton 2000).

Psychologists will often differ in the type of therapy they offer. This will vary in technique and style. This chapter outlines the use of a particular therapeutic approach. The primary basis of such an approach is that which has been outlined by Winnicott (1971), and later developed by Gabbard (1994) and Wallace (1983). The core features of such an approach are:

- The recognition of how the provision of psychotherapy needs to address the level of emotional development in the patient.

- The adjustment of therapeutic technique according to the developmental level of the patient.

The importance of the clinician taking into account the level of emotional development of the patient was addressed by Winnicott (1971), in which he described how for certain patients, the provision of a different experience to that of traditional psychoanalytic therapy was more effective. He termed this *therapeutic management*. These ideas have been expanded upon by Gabbard (1994) and Wallace (1983), who describe the importance of adapting the therapeutic technique to the level of ego development in the patient. This would include those patients whose fragility in ego strength is due to their present psychiatric illness. In terms of what this means for clinical work, the team will need to recognise certain key factors that are applicable to a psychiatric intensive care setting:

- Psychotherapy should be more *supportive* (Wallace 1983), in the sense of supporting the building up of ego resources in the patient.

- The therapist should be cautious not to unravel the fragile defences the patient is employing, and hence contribute to the patient regressing. (Regression is a term employed to describe a defence mechanism in which, in the face of anxiety, a person returns to an early level of emotional functioning.)

- The emotional needs of the patient should be taken into account. Some of these needs may not be consciously recognised. One of the key emotional needs that has been outlined in work with such patients is the need for *containment*. This will be outlined in more detail below.

In terms of the above-mentioned descriptions, an important aspect of the therapeutic work is to keep the notion of *emotional vulnerability* in mind. In a short-term setting, this will assist the therapist to formulate a therapeutic strategy that will be meaningful for the patient. This can enable the patient to have some emotional space in the intensive care setting, to feel understood and contained.

However, difficulties with forming a therapeutic rapport are also part of the challenge for the therapist working with patients on the unit. Many of the difficulties found in therapeutic work in the psychiatric setting have been highlighted in Chapter 6B. It may be useful to expand on some other concerns which occupy the therapist working on the intensive care unit.

The involuntary patient

Patients admitted on to the PICU have been sectioned in accordance with the Mental Health Act. Szasz (1998) described how the essence of the sectioning process included

'… the legal and/or physical ability to restrict another'. Inherent in this process is the experience for the patient of some degree of coercion to treatment. The recognition of the involuntary basis of treatment and the patient's experience of such a process is essential for treatment care. Much of this has been described in Chapter 6B.

Some further considerations

Patients may appear resistant to making emotional contact with the therapist. There may be a refusal to attend sessions, or little initiative taken in therapy. The initial reaction may be to see this as an inherent basis of the mental illness. However, it is also important for the therapist to consider the patient's withholding in the sessions as a possible reaction to the involuntary basis of the treatment. In a sense, the therapist's difficulty with engaging the patient in treatment may be the patient's only sense of control in the treatment in which s/he feels disempowered. The patient may also fear that in revealing these feelings, their stay on the unit may be prolonged. The therapist may need to spend time within the sessions addressing these issues with the patient, and attempting in the process to build therapeutic rapport.

Patients may be in need of the physical holding inherent in the secure environment of the unit. This may leave patients with a belief that their anxieties or inner emotional states are unmanageable to themselves and those around them, and hence reason for their admission to the unit. Patients may experience the involuntary basis of the treatment as a 'locking away' due to their inner sense of chaos, or external behaviour. One important aim in psychotherapeutic work is to recognise that, for certain patients, a difficulty in making emotional contact may be due to the patient's deep sense of believing that they cannot be contained. A central role in psychotherapy would be to offer the patient the emotional space in which s/he may begin to experience his/her feelings and emotional states as bearable and tolerated by the therapist (Docker-Drysdale 1991, Winnicott 1971).

The violent patient

Violent patients pose a considerable challenge to the team on the intensive care unit. The psychologist working psychotherapeutically with such patients forms an integral role in the treatment of such patients (Goldstein 1999). Violence may be the by-product of severe mental illness that will need particular pharmacological action. However, the psychologist may be able to point out to the team some of the *psychological* factors involved in patients' proneness to violence. Many patients who have admissions to acute psychiatric services have long-standing difficulties with containing their own feelings, which are hence turned into some form of action outside themselves. This action may include aggressive and violent behaviour. From a developmental perspective, an understanding of this would include the idea that, since early development, the patient has given up in despair of believing that their emotional states could be understood or managed by the environment around them (Docker-Drysdale

1991). This breakdown in feeling understood, as well as the concrete expression of feelings through actions, is important for the therapist to consider in the treatment of such patients.

Another important element of the psychological approach to the management of violent or aggressive patients is to understand their underlying feelings of rage and anger. An investigation of the developmental history of the patient may give an indication of some of the antecedent features in the person's life that have left them feeling so angry and enraged. Such an approach would recognise that the manifestation of violence would constitute a long-term building up of feelings that have their origin in some form of environmental failure and/or abusive experience (Miller 1987, 1995, Winnicott 1975). This approach would counteract a tendency to consider the patient's violent behaviour as only a manifestation and by-product of mental illness.

Psychologists may utilise a number of psychological techniques to contain the patient and prevent the disruption of violence; much of this is described by McKenzie (2000). An important element in the employment of interventions to assist patients with the management of violence would be to give patients the opportunity to experience ways of managing their own feelings and urges. The significance of this is to strengthen the patients' coping skills, but also in the process to help patients to develop a growing sense of internal capacities and resilience. Specifically, certain behavioural techniques, such as anger and anxiety charts, may prove effective in such cases.

It should be recognised, however, that the effectiveness of such psychological intervention is dependent partly upon the patients' capacity and willingness to use these interventions. An example of this would be the patients' willingness to consider managing their own violent urges, rather than relying on external containment such as drugs or control and restraint to manage their violence for them. For those patients who lack the abstract cognitive capacities to think about this, or who may on a deeper emotional level fear their own unmanageable feelings so much, the expectation of the staff for the patients to use such techniques may be premature.

Linked to this is the therapist and staff's willingness to work with violent patients. The emotional impact on staff members of violence and violent patients is a central element in the treatment of such patients (Goldstein 1999). Staff should feel supported and safe enough when expected to undertake this work, and the constant monitoring of countertransference to the patient is important (Docker-Drysdale 1991).

The suicidal patient

Many admissions to intensive care units include patients who are actively suicidal, or remain a high risk for suicide. Other patients may become suicidal as their mental illness is treated and insight returns. Intensive care units formulate effective and structured treatment plans in the management of the suicidal patient. This may include the implementation of high levels of observation and the consistent monitoring of patients' behaviour and mental state. The highly stressful nature of this form of patient treatment for the multidisciplinary team is recognised by many staff. It is important, then, that staff working with suicidal patients are given the opportunity to share their experiences and feelings about this work. Psychologists can offer support to staff in the form of support groups or one to one supervision sessions. This offers staff the opportunity to talk about the emotional impact that such patients evoke and can hopefully have a containing function for the staff member, who then may feel more able to manage another shift and session with the patient. This can also prevent staff acting-out, such as in anger, and even in certain cases a high turn-over, with many resignations from the unit (Hinshelwood 1999). Staff may also fear allowing themselves to get too close emotionally to the suicidal patient, for fear of the patient dying, and the emotional consequence of this for the staff member.

Psychologists wanting to include such staff support groups on the ward would need to recognise the possibility of the ambivalence that some staff members may feel about joining such groups. The necessity for some staff to maintain a particular 'professional' image in front of peers, and the fear that staff may experience at becoming too vulnerable in a group, should be considered. Furthermore, for those psychologists actively involved on the unit, the capacity to take on such a leadership role in the group may be seen as a possible boundary impingement. Outside facilitation may hence become a viable option.

The importance for staff members to feel able to recognise and manage the feelings that the suicidal patient evokes will influence the overall treatment of the suicidal patient. There are techniques that therapists and staff members can use to challenge suicidal thinking and behaviour. However, more important than any one technique is the facility for patients to meet a therapist/staff member who is able to cope with the range of feelings that the patient may communicate (verbally or non-verbally).

This applies to cases of self-harming as well, although self-harming has its own potential difficulties that are in certain ways unique to suicidal patients. Self-harming as a challenging behaviour is also found in many intensive care settings. Many such patients have had numerous hospital admissions and evoke very strong feelings in the staff who manage their care (Hinshelwood 1999; Chapter 6B). Generally, this may include negative feelings and a move towards moral judgement (Hinshelwood 1999). The capacity to offer such patients a meaningful and therapeutic stay on the ward is challenged by their often frightening and disturbing behaviour or feelings. Ongoing staff discussions and feedback about such patients is essential.

Coming to terms with admission and illness

As described in the section on family dynamics, the emotional impact of facing mental illness is crucial for the psychologist to address. For the person admitted on to the unit, the reality of facing a psychiatric diagnosis and admission on to a locked ward can stir an array of feelings. The psychologist would need to consider the psychological impact of the admission on the individual patient. *This becomes important in terms of how much the patient is able to accept the reality of their mental illness.* Patients may differ in this respect, and an integral role for the psychologist in individual sessions could be to assess the level of this acceptance of the illness. Some reactions the patient may experience in the struggle to come to terms with the diagnosis and treatment can be important to consider in the management of the patient on the intensive care unit and in referral back to the referring ward.

- The psychiatric team may be faced with patients who seem to have *poor insight* into their condition. They may deny the presence of mental illness, or minimise the extent to which they are ill. This lack of insight may be seen by the team to be a by-product of the illness; the psychological approach would be to consider the possibilities of *denial* and *avoidance*. The patient may utilise defences such as these and it is important to consider how emotionally painful and frightening it can be to face the reality of such an illness.

- The psychologist may aid in uncovering some underlying reasons for this reaction by the patient, such as the role of the often socially unacceptable stigma of the illness. For patients, such as those who had high levels of social and occupational functioning, the label of psychiatric patient may be very difficult to acknowledge.

- An important aspect to facing this label may be the experiencing of feelings of self-loathing or shame. Bradshaw (1991) has described shame as linked to a person's sense of feeling there is something defective about themselves. The psychological aim may be to examine such feelings, and the impact of the mental illness on self-esteem.

- Some patients may go through a period of depression following admission to the unit and coming to terms with the reality of the mental illness. Rather than denying the extent of the illness, these patients may experience feeling emotionally stuck and unable to move forward. They may be left with a sense of loss and hopelessness. The psychologist may need to help the multidisciplinary team become aware of this form of reactive depression, which may at times be confused with mental illness and hence overlooked in the management of the patient.

- In other cases, admission to the unit may be one of several psychiatric admissions to acute psychiatric services. Patients may respond well to acute management, but may become more vulnerable when the recognition sets in of having been so ill again. This may become a crucial time for psychological work, when the patient is particularly emotionally vulnerable. Patients may feel unable to bear living with another relapse. This is often found in the cases of patients with good premorbid functioning, and in those patients who had assumed that they would not become ill again. Patients may have the insight to recognise how much their functioning has declined, and how different they may feel from those around them. The ability for the intensive care unit to offer psychological treatment, in which these issues can be addressed and worked with, is crucial. Patients may be able to do this in their individual therapy sessions, as well as in group therapy sessions. It is also important for the referring wards who have admitted the patient to the unit to have an idea of how best to continue this psychological work after discharge from the intensive care unit.

CONCLUSION

The aim of this chapter has been to highlight some important features of psychological work in psychiatric intensive care settings. The recognition by the team of psychological factors inherent in the process of patient care have been outlined. The essential aspect of this outline has been the recognition of how patients admitted to and treated on the unit have an emotional experience and reaction to their illness and care. The aim of the psychological work is to bring these features to the fore, and to address them with both the patient and the multidisciplinary team. The psychological work begun on the unit can hopefully be continued once the patient is back in the referring ward, so that the patient has a sense of continuity in terms of psychological care.

REFERENCES

Bradshaw J. 1991 Homecoming. New York: Piatkus

Clinton C. 2000 Unpublished Survey, Pathways PICU. Goodmayes Hospital, Essex

Docker-Drysdale B. 1991 The Provision of Primary Experience: Winnicottian Work with Children and Adolescents. New Jersey: Jason Aronson

Gabbard GO. 1994 Psychodynamic Psychiatry in Clinical Practice. Washington, American Psychiatric Press

Goldstein MJ. 1999 Psychological Approaches to Management of Violence. Paper delivered at Management of Violence Workshop, James Fawcett Centre, King George Hospital, Goodmayes, Essex

Hinshelwood RD. 1999 The difficult patient. Br J Psych 174: 187–190

Kaplan HI, Sadock B, Grebb J. 1994 Synopsis of Psychiatry. 7th edn. Baltimore: Williams & Wilkins

Kernberg OF. 1975 Borderline Conditions and Pathological Narcissism. New Jersey: Jason Aronson

Kings Fund Briefing – What is clinical governance? February, 1999

Mervis J. 1999 Workshop on Loss and Grief. Presented to Mental Health Professionals at Tara Hospital, Gauteng, South Africa

Miller Alice. 1995 The Drama of Being a Child: The Search for the True Self: London, Virago

Miller Alice. 1987 For Your Own Good. London: Virago

Szasz T. 1998 The Involuntary Patient. Br J Psych 15: 216–225

Wallace ER IV. 1983 Dynamic Psychiatry in Theory and Practice. Philadelphia: Lea & Feliger

Winnicott DW. 1971 Playing and Reality. New York: Basic Books

6B

PSYCHOLOGICAL APPROACHES TO LONGER-TERM PATIENTS PRESENTING WITH CHALLENGING BEHAVIOURS

Brian M McKenzie

INTRODUCTION

Patients identified by the treating services as presenting with 'challenging behaviours' or having 'challenging needs' are often to be found in PICUs, other low secure units and on open wards. Severely disturbed behaviour posing a risk to the treating teams or other patients often co-exists with the acute and chronic forms of psychosis. Therefore on many occasions the intensive care of psychotic patients is, *de facto*, the management of challenging behaviours.

A wide range of behaviours may be construed as challenging. Aggression to people or property generally instance the greatest concern. However, it is perhaps the case that any behaviour sufficiently persistent or disruptive might be defined as challenging. Common examples in psychiatric settings are:

- Non-compliance with medication.

- Extreme withdrawal on the ward.

- Physical violence to staff, other patients or property.

- Sexual aggression.

- Self-harm.

- Firesetting.

- Persistent verbal abuse.

The task of treating patients with a combination of psychotic and behavioural disorder can further be made even more difficult by the fact that other dimensions of the patient's life may equally show impairment. Shepherd (1999) defines the challenging behaviour group as a combination of severe and intractable clinical symptoms, a range of behavioural problems and profound social dislocation. One might add problems of degradation of living skills and perhaps disorders of personality. Whatever the ultimate conception of this group, the combination of psychosis, not being able to manage emotions or frustration, hostility and social alienation will be a common experience to practitioners working in this field.

Challenging behaviour is not a new phenomenon. Individuals with these characteristics were described in a survey of repeated admissions to psychiatric facilities 25 years ago as the 'new long stay' (Mann and Cree 1976). A more recent national audit has indicated that, if anything, this group had increased in size within UK National Health Service psychiatric facilities (Lelliott and Wing 1994). They pose both short- and long-term problems but invariably their treatment requires intensive resources over the longer term. The difficulty in treating this group is perhaps seen in the fact that many patients having this combination become revolving door patients (Lelliott and Wing 1994).

This chapter concentrates on psychological approaches to conceptualising and managing the behavioural problems this group brings. The other aspects of their need, especially the psychotic dimension, are not directly touched upon. However, it should be stressed from the outset that the problems overlap greatly and psychological treatment responses *must interconnect with medical, nursing and social interventions* if any success is to be hoped for. Furthermore the reinforcing nature of the multilayered needs of this group demand that psychological treatment occurs simultaneously at *individual and systemic levels*.

Instead of focusing on a specific form of challenging behaviour, such as sexual aggression, this chapter attempts to draw out general principles of understanding and approach to treatment. Specifically as a starting point patients exhibiting challenging behaviours are conceptualised as bringing three clinical problems to the treating team, i.e.:

- They present highly complex processes of thought, emotion and behaviours which are difficult to understand.

- They pose profound difficulties of engagement.

- They bring pressures to bear on the treatment teams.

The chapter divides into two sections: Understanding challenging behaviours, and Treatment approaches.

UNDERSTANDING THE COMPLEX PATTERNS OF THOUGHTS, EMOTIONS AND BEHAVOURS THAT MAKE UP CHALLENGING BEHAVIOURS

Many of the patients in this group act in such a way as to tax the understanding of the team. Their behaviour often seems beyond the comprehension of ordinary insight. There is a resulting temptation to place the behaviour in the realm of psychotic disturbance and thereafter disregard any need for any functional or psychological analyses of the behaviour. It is true that there might be very deeply held disturbed beliefs underlying the behaviour, seemingly profoundly at odds with reality. An example might be the belief that a member of staff is attempting to poison that patient.

However many disturbed behaviours seem to reflect psychological or emotional processes that are not directly part of a psychotic process or are disinhibited by the psychosis. Consider the following example.

Case history

A's diagnosis was unclear. She appeared mildly thought-disordered at times and had made a serious suicide attempt. She had also been violent to staff and generally presented angrily and assertively. The staff would attend and use de-escalation techniques that would calm her. She would apologise and a genuinely positive interaction would ensue. Any difficulties and concerns she had would be resolved to the best of the parties' abilities. She would return to her room feeling exhausted and saying that she wished to sleep. Some hours later she would emerge in a furious and abusive state, forcing intervention from the nursing team, often leading to restraint which would damage relationships. When calm enough to be interviewed she could only say that she had felt suicidal while lying down. She could not elaborate any further.

The intense violence of her presentation after a positive exchange seemed puzzling. However simply from the short description above a number of hypothesis could be proposed for her seeking conflict as shown below.

Some possible reasons for challenging behaviour

- She was seeking more positive attention.

- A more paranoid view of staff had set in.

- Her anger had not been properly resolved.

- She could not tolerate being alone.

- She did not like having a good relationship with staff.

- She could not tolerate her suicidal feelings.

This list is far from exhaustive. However it makes the point that there are at least a number of areas that might provide a lead for a functional analysis of the behaviour. Recent developments in a number of psychological theories might provide a basis for these hypothesis; *understandings of personality disorder put forward in the cognitive–behavioural theory, attachment theory*, and *developments in therapeutic communities*. These are set out directly below.

Before turning to these developments it should be stressed that at the basis of the psychological approaches is the understanding that *all behaviour is fundamentally interpersonal*. Challenging behaviour is therefore to be understood within its interpersonal context.

Concepts from modern cognitive therapy

Cognitive therapists have traditionally put forward the view that situations, thoughts, emotions and feelings are closely connected. Thoughts are seen to play a primary role in interpreting events and regulating emotional responses. Disturbances in thought are thereby seen as critical in maintaining disturbances of emotion. A prime example is an 'automatic thought'. An example might be the thought 'I'm useless' which occurs whenever something goes wrong in the individual's life. Such negative automatic thoughts displace the possibility of more positive thoughts, for example, 'everyone has failures, let me try again'.

Furthermore thought patterns play a fundamental role in interpreting events, often skewing our perception. Beck (1996) lists a number of faulty thought processes.

Faulty cognitive styles

- All or nothing thinking.

- Catastrophising.

- Personalising.

- Negative focus.

- Living by fixed rules.

- Jumping to conclusions.

Sets of automatic thoughts, self-statements, perceptual distortions and faulty cognitions may become organised into cohesive wholes. These are called schemas. Schemas provide an organising focus for experience, rules and beliefs. They therefore act in an executive manner. Maladaptive schemas are seen as the self-reinforcing basis of disturbances in behaviour. An example of a maladaptive schema and the connection to disturbed behaviour might be seen below.

Case history

B was referred with a problem of repeatedly getting into fights in social situations. He had a history of ridicule and rejection at the hand of his father and being bullied and teased at school. Ultimately he had fought back and developed a reputation for violence. Now when he walked into a social situation he felt tense and aroused with the expectation of confrontation. Any glance from other men he interpreted as being a challenge and a threat. He would brood on this matter, believing he could not let this challenge pass as it would mean he was less than a man, in fact he was worthless. This thought would lead to him feeling bad about himself. Ultimately he would react angrily and challenge his perceived rival. If a fight ensued all negative thoughts and feelings would be lost.

One can see a reinforcing relationship between expectation and perception of the situation, beliefs about self, emotions and behaviour. B would mistakenly read perceptual cues and would reach faulty conclusions about himself. Further his aggression resolved his bad feelings about himself.

'It is the consistent failure of schemas to manage feelings relating to interpersonal functioning that cognitive theorists believe define personality disorder' (Beck and Freeman 1990, Beck 1996). They put forward the view that certain maladaptive schemas correspond to the various personality disorders. This is outlined in Table 6B.1.

Table 6B.1: Cognitive analysis of personality disorders

Personality disorder	Automatic thoughts	Strategy
Dependant	I am helpless	Attachment
Avoidant	I may get hurt	Avoidance
Passive –aggressive	I could be stepped upon	Resistance
Paranoid	People are adversaries	Wariness
Narcissistic	I am special	Self aggrandisement
Histrionic	I need to impress	Dramatics
Obsessive – compulsive	I cannot make mistakes	Perfectionism
Antisocial	People are there to be taken	Attack
Schizoid	I can't allow myself to be close	Isolation

Problems of internal control

Beck and Freeman go on to further develop the concept. Patients with personality disorder have a maladaptive schema that attempts to control internal feelings and external interpersonal events. *When the maladaptive schema fails the result is profound levels of anxiety.* The individual then attempts to rectify the situation with further disturbances in affect, behaviour and cognition in a desperate attempt to re-establish control. The authors refer to this *as problems of internal control* (Beck and Freeman 1990). In cases of severe disturbance of personality or of behaviour these authors argue that the maladaptive schemas are coupled to disorders of internal control. *In doing so it would appear that they have put forward a conceptual framework capable of* understanding *the basis of challenging behaviour.*

Emotional dysregulation and affect intolerance

A very similar concept is put forward by Linehan in her study of self-harm in borderline personality disorder conditions. She argues that the core problem is *affect intolerance* Linehan (1993). Certain feelings are unacceptable to the borderline patient and the patient embarks on a disturbed process of behaviour, *or substitution of different affects*, to minimise the effect of these feelings. Such behaviours are frequently seen in self-harm. Linehan (1993) refers to this process as *affect intolerance or emotional dysregulation.* Such processes might be seen in the following examples.

Case history

C had made a number of serious attempts on her life and severe acts of self injury. She stated she did this to get rid of persecuting memories of serious sexual, physical and emotional abuse she had suffered as a child. These thoughts brought on 'black feelings' of which she could identify self-hatred. They made her feel terrible. Harming herself brought relief.

C appears to substitute physical pain, which she was in control of, for psychic pain.

Case history

D would glance over at the nursing station and try to catch the eye of a nurse busy at work. The nurse would look away and return to her paperwork. This would arouse feelings in D of rejection and exclusion. D would then knock on the door of the nursing station, sometimes angrily, and demand something in the nurse's ambit, for example an escorted trip to the patients' bank. The nursing staff, often under pressure, would indicate that nothing could be done that shift. An angry altercation would follow and D would storm off to D's room where D would brood about the injustice of the matter. Later in the afternoon D would explode violently at a seemingly trivial incident with a ferocity which took staff aback.

Here we can see an entrenched schema which appears to organise D's perception and cognition to cue into any behaviour which may be taken as rejection. Such feelings could not be tolerated and could only be worked out through the explosion of anger and the taking of revenge. The above example perhaps opens up an understanding of a distorted schema that might coincide with a dependent personality disorder. Although the behaviour on initial glance seems simply violent, an analysis based on emotional dysregulation and problems in internal control now suggests itself. Furthermore if one accepts a concept of *affect substitution* the treatment team has the beginning of powerful tools to understand the seemingly paradoxical behaviour of challenging behaviour patients.

Concepts from attachment theory

Ainsworth (1969) indicates that around 4% of infants show a pattern of attachment that might be defined as insecure or disorganised. These infants are profoundly affected by separation from the primary caretaker and cannot sustain any purposeful or organised pattern of behaviour during their absence. Furthermore following separation these children show disturbed patterns of re-establishing and showing attachment. It is postulated that they become the future generation of borderline patients. It has also been shown that these children tend to have been subjected to major parental failure (Fonagy *et al* 1997).

The same authors make the point that the disturbed bonds and the behaviour that marks that which become set between child and caretaker transfer or are carried as a model of interaction to adulthood. Relationships with members of caring staff of social institutions would therefore become characterised by disturbed patterns of attachment. Furthermore the absence of a containing relationship or attachment on the ward might lead to disturbed and disorientated behaviour.

Ainsworth *et al* (1978) identified the following insecure attachment patterns in infants:

- *Avoidant*, *in which attachment figures are avoided.*

- *Ambivalent*, *where there is distress on separation and failure to settle on reunion.*

- *Disorganised*, *where there is extremely disorganised and disturbed behaviour in the context of having no attachment strategy.*

George *et al* (1996) identify three corresponding adult states of mind:

- *Dismissing*. *Attachment-related behaviour or the need for attachment is dismissed.*

- *Preoccupied*. *There is a preoccupation with attachment failures.*

- *Unresolved*. *This group shows a striking lack of ability to think about attachment.*

To summarise, attachment styles might be conceptualised as

- *Secure.*

- *Avoidant/dismissing.*

- *Ambivalent/preoccupied.*

- *Disorganised/unresolved.*

Disturbances in attachment might underlie what appears to be very disturbed behaviour on the ward. The overly isolated and schizoid patient may be acting out an avoidant/dismissing attachment pattern. Similarly the ambivalent or preoccupied patient may show disturbance when left unsupported.

The following example may make the unresolved or disorganised pattern clear.

Case history

E had a long-standing pattern of repeated absconding, angry outbursts in which verbal abuse and damage to property occurred, as well as times occasioning minor physical violence. Although deemed to be chronically psychotic, this side appeared not to trouble E unduly. Many behavioural programmes had been put into place without much success. E's keyworker unflaggingly tried to keep a rapport going but was little rewarded, as E would rarely stay any length in conversation. E could be loquacious, although this could end unpredictably. E seemed an impulsive law unto himself.

A behavioural contract was suggested and presented, leading to E storming out of the room in anger. E returned an hour later and said he would sign it. The contract set clear goals but tolerated a level of failure. It also required regular update and brief feedback sessions that emphasised positive reinforcement. Much to the surprise of the team E began to use this contract to relate to all staff members. It appeared that E had found a useful and safe way to relate. E became far less verbally abusive.

Concepts from therapeutic communities

Problems in dependency

Experiences in therapeutic communities have led to useful understandings in disturbed ward behaviour. Green (1986) makes the observation that often violence on the ward is preceded by a period in which relationships between staff and patients appear to be getting better. He explains this as a period in which there is an opening up in the emotional relationship towards each other. However, this openness upsets the psychological equilibrium of the patient and exposes the individual to intolerable feelings of both intrusion and exclusion. The good relationship must then be damaged.

This is closely related to the '*core complex*' described by Glasser (1979). He emphasises that the severe anxieties associated with separation and with suffocation or disregard for the individuated self can rapidly alternate, leaving the carer with seemingly contradictory disturbances in behaviour.

Problems in interpersonal/functioning

Campling (1999) identifies a number of related problematic dynamics that work against a positive therapeutic relationship. The first is hostile dependency. This occurs when the patient, experiencing dependency needs, feels them to become overwhelming and has to relieve them by attacking the carer. This in turn leaves the patient anxious, more vulnerable and more dependent.

The second dynamic she identifies is one of envy. This is a strong hostile wish to destroy any good qualities in the person trying to care for them. A third related concept outlined by Campling is the negative therapeutic reaction; an attempt to sabotage everything that points to success. Another quality that she feels requires urgent attention in therapeutic communities is deceitfulness. This she states often covers up more profound feelings of emptiness and shame and neglect.

Summary

The concepts of affect intolerance, affect substitution, disorders of attachment behaviour and disorders of dependency give strong tools to the practitioner in understanding the development of disturbed behaviour on mental health wards. These concepts again become very relevant in the two following sections.

Problems in engagement

It is extremely rare with patients exhibiting challenging behaviours for the patient to sit down with a member of the treating team, agree that he or she has a problem behaviour, and ask for help and guidance from the therapist. However the collaborative nature of goal setting is one of the most important features of any therapy (Beck *et al* 1979).

Understanding the marked resistances of this group is therefore important. In discussing the cognitive–behavioural treatment of personality disordered patients, Beck and Freeman (1990) have commented that the course of cognitive therapy is far more complicated when there is a combination of behavioural disturbance with mental illness or personality disorder.

> One of the most important treatment considerations in working with personality disordered patients is to be aware that therapy will evoke anxiety because individuals are being asked to go far beyond changing a particular behaviour or reframing a perception. They are being asked to give up who they are and how they have defined themselves for many years. (Beck 1990, p 9)

Furthermore not only is the patient's behaviour inextricably bound up in defending their self-concept, but it is also defined in opposition to the treating team from whom they have long been alienated. This alienation may have little to do with the treating team. Campling (1999) working in therapeutic communities indicates that patients with severe personality disorders, presumably because of grossly inadequate parenting, have no basis for trusting that people in caring positions have their welfare at heart. Key figures, Campling says, may have neglected and abandoned the patients in the past. These relationships become prototypes for future relationships with authority figures, undermining the treating team.

While the above observations are findings in respect of personality disorders, the situation appears, if anything, more pronounced in challenging behaviour. It might be a trite observation but unless these factors are understood the most technically sound interventions might fail. The following example might illuminate this. Here the team attempted to use behavioural principles to positively reinforce the desired behaviour of non-aggressive behaviour.

Case history

F had a long history of intimidation and property damage. His aggressive behaviour continued with frequency on the ward. The team decided on a plan to impose strict boundaries with respect to his verbal and physical aggression. Alongside this was a programme of positive reinforcement. F was known to enjoy socialising at a hospital social centre. The shift was divided into short time periods. For every period he achieved free of aggression he would be rewarded with time to visit the social club. This was to act as the primary reinforcer. Help on adopting different strategies to the verbal and physical aggression he had employed in the past was taken up in regular keyworker sessions.

When the plan was presented to F by the team his reply was, 'I know what you are up to. You can F off. There is no way I am going to work for my ground leave. You and your behavioural programme can get stuffed.'

It should be noted that staff had been careful not to mention the phrase behavioural programme but clearly he knew exactly where the team was coming from. Hence the proposal and rejection of the behavioural programme became part of the problematic interaction and not part of the solution.

Understanding the genesis of the resistance or breakdown in the therapeutic relationship is extremely complex. However, again, the approaches adopted by attachment theory and issues of problems of dependency are highly pertinent here. One need only think of the avoidant/dismissing style of attachment and the problem in forming a working relationship. The central point to be taken is that all insecure forms of relating are fragile and riven by anxiety. In cases where there is an accompanying psychosis these anxieties must be profoundly magnified. Furthermore if patients are able to form relationships these will be, in part, marked by destructive acting out. All the above factors undermine the collaborative therapeutic relationship.

Pressures on the treating teams

The treating team is in a complex relationship with the patient. In this interaction perceptions of patient behaviour and the thresholds of acceptance vary. A judgement of whether a patient is presenting with challenging behaviour will in part depend on how much the team is put under stress or pressure by that patient, or by other parts of the system.

Consider the example below.

Case history

G had been on an acute ward for a number of months. Several attempts had been made to re-establish him in the community but all had failed through his verbal and sometimes physical aggression. On the ward he remained a difficult to manage patient, being frequently verbally aggressive and physically destructive. He also wished to dominate the patient group, often demanding to watch his television programme despite others wishing to watch another. One evening in a conflict about who had the right to choose which channel to watch, he became so aroused that he broke the television set. This was nothing new to the staff group who was inured to him by this point. However, at a ward meeting the rest of the patient group was so angry and voiced such complaints about G that the staff group then decided to refer him to a challenging behaviour unit.

As can be seen in the above example the threshold and impetus for referring Mr G as a 'challenging behaviour patient' emerged with the pressure applied by another part of the system, i.e. the patient group. This process reflects a very central aspect to understanding challenging behaviour: challenging behaviour patients place pressure on staff teams, directly or indirectly. Understanding the nature of these pressures and the anxieties held by treatment teams often identifies the necessary focus of treatment. However pressure on teams often leads to the team becoming polarised and unable to pursue clear therapeutic strategies.

Subjective pressures and their responses

The behaviour of certain patients impacts emotionally on individual members of the treating staff, thereby communicating itself to the treating group. The following examples, though not exhaustive, are commonplace in challenging behaviour wards.

- *Attack on the relationship with the staff.* One may start with the psychoanalytic view expressed by Jeammett (1999) who, working with disturbed adolescents in an in-patient setting, sees challenging behaviour invariably as representing an attack on the therapeutic setting and ultimately on the people who are caring for the patient. An act of destructive behaviour often seems to undo the hard work put in by the team and breaks trust and confidence in the patient–carer relationship. Staff may feel angry and want to reject the patient in turn.

- *Undermining of team therapeutic confidence.* These patients often create a situation where, whatever the staff does, they 'fail'. Patients often vacillate between opposite demands, criticising staff for not meeting their needs at the particular point they are at. Attempts to rectify the immediate demands result in criticism that the other side of the continuum is ignored. One such potential impasse is seen in unresolved dependence–autonomy needs (Green 1986). An example of this might be seen in the following:

Case history

H's admission had come about after violence to staff on an open ward. On the ward H kept up a steady barrage of hostility for many weeks, flouting a number of ward rules and agreements made by her. H demanded that a date be set for discharge. On the other hand a reading of H's history indicated that it was just such the setting of dates that precipitated the worst violence on staff members.

Staff felt bewildered and at odds with each other. Their ability to manage and therapeutically help the patient felt undermined.

- *Raising staff levels of anxiety.* 'Challenging behaviour' patients can easily raise levels of personal anxiety in staff, either through direct threat or by acting in such a way that their behaviour exposes staff to censure. The following example illuminates the point.

Case history

J had started to see the ward psychologist. She had a prolonged but not severe psychosis. The psychologist (perhaps incorrectly) had begun to challenge some of her avoidance of her own emotions, leading to some anger in J. Later that day she made loud allegations that he and other members of staff had made sexual advances towards her. She was clearly sexually vulnerable and slightly disinhibited. Although retracted, these allegations led staff members to feeling anxious and unable to engage in treatment.

Intrinsic structural pressures

The pressures described above have their origin in the patients' behaviours. However it is a very important principle to keep in mind that from the patients' subjective perspective these behaviours are often entirely with reason. In part this may have to do with their history and this was discussed particularly in the previous section. However, it is also important to keep in mind that the context of being on a ward, particularly a locked ward, is a ready source of tension and may go some way to explaining the above difficulties in staff and patient interaction.

These conditions are clearly outlined by Cahn (1998).

- The ward is most often part of an infrastructure for medical treatment. Accordingly the institution is expected to operate with the objectivity and rationality that characterises medicine. Tensions therefore inevitably arise with the subjective aspects or needs of the patient. These are characterised by emotionality, irrationality and ambivalence, all of which fail to follow the expected orderly course of treatment.

- Admissions are seldom made voluntarily. The ward therefore takes on a law and order function that is only partly explicit and this is in tension with the subjectively perceived needs the patient.

- Patients who have exhibited a great deal of violence are often admitted into a PICU/ challenging behaviour ward. The ward is therefore required to contain and control this violence which becomes a policing functioning. Again this produces a tension with the subjective needs of the patient.

- The ward must often accept all patients referred. Hence patients are very different in terms of age, outlook and social interactions. The equilibrium of group life is often under enormous stress.

- Often there is no mutual agreement on treatment. Staff have no choice of whether to work with someone or not and vice versa. Interpersonal tensions might therefore be generated.

It is clear that if the team does not guard against these structural tensions the subjective aspect of the patient can be devalued. If this occurs, Cahn argues, the experience of staff is very much drawn into the problem of devaluation. If the patients feel devalued it would be easy to identify the staff as the devaluers and in reprisal devalue any work done by staff.

Unless these tensions and pressures are taken into account and managed at a systemic level they will lead to an elevation in the disturbance of behaviour at ward level and impede therapeutic engagement, with medical, psychological and social treatments.

TREATING CHALLENGING BEHAVIOURS IN WARD SETTINGS

If the above analysis is correct, then psychological approaches should, as a starting point, focus on the goals summarised below:

- Contribute interventions that aim at understanding the complex thought, emotion and behavioural processes that underlie the difficult cycles of interaction that exist between treating staff and the 'challenging behaviour' patient. This would include both understanding the patient and contributing to the engagement of the patient.

- Help develop the integrated treatments.

- Help develop structures and processes of communications that go some way to ameliorating problems in team cohesion and ward tensions and pressures.

- Contribute to the general understanding of the impact of patients on staff members and act supportively towards treating staff members.

The following sections of the chapter attempt to address practically the above goals by looking at current practices in associated areas.

Cognitive–behavioural approaches to challenging behaviour

Identification of problematic schemata

Beck (1996) suggests therapists should collect information from various sources indicating the automatic thoughts, beliefs and self-concept the patient lives by. Beck suggests that the first cognitive approach should recover automatic thoughts, the almost instantaneous sense the patient makes of a situation. An example of it might be 'staff don't care for me'. Generally from there the therapist must elicit the distorted cognitions built into or making up the automatic thought. An example may be a number of 'conditional assumptions' or distorted beliefs about interpersonal functioning, such as 'If I'm not liked I am worthless.'

Distorted cognitions that make up a schema

The following cognitions may be elicited, which could be organised into a coherent schema

- 'If they don't pay attention to me they don't like me.'

- 'I cannot bear not to be liked.'

- 'If I'm not liked I am worthless.'

The therapist then has the task of translating these underlying interpersonal beliefs as they form the basic motivations of maladaptive interpersonal strategies. This, as discussed above, is in itself a difficult process. Beck (1996) recommends the use of cognitive probes. This is a method in which the therapist and patient identify incidents that illuminate the problems and clearly focus on a particular actual incident. Beck (1990) suggests the use of imagery to re-imagine the experience and recover the automatic thoughts.

Identifying problematic thinking styles

In addition to maladaptive beliefs and thoughts cognitive therapists, as discussed above, focus on distortion in thought. Linehan (1993), working with borderline personality disordered patients, identifies a number of problematic thinking patterns. These include: arbitrary inferences, (conclusions based on insufficient evidence), exaggeration, inappropriate attribution of all blame and responsibility for negative events on oneself, inappropriate attribution of all blame and responsibility for events to others. Catastrophising, (unrealistic expectation or pessimistic predication based on selective attention to negative events in the past), predominate with this group.

Countering problematic beliefs and patterns of behaviour

The beliefs underlying disturbed behaviour then need to be challenged. A variety of techniques can be identified: discussion, re-attribution, use of homework and adducing empirical evidence for such judgements. Linehan (1993) has developed what she believes are core skills needed for the borderline patients. These seem equally appropriate with challenging behaviour patients.

Mindfulness skills. These essentially are based on teaching the patient to take a non-judgmental stance and to observe their own behaviour, that is, what are the events, emotions and behavioural responses.

Distress tolerance skills. Emphasis here is on learning to bear pain and the ability to tolerate and accept distress. Distress tolerance can lower impulsive and reactive destructive behaviour. Many cognitive skills are put into place, such as not catastrophising or being over-judgmental.

Emotional regulation skills. Linehan indicates that many borderline individuals are affectively intense and labile and argues that they would benefit from learning to regulate affective levels. She suggests that the emotions are initially validated, then that they are identified and labelled, again from the patient's perspective. Thirdly the patient is taught to understand the function and the connection between the emotion and destructive behaviours.

Interpersonal skills. These are similar to those taught in assertiveness or interpersonal problem-solving classes.

Self-management skills. Behavioural targets are set with realistic goals, self-monitoring and carrying out contingency management skills.

Approaches to the problem of engagement

Therapeutic contracting

Campling (1999) makes the point that one of the main differences between working psychotherapeutically with more disturbed patients in comparison to less disturbed patients is that one cannot take the therapeutic alliance for granted. The relationship cannot be left to develop, and mistrust needs to be analysed as it arises. Trust is to be created and the therapeutic alliance built up in a way that is tangible and understood by the patient. She suggests the following:

Suggested preparation for engagement on the ward (Campling 1999)

- Take time in the assessment phase to look at the patient's fears about therapy.

- Make it clear that progress will be slow and sometimes matters will become worse.

- A therapeutic contract should be established that spells out the staff responsibilities, the patients' responsibility and the need to work in partnership.

An interesting experiment in partnership occurred in the 1980s at the Littlemore Hospital in Oxford. The Eric Burden Community and Young Adult Unit was set up. Its admission criteria were very similar to those which might be established for a challenging behaviour unit today, i.e.

- Diagnosis of a functional psychosis or borderline personality disorder.

- Normal intelligence.

- No or partial response to conventional medical treatment.

- Breakdown of social network.

Anyone on a young adult unit case register had the right to request admission. The patients had the right to set the level of medication and manage the thresholds of symptoms to those that they felt were acceptable. It was not the staff's role to eliminate delusions or hallucinations. Clear emphasis was placed on communalism as a strong cultural value on the ward. It was found that psychotic patients used her therapeutic community in much the same way as personality disordered contemporaries elsewhere (Pullen 1999).

Therapeutic forbearance

Holmes (1993) describes secure attachment as when an individual is in proximity to his attachment figure he or she feels safe and can engage in exploratory behaviour. This is important for the therapeutic relationship between patient and therapist. The attitude of the therapist may contribute to the patient's progress from insecure to secure attachment to the treating team. The team, like a good mother, picks up cues from the patient's affect or behaviour, and feeds them back to him in an appropriate way.

Motivational interviewing

Motivational interviewing is an approach to develop a therapeutic alliance, originally developed in the addiction services, particularly with problem drinkers (Miller and Rolnick 1991). The approach evolved out of Rogerian principles in that the critical conditions for change are accurate empathy, non-possessive warmth and genuineness. The therapist role in this view was not a directive one providing solutions. Confrontation is seen as counterproductive.

Miller and Rolnick (1991) argue that the fundamental goal is to let the patient consider both advantages and disadvantages to change. The patient should therefore experience ambivalence.

- To express empathy.

- To develop discrepancy i.e. for the patient to look at both sides of the problem – positive and negative features.

- To avoid arguments.

- To 'roll with' resistance.

- To support self-efficacy.

Box 6B.1 Principles of motivational interviewing

Alongside this they outline a number of traps to avoid: avoiding confrontation and denial, avoiding what they call the 'expert trap', avoiding the labelling trap and avoiding a premature focus trap. The motivational interviewing techniques are entirely appropriate for this highly resistant group and should inform any approach to working with challenging behaviour patients.

Approaches from dialectical behaviour therapy

Linehan (1993), working with borderline patients, articulates a view she calls 'dialectical behaviour therapy'. The 'dialectic' can be described as trying to hold in mind a balance of both where the patient is struggling and the reasons for his or her difficult behaviour, as well as, the goals of less destructive behaviour. In defining what is distinctive about this approach she states

> the most fundamental … is the necessity of accepting patients just as they are within a context of trying to teach them to change. The tension between patients' alternating excessively high and lower aspirations and expectations relative to their own capabilities offers a formidable challenge to therapists. It requires moment to moment changes in the use of supportiveness and acceptance versus confrontational and change strategy. (Linehan 1993, page 10)

In addition to the focus on acceptance, Linehan emphasises treating 'therapy-interfering behaviours' as legitimate aims of treatment. Linehan identifies three groupings of behaviour that interfere with therapy:

- *Inattentive behaviour.* This includes not attending, attending late, taking substances before coming to the session, having feelings or behaviours which preclude therapy.

- *Non-collaborative behaviour.* Being oppositional, distracting and digressing.

- *Non-compliant behaviours.* These include failure to carry out agreed tasks.

These she says should be taken up and treated cognitively and dialectically. This serves to provide a useful approach to challenging behaviours.

Constructive institutional responses

Defining tasks and boundaries

Roberts (1994) has explored failing organisations within the NHS. She establishes a number of common problems including vague task definition, defining methods instead of aims, avoiding conflict over priority, confusing tasks with aims and failing to manage boundaries. It might be argued therefore that central to the successful running of a challenging behaviour ward is for the management team to define the primary task, the subordinate tasks and the systems to manage them.

The primary task. The concept of a primary task can seem to be an over-simplification given the complexities that challenging behaviour patients bring. However as a starting point it is invaluable. In this respect Miller and Wright (1967) describe establishing the primary task as a useful concept which allows the team to explore ordering of multiple activities. If one conceptualises challenging behaviour as the breakdown of the ordinary treatment relationship, then the primary task is to re-establish a working patient–carer relationship. The tasks of addressing specifically the disruptive behaviours and underlying psychological problems that disrupt the relationship then become clear. This conceptualisation has become much more prevalent in the treatment of personality disordered patients where 'therapy disruptive behaviours' form legitimate and initial focuses for treatment, rather than reasons for exclusion from treatment (Campling 1999, Linehan 1993, Beck 1996, Beck and Freeman 1990).

Tasks understood by the organisation. Lawrence (1977) described how in any institution there can be task confusion. He distinguishes between them as follows:

- *Normative primary task*, which is the formal operationalisation of the organisation,

- *Existential primary task*, which is the task people from the enterprise believe they are carrying out,

- *Phenomenal primary task*, which can be inferred from people's behaviour and of which they may not be consciously aware.

If there is task confusion the treating team can be split with arguments. The following example hopefully shows how severe challenging behaviour patients can stress the organisation's definition of itself.

Case history

K was an extremely angry woman who could be physically violent and physically destructive to property. A psychiatric report identified a long psychiatric history the presence of personality disorder and was equivocal as to the presence of psychotic features.

She was admitted to the challenging behaviour ward. After an initial assessment the psychiatric team identified mood instability and she was treated accordingly. The psychologist attempted to take up her intense feelings of rage and work in anger management or appropriate expression of anger. The nursing team, however, experienced the full force of her daily anger, deviancy and non-engagement. They rapidly adopted a defensive position in which the best option was to avoid confrontation with K during the shift. The phenomenal task became of increasingly avoiding her altogether. Soon very powerful arguments began to develop between various elements of the team as to the purpose behind her continuing stay on the ward. Little understanding of each other's position could occur. The normative and existential tasks had become increasingly shunned.

In this example a clear definition of the ward task as restoring the treatment relationship and dealing with the behaviours that prevent the formation of such a relationship would help prevent splits in the team and enable treatment to start.

Therapeutic structures at ward level

Systematically Cahn (1998) considers that intervention or organisation should occur at three levels. The entire institution is regarded as a therapeutic system or environment with each level needing to contribute to the primary task.

The managing group. Here the task must be to endeavour to create and keep open an environment in which therapeutic processes can take place. This should be in part to define tasks and structures and to support the subgroups.

Ward structures and treatment teams. The ward constitutes a boundaried environment in which the patient should be given concrete, tightly drawn and firm rules. This provides security.

Staff–patient ward groups. Most therapeutic communities stress the need for regular meeting of staff and patients (Byrt 1999). The principle seems important for all ward groups, in particular in the light of the structural pressures outlined above. Cahn (1998) says that ward meetings should represent the entire ward with all its subgroups. Patients should be free to bring up subjects of their own. The group leaders must often provide structural help. As far as possible collaboration needs to occur and agreements drawn up that staff and patients can become partners. In practice there needs to be agreed minute-takers, chairpersons and a formal process for decisions to be taken to the appropriate hospital manager/clinician if the matter cannot be dealt with at the ward meeting.

There clearly needs to be communication between each level.

Integrative treatment approaches

The task of the ward should be discussed and integrated. There is a constant stress on this and the focus for the psychological practitioner is to suggest means of integrating and communicating the primary task of the ward and to explain how that translates in respect of the patient. Some useful therapeutic approaches can be adopted that strengthen this goal and the tasks outlined above.

The RAID programme for challenging behaviour

One method for maintaining a positive style by all treating staff in the face of difficult behaviours is the adoption of the RAID programme. This is a programme developed by Davies (1993).

RAID is an acronym standing for 'Reinforce Appropriate (Behaviour), Ignore Difficult or disruptive (Behaviour)'. Focus is placed on the positive aspects of the patient's behaviour while de-emphasising the more disruptive. This creates an environment in which more positive interaction occurs and helps the staff think positively of the patients despite the difficult behaviours exhibited by them. Reinforcing positive behaviours makes future positive action more probable and builds on the patients' sense of competence. Ultimately therefore success on the ward should strengthen the relationship between the staff and the patient.

Davies (1993) identifies an essential stance to be maintained by the treating team.

- Staff should not focus on disruptive behaviour and its consequences.

- Staff should be ready to reinforce the next appearance of appropriate behaviour even if it comes very soon after disruptive states. Even on wards containing the most difficult or disruptive patients they will be behaving appropriately for 85% of the time. The temptation for staff, of course, is to focus on the remaining 15% of time during which the patients cause trouble, thereby unconsciously reinforcing this mode of personal interaction. The task of the staff is to positively reinforce every time the patient behaves appropriately.

- Identify and target appropriate behaviours – situations such as talking to others, watching TV, smiling, cooking, playing, doing repairs, eating appropriately, using the bathroom appropriately and sleeping.

- By reinforcing these appropriate behaviours Davies (1993) argues that the inappropriate behaviours diminish in frequency.

Box 6B.2 : Principles of the RAID approach

Psychosocial nursing

A particularly appropriate means of establishing the basis of positive interaction with patients is the development of psychosocial nursing. The aim of this approach is to strengthen social functioning. Essentially the stance taken by nurses is to maintain in mind a view of the patient's potential capabilities and encourage and foster responsibility for putting these abilities into action, rather than assuming the patient to be ill. The following example might make this process clear.

Case history

L was constantly wrapped up in concerns about other patients, often approaching staff with these worries and asking for advice. However, she could rarely think of her own emotions and needs. Staff formulated the response of asking her what her feelings were in relation to the problem, and encouraged her to try to develop her own plan of action.

INTEGRATING TREATMENT

Functional analysis

This is based upon an understanding of challenging behaviour as disorders of attachment, dependency and emotional dysregulation. To do effective work at this level it is necessary to perform a clear functional analysis of the behaviour. Once the problem is established intervention needs simultaneously to be integrated at the level of individual and ward approaches, and to make sure there is the least possible contradiction. Consider the following example.

Case history

M had a long history of emotional instability and self-injurious behaviours, some quite severe and life threatening. After a number of ups and downs she appeared to make a concerted effort to re-establish a more normal pattern of life. Things improved and she went for a number of visits to her sister who was married. One evening her sister and husband had an intense and lengthy argument. Nothing negative was expressed to or about M.

She returned to the ward saying all was well. She went to her room and took an overdose of anti-depressants. She reported their argument of the weekend had upset her. On closer questioning she indicated that at the time of the argument she had felt very alone and had decided to take the tablets. Clearly she had been storing tablets for some time. One knew from past treatment that she self-harmed when feelings became unbearable and often these had to do with feelings of anger and rejection.

The first step is to gain a very clear and detailed understanding of the whole chain of the behaviour, its antecedents and consequences. Linehan (1993) calls this 'chaining'. She argues that a clear analysis of a whole chain of an episode of disturbed behaviour must be made; understanding the trigger, the underlying cognitive, affective and behavioural schemata. Similarly Beck and Freeman (1990) suggest an analysis of the view of self, view of others, one's own negative beliefs and basic strategies. The latter authors call these flow charts.

If one couples this with the understanding brought by the concepts of affect intolerance, disturbances of internal control, problems in dependency and disturbances of patterns of attachment, then the approach of functional analysis provides an extremely powerful method of understanding the behaviour.

Using this as a basis one can postulate that the argument between M's sister and brother-in-law is the trigger for the behaviour. M's perception is that she is ignored and excluded. This re-awakens powerful feelings of rejection which are not tolerable. M then takes the overdose. This paradoxically is a matter of psychological or emotional survival. The focus of treatment is needing to tolerate pain and anxiety associated with feelings of rejection. This can be addressed in individual treatment. Furthermore the patient needs to be taught more appropriate means of expression. This is most probably done best at ward level on a daily level, perhaps using the RAID approach. The ward can also do supportive work at community group level, countering the strong cognitions of rejection. Intensive work needs to be done on maintaining relationships both at ward and individual levels.

The following flow chart (Figure 6B.1) provides an example of an integrated approach to treatment.

CONCLUSION

Figure 6B.1 shows how chronically disturbed behaviour could be managed on a ward. The approach also hopefully allows for an integration of thoughts from different theoretical standpoints. The ultimate emphasis of this chapter is how to

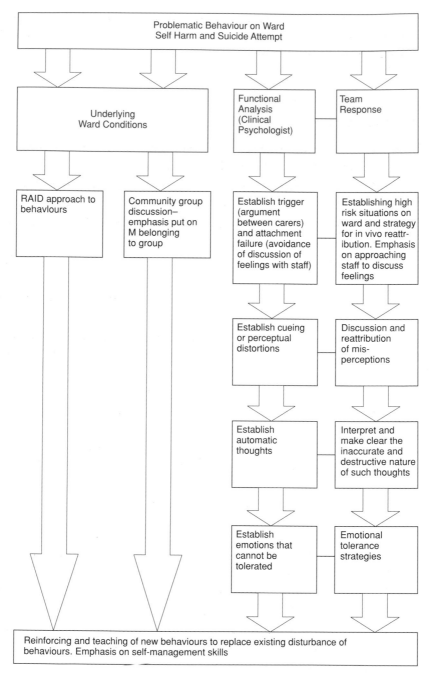

Figure 6B.1 – An example of treatment of challenging behaviours at ward level

understand the powerful processes that undermine the working patient–carer relationship and adopt treatment approaches aimed specifically at re-establishing the relationship. Once established many of the problems this group faces can then be effectively treated.

REFERENCES

Ainsworth M. 1969 Object relations and dependency and attachment: theoretical review of mother infant relationship. Child Development 40: 969–1025.

Ainsworth M, Blehar RM, Waters E *et al.* 1978 Patterns of attachment: a psychological study of the strange situation. Hillsdale HJ Lawrence, Erlbaum Associates

Beck AT, Rush J, Shaw B, Emery G. 1979 Cognitive Therapy of Depression. New York: Guilford

Beck AT, Freeman A. 1990 Cognitve Therapy of Personality Disorders. New York: Guilford Press

Beck JS. 1996 Cognitive therapy of personality disorders. In: Salkovskis PM (ed.) Frontiers of Cognitive Therapy. New York: Guilford

Byrt R. 1999 Nursing: the importance of the psychosocial enviroment. In: Campling P, Haig R (eds) Therapeutic Communities Past, Present and Future. London: Jessica Kingsley

Cahn T. 1998 Beyond the treatment contract: psychoanalytical work in the public mental hospital. In: Pestalozzi J *et al* (eds) Psychoanalytical Psychotherapy in Institutional Settings. London: Karnac

Campling P. 1999 Chaotic personalities: maintaining the therapeutic alliance. In: Campling P, Haig R (eds) Therapeutic Communities Past, Present and Future. London: Jessica Kingsley

Davies W. 1993 The RAID Programme for Challenging Behaviour. Leicester Association for Psychological Therapies

Fonagy P, Target M, Steele M, Steele H. 1997 The development of violence and crime as it relates to security of attachment. In: Osojsky (ed.) Children in a Violent Society. New York: Guilford Press. 150–177

George C, Kaplan N, Main M. 1996 Adult Attachment Interview 3rd edn. Unpublished Manuscript, Dept. of Psychology, University of California, Berkeley

Glasser, M. (1979) Some aspects of the role of aggression in the peversions'. In: I. Rosen (ed.) Sexual Deviation. London: Oxford University Press

Green A. 1986 On Private Madness. London: Karnac

Holmes J. 1993 Attachment theory: a biological basis for psychotherapy. Br J Psych 163: 430–438

Jeammet P. 1999 Links between internal and external reality in devising a therapeutic setting for adolescents who present with serious conduct disorders. In: Amastasopoulous D, Laylou-Lignos E, Wadder M (eds) Psychoanalytic Psychotherapy of the Severely Disturbed Adolescent. London: Karnac

Lawrence. 1977 Management Development. Some ideals, images and realities In: Coleman AD and Geller MH (eds) Group relations reader No. 2. Rice Institute, Washington

Lelliott P, Wing JK. 1994 A national audit of new long stay psychiatric patients. II: Impact on services. Br J Psych 165: 170–178

Linehan M. 1993 Cognitive Behavioural Treatment of Borderline Personality Disorder. New York: Guilford

Mann S, Cree W. 1976 New long stay psychiatric patients: a national sample survey of fifteen mental hospitals in England and Wales 1972/1973. Psychol Med 6: 603–616

Miller EJ, Wright AK. 1967 Systems of Organisation: The Control of Task and Central Boundaries. London: Tavistock

Milner WR, Rolnick S. 1991 Motivational Interviewing: Preparing People to Change Addictive Behaviour. New York: Guilford

Pullen G. 1999 Schizophrenia: hospital communities for the severely disturbed. In: Therapeutic communities Past, Present and Future. Campling P, Haigh R (eds) London: Jessica Kingsley Publisher

Roberts VZ. 1994 The organisation of work: contributions from open system theory. In: Obholzer A and Roberts VZ (eds) The Unconscious at Work. London: Routledge, pp. 28–38

Shepherd G. 1999 Social functioning and challenging behaviour. In: Meuser KT, Terrier N (eds) Handbook of Social Functioning and Schizophrenia. Massachusetts: Allyn and Bacon

7

SECLUSION

Roland Dix, Christian Betteridge

INTRODUCTION

Whether or not seclusion has a place within the treatment of the mentally disordered is possibly the longest running debate concerning any issue in the history of health care (Mason 1994). The use of seclusion is at least 2000 years old and many of the related questions have remained consistent, surviving to the modern day. It is not the intention of this chapter to re-describe the moral, ethical and legal paradigms that have punctuated much of seclusion's history. The focus here will be to provide: an overview of the history of seclusion, its value or otherwise; alternatives, and the necessary supporting policies for its use; and finally, to offer a practical framework within which seclusion may be considered in the context of psychiatric intensive care units (PICUs).

'The forcible confinement of a patient alone in a room for the protection of others from serious harm' (MHA Code of Practice 1999).

Box 7.1 Definition of seclusion

Seclusion is widely used throughout the world (Mason 1994). Not surprisingly, different cultures have different attitudes and, as a result, different variations on the use of seclusion. While it would be unwise to ignore the experiences of other countries, the theme of this chapter will be the use of seclusion in the UK.

No attempt to deal with the use of seclusion can be completely divorced from the simple question of whether seclusion should be used or not. To do so, would deny the emotive nature of the issues innate to the subject. Having recognised this, the authors will not offer a definitive view as to whether PICUs should have seclusion, but will rather provide a balanced guide to thinking, informing the decision-making process for anyone planning an intensive care service. The arguments for and against the use of seclusion will be apparent throughout the chapter.

HISTORY OF SECLUSION

It is difficult to define an era that marks the birth of seclusion in the management of mental disorder. The ancient Greeks had rooms designed to entice the mentally ill patient to sleep so that they would dream their way back to sanity (Wells 1972).

In the Middle Ages and the Renaissance, different religions attached their own meanings to the disordered mind and the extent to which severe methods of management featured, including the use of seclusion, varied considerably (Mora 1967). The eighteenth and nineteenth centuries included a shift towards the institutional model for the housing of the insane, and with it brought the use of seclusion that more closely resembles modern-day methods, i.e. for management of the most disturbed behaviour. During the 1790s Philippe Pinel demonstrated that his asylum, the Bicêtre in Paris, could operate without a profound reliance on the use of seclusion and restraint (Renvoize 1991). Pinel was confident that, with the correct method of communication, paying attention to the in-mates' individuality and self-respect, few restraints were necessary (Hunter and Macalpine 1963). While it is apparent that Pinel had stumbled on the value of de-escalation, it is difficult to overlook the use of the term 'few' which clearly signals that physical confinement was still deemed unavoidable in some circumstances. In Britain, William Tuke, a layman superintendent of the Retreat Asylum in York, also advocated a more humane approach based on his Quaker 'moral therapy' philosophy. 1892 saw an interesting debate about the use of seclusion when another Tuke cited the British pioneer, of non-restraint John Conolly:

> 'If Conolly attached too much importance to this mode of treatment (*seclusion*), the other extreme, of regarding the padded room as never useful, is a very questionable position to take' (Angold 1989).

It is difficult to avoid the feeling that in the dawn of the twenty-first century this debate is no nearer to a conclusion. The latter half of the nineteenth century saw increased attempts more clearly to legislate for the legal and conceptual underpinnings of mental health care. There emerged several consistent themes, often in conflict with each other, attempting to improve the experience of the patient while at the same time addressing the fears of society. A number of attempts were made to balance the determined efforts by the medical profession to claim the scientific high ground, with those of the law makers, who argued that mental health care was a legal rather than medical concern (Rogers and Pilgrim 1996). While this situation focused on the humane treatment of the patient in varying degrees, by and large, the experience of the patient remained unchanged with the continued and unregulated use of mechanical restraint and seclusion.

During the 1920s there was growing concern about the conditions in many psychiatric hospitals for staff and patients alike. Staff were expected to work 14 hours a day with only half a day off per month. In September 1922 tensions reached such a pitch that staff and patients of the Nottinghamshire County Mental Hospital joined forces in fighting against police who were sent there to restore order (Nolan 1993). In 1923 an inquiry at Hull Asylum reported on the lack of privacy, dirty conditions – patients having to bath in the same water and most worryingly 'patients being confined in dungeons for long periods of time'. Conditions for all within many of the institutions during the early 1920s left little time or interest in singling out the use of seclusion for debate, amongst what appeared to be far more important concerns. In 1923 Dr Montague Lomax published his *Experiences of an Asylum Doctor*. It was highly critical of the conditions in many institutions, the appalling arrogance and behaviour of many medical superintendents and also the barbaric methods of treatment including the use of seclusion. A storm of debate resulted from the book's publication. Even amidst aggressive attempts by medical superintendents to discredit Dr Lomax, the Royal Commission recommended wide-reaching improvements which included limiting patient seclusion to certain clearly defined circumstances. Also, the patients had to be carefully monitored whilst in seclusion (Nolan 1993). This was possibly the first appearance of standard regulation on the use of seclusion.

The outbreak of war in 1939 preoccupied much of the 1940s. Mental hospitals, as far as it was possible, were emptied to accommodate the wounded. This also resulted in a renewed interest in the science of mental illness, in particular the use of electro-convulsive therapy for the treatment of shell shock and depression (Merskey 1991). Another addition was the introduction of psychotherapeutic techniques. Even with these innovations the widespread and unregulated use of seclusion continued. This is chillingly illustrated by the personal accounts of nurses working in hospitals during the 1940s, collected by Nolan (1993). One nurse recalls:

'Patients were subjected to hours and hours of endless boredom in the airing courts. . . . We counted patients in and out . . . In side rooms, there were patients locked up for weeks on end; the staff had become so used to the screaming of these patients that they totally ignored it.'

The 1950s saw the introduction of chlorpromazine, hailed by many as a miracle cure for psychosis. Even though the true efficacy of chlorpromazine remained in debate, a new era had dawned with many hospitals opening their doors during the 1950s and 1960s. Many wards now had open-door policies with new freedoms given to many patients, however, for a significant minority of patients locked wards and seclusion continued.

In 1983, a new Mental Health Act (MHA) resulted in the publication of a MHA Code of Practice in 1990, which made a determined attempt to regulate finally the use of seclusion. The Mental Health Act Commission (MHAC) was appointed to support the 1983 Act and to prevent the re-emergence of mental hospital brutality scandals that riddled the 1970s. In spite of this, the 1992 *Cutting Edge* television documentary had again exposed appalling practice involving seclusion at Ashworth Special Hospital, as they had done at Rampton 12 years earlier (Department of Health 1992). The vice chair of the MHAC was forced to concede the Commission had failed where investigative journalism had succeeded (Rogers and Pilgrim 1996).

The 1970s to 1990s have been characterised by a massive increase in debating the moral, practical and conceptual issues attached to the use of seclusion. A snap-shot survey of the professional press in 1999 showed 314 papers containing the word 'seclusion', highlighted in three popular databases. During the past 20 years a number of often polarised arguments have been advanced resulting in some cases in the abolition of seclusion altogether in many hospitals (Whittington and Mason 1995). As far as PICUs are concerned, Beer *et al* (1997) in their survey found that of 110 PICUs in the UK, 40% had no seclusion room. Of those that did have seclusion, 15 units admitted to having no written policy on its use.

Even today, apart from the academic debate, the press has also recorded deaths of secluded patients. In America, the use of mechanical restraint and seclusion remains a routine procedure in many modern psychiatric hospitals (Hamolia 1995). Appelbaum (1999) reported on 142 deaths in American seclusion rooms between 1988 and 1998. While allowing for the Americans favouring seclusion compared with their European counterparts, it is interesting that the House of Representatives (1999) has recently introduced a bill entitled the 'Patients Freedom from Restraint Act 1999'. It appears that unease surrounding the use of seclusion has even penetrated the long held hard line of many states of America. In Britain the famous and disturbing case of the death in seclusion of Orville Blackwood left the panel of inquiry concluding that a 'macho culture' existed around the use of seclusion in Broadmoor Special Hospital, as well as a critical lack of operational procedures (Prins 1994).

Amidst the often passionate and polarised arguments presented by supporters and opponents of seclusion, one thing is clear. Seclusion continues to be used in many hospitals and when staff are in the position of having to manage serious aggression, they are often reduced to few options. This point was succinctly made by Mason (1994) who concluded his international review of seclusion with the following comments:

> 'When the patient is no longer susceptible to the paradigms of treatment, when they are in the throes of assault, when they are combatant – there remain only four things one can do: seclude them, restrain them, medicate them, or pass the problem on to some one else (transfer them).'

The remainder of this chapter aims to illuminate a path through the maze of argument surrounding the modern day use of seclusion, that will guide the thinking of PICU staff.

FACTORS THAT AFFECT THE MODERN DAY USE OF SECLUSION

Opponents of seclusion are rapidly growing in numbers and as we will see later in this chapter, arguments for its abolition are profound and diverse. Seclusion continues to hold a precarious position in modern psychiatric hospitals and its continued use is under close scrutiny. The survival or demise of seclusion depends upon clear and honest analysis of what factors affect its use. Furthermore, alternative interventions and their impact on seclusion rates need to be examined. There has been an identified lack of available guidelines for making decisions regarding seclusion (Outlaw and Lowery

1992). If seclusion has a future in modern psychiatric practice, evidence based policies for its implementation must be utilised.

Patient behaviour

Patients in psychiatric hospitals can display a wide diversity of challenging behaviours. The decision to implement seclusion is a complicated process fraught with problems. Much of the empirical literature reveals alarming variations in the rationale offered for the use of seclusion. Angold (1989) noted violence, in particular interpersonal violence toward staff, to be the most common rationale for seclusion. Likewise, Tooke and Brown (1992) found that both staff and patients viewed not only destructive, aggressive behaviour but also inappropriate sexual behaviour as the main reasons for seclusion. A review of ten studies undertaken by Soloff et al (1985) concluded that seclusion was most frequently used to contain disruptive, agitated or excited behaviour. Also it was the clear belief of the staff that much of the behaviour represented a serious risk of escalation into actual violence. The conclusion of this extensive review was that early use of seclusion dramatically reduced the incidence of actual violence.

Morrison and Lehane (1996) concluded that physical assaults on staff were the single most common cause for seclusion, closely followed by: threats to staff, self-inflicted injury, damage to property, disturbed behaviour, physical assault on patients, threats to patients and self seclusion. Moreover, physical assaults on staff and patients only accounted for one-third of the total episodes of seclusion. Surprisingly, the majority of episodes were precipitated by non-violent behaviours (Morrison and Lehane 1996).

During a year-long study of the use of seclusion and restraint in 82 medical centres in America, the primary reason given for its use was disruptive behaviour disturbing the ward environment, not necessarily violent behaviour itself. Closely following in descending order were patient agitation, physical and verbal aggression (Betemps et al 1993).

Ward characteristics

General ward characteristics and non-behavioural patient profiles have also proved to have had a significant impact on the use of seclusion. Staffing levels in particular have been the focus of many studies which have consistently found a strong correlation between increased staffing levels and reduced incidence of seclusion (Outlaw and Lowery 1992, Morrison 1995). Craig et al (1989) found that staffing levels, education and experience in dealing with disturbed behaviour made a significant impact on the use of seclusion. De Cangas (1993) linked staffing levels to frequency of seclusion, however, factors rated more highly were unit layout, degree of crowding and conflicting personalities.

Attitudes and culture

There is good evidence that the attitudes and general ethos of staff groups are significant in the use of seclusion. Indications that staff are reluctant to be self critical with regard to seclusion have been presented. De Cangas' (1993) found that staff viewed seclusion use to be more affected by unit factors than variations in their own attitude and performance. In contrast, De Cangas and Shopflocher (1989) recorded that nursing staff held a positive attitude towards seclusion, were open minded about its implementation and believed that it was an effective intervention. Steele (1993) surveyed staff attitudes in four hospitals and revealed that 80% of staff claimed to refuse to consider seclusion until verbal intervention had been attempted and had failed. The majority of staff viewed seclusion as a last resort which had some therapeutic benefit.

Further evidence of the importance of staff attitude was presented by Gerlock and Solomons (1983) who established a correlation between staff attitude, ward culture and the frequency of seclusion. Tolerance levels towards disturbed behaviours, anxiety levels, the need to control behaviour because of low staffing levels as well as perceptions of the therapeutic benefits of seclusion were all highly significant. Considering the literature concerning attitudes, it is clear that some staff teams are more motivated towards proactive interventions that can de-escalate behaviours which would otherwise warrant seclusion. Reasons for failing to engage in proactive intervention are offered by Morrison (1990) who argues that nurses are too often engaged in non-clinical tasks, resulting in lost opportunities to prevent escalating behaviour which culminates in seclusion. It is reasonable to hypothesise that units with a positive attitude towards seclusion as a therapeutic treatment and low motivation towards creative interventions will undoubtedly have higher rates of seclusion.

Non-behavioural patient characteristics

Correlations between seclusion and non-behavioural patient characteristics such as gender, age and race have been established. Soloff and Turner (1981) found an alarmingly disproportionate number of black patients were being secluded. Lack of communication and cultural understanding between predominantly white staff and black patients was one proposed explanation. However, in a follow-up study 4 years later, Soloff *et al* (1985) found that young patients were secluded more often than older patients and that race and gender bore no significance. More recent British studies have shown that black people were over-represented in seclusion rates, were given higher doses of medication and tended to spend longer in hospital than white patients (Browne 1997).

Swett (1994) found slightly higher seclusion rates for males than for females but again confirmed being younger (under 35) was much more likely to result in seclusion. In terms of general patient characteristics, it is difficult to make confident assertions about their relevance to seclusion, although there appears to be more than enough evidence to think seriously about perceptions of age and race.

Summary of important factors that affect the use of seclusion

To conclude our analysis of important factors a number of clear themes emerge. The literature has identified a deficit of descriptive accounts of the nature and degree of verbal and physical violence that precede seclusion. The lack of empirical data that describes the intricacies of violent behaviour has serious implications for future practice. Indeed, Breakwell (1997) strongly supported careful monitoring of patterns of violent behaviour for the purposes of future clinical predictions and practice. Without better data on details of aggressive behaviour that are deemed to warrant seclusion, much of the decision making process will be left to individual staff. Finally there are many other variables, for example staff attitude and perceptions of age and race, that simply should not be involved. Anyone planning to use seclusion should assign serious thought to these issues.

- The temptation to justify the use of seclusion purely on the grounds of managing violence is simply not supported by the evidence.

- There is good indication that seclusion is used to supplement staffing levels.

- Staff attitudes are important.

- Levels of training are needed.

- There is no satisfactory explanation for the over representation of non white patients in seclusion statistics.

Box 7.2 Key points

DOES SECLUSION HAVE A PLACE IN CONTEMPORARY PSYCHIATRIC PRACTICE?

The arguments for and against seclusion are complex. Many authors have advanced both evidence and argument to support their particular viewpoint. In order to promote clarity, and provide a context within which to consider the evidence, it is helpful to categorise the debate under three main headings.

- *Morality*: There are those who believe that the use of seclusion is morally wrong. Put simply, it is held that within modern practice the procedure of locking a patient alone in a room, cannot in principle be justified (Hammill 1987).

- *Consequentialism*: Some maintain a consequentialist approach to ethical reasoning; this means that the decision, whether or not seclusion is used, results from a direct appraisal of the potential consequences that might arise for the patient and others (Morrison and Lehane 1995). In other words when faced with extreme aggression the end justifies the means.

- *Treatment*: Some commentators have maintained that seclusion is a useful treatment modality (Orr and Morgan 1995). They do not, in the first instance, overly concern themselves with moral or ethical debate, but rather maintain that the practice can produce positive effects in the mental and behavioural state of the patient.

Box 7.3 Seclusion: Basis of arguments for and against

The moral argument

Within the literature it is not difficult to find examples of powerful condemnation of seclusion. Some commentators have described the practice as an 'archaic, controversial form of tyranny' and 'an embarrassing reality' in the management of mental disorder (Pileete 1978, Rosen and DiGiacomo 1978). The Royal College of Nursing has been quoted as regarding seclusion as an anti-therapeutic intervention that will ultimately become redundant (Topping-Morris 1994). Topping-Morris goes on to suggest that 'as patient advocates, nurses should seek to expose the issue of seclusion as a lingering relic of the past'.

Although the comments listed above are generally representative of the views held by opponents of seclusion, they do not in themselves provide a solid foundation from which to debate. The consistent themes are that seclusion is a very distressing patient experience (Norris and Kennedy 1992, Tooke and Brown 1992), and that it is out-dated and out-moded. These views are fuelled by evidence that patients can perceive seclusion as a form of torture (Chamberlin 1985, Jensen 1985). They illustrate the general unease associated with the notion of locking away disturbed behaviour as a simple method of management. Hammill (1987) asks, 'Why has the practice continued? Is it because it is still easier to isolate an out of control patient behind a locked door, rather than deal with the underlying problem?' Many of these arguments are based on the overwhelming evidence that, when available, seclusion will be implemented with dubious rationale, inconsistently used and its frequency related to many other variables, not necessarily dependent on degrees of violence. These issues have been given appropriate attention previously in this chapter, and from our analysis of factors affecting the use of seclusion, are undeniably valid. The basic core of the moral argument, is that, if one has seclusion as an available option, patients will be secluded inappropriately and suffer extreme distress; staff will not be motivated to develop superior methods of dealing with violence (Drinkwater and Gudjonsson 1989). It is reasonable, therefore, not to have seclusion at all.

The consequentialist argument and alternatives to seclusion

Beauchamp and Childress (1994) defined the application of consequentialism to an ethical debate as 'the right act in any circumstance is the one that produces the best overall result, as determined from an impersonal perspective that gives equal weight to the interests of each affected party'. It is not difficult to see the attraction of this theory for supporters of seclusion as a method for managing violence. Verbal de-escalation, restraint, medication and the use of increased observation in an extra care area, have all been proposed as alternatives to seclusion (Kingdon and Bakewell 1988, Myers 1990, Kinsella and Brosman 1993, Donat 1998). We will examine the evidence for their effectiveness and attempt to balance this with arguments advanced by those who maintain that they do not in every case, provide a preferable alternative to seclusion.

Verbal de-escalation

The value of verbal de-escalation in preventing actual physical assault has long been accepted (Infantino and Mustingo 1985, Turnbull *et al* 1990, Stevenson 1991). Shepherd and Lavender (1999) showed that of 127 violent incidents 50% could be managed with verbal interventions alone. They report seclusion being used in only two of the total incidents. A clinical trial demonstrated a reduction in seclusion use by 50% following the introduction of a model of de-escalation (Morales 1995). Following a change in seclusion policy in a secure unit, Torpy and Hall (1994) found a highly significant reduction in seclusion rates. They suggested that the staff had become considerably more skilled at alternative interventions, in particular verbal de-escalation.

In line with the experience of many mental health nurses, most if not all advocates of de-escalation accept that at best the technique can only dramatically reduce, rather than eradicate physical violence. Some authors point out that verbal de-escalation is a complex process and during interaction the dynamics can easily work in the opposite direction, escalating aggression (Blair 1991, Maier 1996). Soloff *et al* (1985) found in a review of the literature that there was overwhelming empirical support for using seclusion to limit the progression of disruptive behaviour to actual violence. Although seclusion has been advocated as a quick and effective method of preventing progression towards physical assault, it must be accepted that a determined attempt at verbal de-escalation is an obvious first intervention.

Physical restraint

The introduction of control and restraint (C & R) training to a medium secure unit showed several benefits (Parks 1996). Seclusion was used in only 12% of the total number of violent incidents. It was suggested that staff were now in the position to hold a patient safely until either verbal de-escalation or medication could work. This was balanced, however, with an increase in injuries to staff, in comparison to figures before the introduction of C & R. Increased staffing levels are highly significant in reducing seclusion use. One explanation for this could be that if more staff are available then restraint is more readily attempted. Evidence of this is provided by Palmstierna and Wistedt (1995) who showed that increased staff numbers reduce the severity of violent incidents but not their frequency.

Physical restraint as an alternative to seclusion can in itself be a very problematic intervention. While it is permitted in many American states to use four-point mechanical restraint, in the UK restraint may only involve the holding of a person by another (MHA 1999). Betempts and Buncher (1992) showed that some patients spent up to 72.2 hours in a single episode of mechanical restraint in American hospitals. In the UK prolonged restraint has been known to result in sudden death from asphyxia (Paterson et al 1998). Indeed, many of the deaths that actually occur while a patient is in the seclusion room have been correlated with a violent struggle immediately before the patient was secluded (Kumar 1997). The authors work in a PICU without seclusion and we have ourselves experienced situations where the patient continues to fight with staff requiring continued restraint, on some occasions for up to 40 minutes. Mindful of the potential problems associated with restraint, it is reasonable to suggest that, when compared, 40 minutes spent in a seclusion room may be preferable for both the patient and staff than the same length of time spent in physical restraint.

Rapid tranquilisation

Rapid tranquilisation (RT) will be covered in depth elsewhere in this volume so we shall only briefly touch on its relevance to seclusion. The appropriate use of medication has also been proposed as a method of reducing or even eradicating the use of seclusion (Klinge 1994). Not surprisingly, Pilowsky et al (1992) showed that when given intravenously RT had eradicated the need for seclusion. Intramuscular RT has also proved highly effective with only a small minority of cases requiring restraint or seclusion following its use. It is beyond question that rapid tranquilisation is largely effective in calming an agitated, angry and potentially aggressive patient. However, in addition to some delay while it takes effect, its use has also been shown to produce distressing side-effects (Hyde et al 1998) and also correlated with sudden death (Laposata 1988, Paterson et al 1998).

The extra care area (ECA)

More recently the use of an extra care area (ECA) in which a single patient may receive intensive nursing intervention has become a popular method of managing acute disturbance (Kinsella and Brosman 1993, Dix 1995). The principles of the ECA appear to fulfil much of the function of seclusion by removing a patient liable to assault from the general ward population. It also has the advantage of keeping staff in contact with the patient through the aggressive episode so that they develop the enhanced skills necessary for dealing with disturbed behaviour (Kinsella and Brosman 1993). The use of graded observation in concert with the ECA was reported by Kingdon and Bakewell (1988) to have successfully completely replaced seclusion. They report no increase in violent incidents or any cases of refused admission as a result of a new non-seclusion policy.

Again this method is also not without its problems. Kinsella and Brosman (1993) reported on the occurrence of patients receiving positive reinforcement towards disturbed behaviour as a result of the special attention they receive from prolonged use of the ECA. The ECA can also be difficult to staff. In terms of the number of staff needed, there is a danger of creating a ward within a ward (Dix and Williams 1996).

Summary of seclusion alternatives and their consequences

To summarise the seclusion debate within the context of consequentialism, any alternatives to seclusion should be carefully appraised in relation to the problems they present. It is beyond doubt that a combination of the above alternatives has been successful in eradicating seclusion in many hospitals. However, supporters of seclusion continue to argue that it is very easy to maintain a non-seclusion policy, while at the same time failing to recognise the possibility of equally undesirable consequences of alternative interventions. The basic position of this philosophy is that while all possible action should be taken to avoid the need for seclusion, there are rare circumstances in which it remains the least damaging intervention.

- *Verbal de-escalation* is valuable in reducing and managing incidence of assaults, although it cannot eradicate them.

- *Physical restraint* is effective for the immediate management of assault. When used for extended periods, it can be potentially dangerous for the patient and arguably is not preferable to seclusion.

- *Rabid tranquilisation* is effective in the immediate management of disturbed behaviour. There can be difficult delays (unless administered intravenously) in achieving sedation. There is also the possibility of severe side-effects.

- *The extra care area* is effective in containing a patient liable to attack. It can be very expensive in time and resources. There is also a possibility of producing secondary behavioural disturbance in order to maintain intensive contact with the staff.

Box 7.4 Key points: Alternatives to seclusion

The treatment argument

Several authors have produced evidence that seclusion can promote positive mental and behaviour change in the patient (Mason 1993, Orr and Morgan 1995). In short, they advance the argument that, more than just a method of emergency management, seclusion can be an effective treatment. Before we examine some of this evidence, we must clearly state that the concept of seclusion as a treatment is simply not acceptable within the English and Welsh Mental Health Act Code of Practice (1999), where Part 19.16 clearly states that:

'Its (*seclusion*) sole aim is to contain severely disturbed behaviour which is likely to cause harm to others. . . . Seclusion should not be used as part of a treatment plan.'

Most of the support for seclusion as a treatment comes from the USA. Kahn *et al* (1987) concluded that patients who were exposed to low stimulation, mechanical restraint and seclusion experienced a significant reduction in psychotic symptoms. Hamolia (1995) again argues that seclusion can be therapeutic as a result of the patient being contained, removed from the circumstances in which they responded aggressively, and receiving reduced sensory input. She further suggests that: 'Their (*the patients'*) distortions create such psychic pain that seclusion may provide some relief and may be the only place they feel safe from their persecutors'. In addition seclusion is suggested to be a place where the patients can learn to exercise control over their impulses. Sixty percent of the staff surveyed by Steele (1993) felt that seclusion had therapeutic, as well as emergency management value. In a minority of the sample group, some studies of patients' perception of seclusion, have recorded positive comments in relation to the experience of being secluded (Norris and Kennedy 1992). Feelings such as safety, reassurance from the regular observations and the time to reflect in the quiet of the seclusion room were reported.

The major problem with demonstrating that seclusion has any treatment value is the overwhelming evidence that staff and patients perceive seclusion very differently (Plutchik *et al* 1978, Soliday 1985, Heyman 1987, Richardson 1987, Nolan 1989). Staff tend to underestimate the negative experience of the patient, while simultaneously overestimating the positive effects. In addition, it is very difficult to establish a control group of non-secluded patients, who have similar mental and behavioural profiles to those who were secluded and against which therapeutic value may be measured.

To conclude the treatment argument, it is beyond question that the vast majority of patients perceive seclusion as a negative experience. Much of the evidence for positive effects can easily be questioned in terms of its scientific rigor (Whittington and Mason 1995). This modality of 'treatment' is as good as outlawed by the Mental Health Act Code of Practice (1999).

POLICY FOR THE USE OF SECLUSION

During this chapter we have seen solid evidence that the use of seclusion is for the most part a personal affair dependent on the character of wards and their team members. While it may have to be accepted that the very nature of aggression and the use of seclusion in its management will always produce variation in practice, it is inexcusable to maintain the seclusion option without an agreed policy.

Principles of a working seclusion policy

Wherever possible, seclusion should be avoided (Mental Health Act Code of Practice 1999). All other avenues must be exhausted before resorting to this final measure. Professionals faced with the prospect of having to seclude, need to be knowledgeable regarding the legal framework applicable. Furthermore, the policy should be informed by evidence offered in the literature. This necessity may present a degree of discomfort in as much that the policy will need to cater for some potentially sensitive issues, for example staff attitudes, staffing levels and perceptions of age and race.

Legal position: common law

In England and Wales according to Jones's (1999) analysis, two common law authorities are relevant. Firstly, Lord Griffiths viewed one authority as 'Imposing temporary confinement on a lunatic who has run amok and is a manifest danger either to himself or others – a state of affairs as obvious to a layman as to a doctor'. Secondly, Lord Keith outlined the authority to detain and control where someone was mentally ill and likely to harm self or others. This judgment may also extend to the use of seclusion (Jones 1999). The importance of being able to justify detention was emphasised. The common law appears to be at odds with the MHA Code of Practice as it appears to tolerate the seclusion of patient who may present a risk to themselves. This should not, however, be used to supersede the Code.

Mental Health Act 1983

Seclusion is not covered by the 1983 MHA itself, although there is comprehensive guidance in the MHA Code of Practice. The MHA provides no statutory duty to adhere to the Code of Practice (1999). However, as a statutory document, if the Code's principles are not adhered to, then this evidence could be used in legal proceedings. Anyone writing a policy for seclusion should make direct reference to the Code. We will not therefore repeat all its contents on seclusion here. The Code of Practice clearly states that seclusion should be used for the shortest period of time possible, and that it must not be used as a punishment, a treatment, because of staff shortages or because of self harm or suicide risk.

- The sole aim of seclusion is 'to contain severely disturbed behaviour which is likely to cause harm to others'.

Box 7.5 Key point

Unit policies on seclusion should actively incorporate the Code's guidelines by ensuring the safety of the secluded patient in a designated room meeting the MHA Commission's standards for seclusion. Professionals should offer care and support during and after seclusion. The difference between time out and seclusion must be emphasised clearly, the former being an agreed strategy with therapeutic aims and without a locked door.

The evidence and policy making

The published evidence sends clear messages in a number of areas that must be heard by policy makers. They include accounting for varying attitudes of staff, the need to monitor the effects of staffing levels and perceptions of age and race. In addition, accurate records of all patient behaviours and ward environmental factors that preceded seclusion must be kept and regularly reviewed. In terms of audit, the authors suggest the input of professionals divorced from the unit, for both an independent perspective and the credibility of the monitoring process.

The example policy in figure 7.1 incorporates these important issues. It begins with a philosophy statement to which all the staff must contribute and agree. There is also a list of clear statements that must be considered by the decision maker implementing seclusion. These two components aim to minimalise inconsistencies that result from personal attitudes. There are also instructions relating to procedure

The example seclusion form offered in figure 7.2 requires the decision maker to give a clear description of what actually happened and also to consider an assault rating scale of the level of aggression that actually occurred and in the opinion of the staff the level that was prevented by using seclusion. These requirements aim to prevent vague rationale being used to implement seclusion. Moreover they help the staff focus on what level of real threat they are dealing with, hopefully diminishing impulsive reactions while under stress. It is required for staff to describe what alternative interventions were attempted, again promoting emphasis on avoiding seclusion. On the seclusion form, the numbers of staff on duty, the patient's age and ethnicity are also required. This data will provide a solid basis for audit, which will need to occur at least every 6 months. In order to save space the example policy documents suggested here are not as comprehensive as they might be in reality, but they do contain most of the important issues.

Jones Ward PICU Policy for the use of seclusion

Philosophy statement

Seclusion is a serious infringement on a person's civil liberty. It should be avoided whereever possible. It can only be used as a last resort when all other interventions have been tried and failed and for the shortest possible time. Staff must be confident that they can justify the implementation of seclusion.

Seclusion may only be considered when the following conditions are met:

1. The patient is behaving in a way that is likely to injure others in the immediate future.
2. Staff have made a clinical assessment taking into account clinical and actuarial indicators that there is an immediate serious risk of harm to other people.
3. All other interventions have been considered or attempted especially verbal de-escalation including listening skills, negotiation skills aiming for a win/win situation, anger management techniques and diversional activities.
4. The decision maker has carefully considered their own stress levels and ensured that they are not adding bias to the decision to seclude.
5. Seclusion is not being used as a therapy or as a punishment.
6. Seclusion is not being used to manage self harm or suicidal behaviour.
7. Inadequate staff numbers are not influencing the decision to seclude.

Procedure for seclusion

1. Once a patient is in seclusion a designated member of staff must remain within sight and sound of the room at all times.
2. That a member of staff will make a written observation on the seclusion form (see fig 2) of what the patient is doing, at least every 15 minutes.
3. As soon as the risk of serious assault has diminished seclusion should be discontinued. This will be indicated when the patient is verbally/non verbally calm. It is not acceptable for the seclusion record to show that the patient is asleep, lying or sitting quietly on 2 consecutive entries without seclusion being discontinued.
4. Inform the duty doctor immediately that seclusion is commenced who must attend and make an entry in the health record.
5. The need for seclusion must be reviewed by:
   a) 2 nurses every 2 hours
   b) a doctor every 4 hours
   c) a multidisciplinary team including the patient's RMO and ward manager, if seclusion continues for 8 hours.
6. If the need for seclusion is disputed by any member of the team then it should immediately be referred to a senior manager for review.

Figure 7.1 – Suggested policy for the implementation of seclusion

Jones Ward PICU Seclusion Form

Reason for seclusion (terms such as aggression, disturbed in isolation are not acceptable)

_____

_____

_____

From the rating scale (Lanza and Campbell 1991) below record the level of aggression resulting from the patient's behaviour by entering the appropriate number in the boxes provided

Level actually demonstrated =   ARS Number ☐

Level that was assessed to be
likely if patient was not secluded =   ARS Number ☐

     Assaultive Rating Scale (ARS)
     1. Threat of assault but no physical contact
     2. Physical contact but no physical injury
     3. Mild soreness/surface abrasion/small bruises
     4. Major soreness/cuts/large bruises
     5. Severe lacerations/fractures/head injury
     6. Loss of limb/permanent physical injury
     7. Death

Describe the interventions attempted to avoid seclusion

Seclusion Details

Time In Seclusion ☐   Time Out ☐   Number of Staff on duty ☐

Name of person making the decision to seclude _____

Patient Name _____ Sex _____ Ethnicity _____ Age _____

Name of Staff Member observing _____

     Time   Observation

     _____   _____

     _____   _____

     _____   _____

     _____   _____

     _____   _____

Please attach any continuation sheets

Figure 7.2 – Suggested seclusion form

CONCLUSION

PICU numbers are increasing (Reed 1992, Dix 1995). In line with the Reed Committee's (1992) recommendation, most if not all local mental health services will soon have access to PICUs as part of their standard in-patient provision. By definition, the PICU will often be the facility that has responsibility for the most disturbed patients (Pereira *et al* 1999). Already many of these units house the only seclusion room in the hospital. There may be a danger of complacency amongst service managers resulting from the notion that seclusion has been hidden away in corners of PICUs, rather than in view of all patients and staff in every general adult ward. In the 40% of PICUs without seclusion rooms (Beer *et al* 1997), it is beyond question that it is possible to operate without them. We have seen throughout this chapter that seclusion continues to be an enormously complex issue. To date, the polarised positions held by many commentators have not been helpful in progressing into the new millennium with any more clarity than the last. Supporters and antagonists of seclusion often leave confusion in their wake. Much of the published analysis is undertaken from an academic foundation which often leaves unanswered questions for staff who actually face violence on a daily basis. To break from this tradition, the authors will conclude with thoughts based on first hand experience of dealing with aggression both with and without seclusion.

The commissioning in 1994 of 'Greyfriars Ward' general adult PICU in Gloucester, England marked the end of a 157-year history of seclusion in Gloucestershire's mental health services. To assist with this chapter the authors reviewed all the violent incident forms generated over the past 6 years of PICU operations. We could only find two incidents during which seclusion may have been useful compared to the interventions used. Both cases resulted in 40 minutes of difficult restraint. During a discussion with the rest of the staff team, all were agreed that, if available, seclusion may have been useful in these two situations. However, it was also unanimously accepted that if the ward had a seclusion room, it would be very likely that the actual incidence of seclusion in 6 years would have been many more than two.

While we accept that PICUs in medium- and high-secure hospitals may find increased examples of situations where it could be argued seclusion might be useful, the challenge for PICU staff may be in deciding if it is worth maintaining the use of seclusion for the management of extreme situations, the frequency of which can be as few as twice in every six years, against the cost of its negative effects. These can very easily include the seclusion of patients unnecessarily and the tendency of seclusion to stunt the growth of more creative and sophisticated methods of management.

REFERENCES

Angold A. 1989 Seclusion. Br J Psychiatry 154: 437–444

Appelbaum P. 1999 Seclusion and restraint: congress reacts to reports of abuse. Psychiatric Services, 50: 881–885

Beauchamp T, Childress J. 1994 Principles of Biomedical Ethics, 4th edn. Oxford: Oxford University Press

Beer D, Paton P, Pereira S. 1997 Hot beds of general psychiatry: a national survey of psychiatric intensive care units. Psychiatr Bull 21: 142–144

Betemps E, Buncher M. 1992 Length of time spent in seclusion and restraint by patients at 82 VA Medical Centres. Hosp Community Psychiatry 43(9): 912–916

Betemps E, Somoza E, Buncher C. 1993 Hospital characteristics and staff reasons associated with use of seclusion and restraint. Hosp Community Psychiatry April 44(4) 367–371

Blair DT. 1991 Assaultive behaviour: does provocation begin in the front office? J Psychosocial Nursing Mental Health Services, 39: 21–26

Breakwell G. 1997 Coping with Aggressive Behaviour. Leicester: BPS Books

Browne D. 1997 Black People and Sectioning, London: Little Rock

Chamberlin J. 1985 An ex-patients response to Soliday. J Nervous Mental Dis 173(5): 288–289.

Craig C, Ray F, Hix C. 1989 Seclusion and restraint: decreasing the discomfort. J Psychosocial Nursing Mental Health Services 27(7): 16–19

De Cangas J, Shopflocher D. 1989 The practice of seclusion and factors affecting its use. In Chi-Hui (Kao) Lo (eds) Proceedings of the Sigma Theta Tau International Research Congress. Advances in International Nursing Scholarship Taipei: Sigma Theta Tau, p. 83

De Cangas J. 1993 Nursing staff and unit characteristics: Do they affect the use of seclusion? Perspectives in Psychiatric Care 29

Department of Health. 1992 Report by the Committee of Inquiry into Allegations of Abuse at Ashworth Special Hospital. London: HMSO

Dix R, Williams K. 1996 Psychiatric intensive care units: a design for living. Psychiatr Bull 20: 527–529

Dix R. 1995 A nurse led psychiatric intensive care unit. Psychiatr Bull 19: 285–287

Donat D. 1998 Impact of a mandatory behavioural consultation on seclusion/restraint utilisation in a psychiatric hospital. J Behaviour Therapy Experimental Psychiatry 29: 13–19

Drinkwater J, Gudjonsson G. 1989 The nature of violence in psychiatric hospitals. In: Clinical Approaches to Violence, eds: Howells K, Hollin C Chichester: John Wiley, 287–307

Gerlock A, Solomons H. 1983 Factors associated with the seclusion of psychiatric patients. Perspectives in Psychiatric Care 21

Hammill K. 1987 Seclusion: inside looking out. Nursing Times, 4 February, 38–39

Hamolia C. 1995 Managing aggressive behaviour. In: Principles and Practice of Psychiatric Nursing 5th edn, Eds: Stuart G, Sundeen S, St Louis: Mosby, pp. 719–741

Heyman E. 1987 Seclusion. J Psychosocial Nursing Mental Health Services 25(11): 8–12

House of Representatives. 1999 10th Congress 1st Session Ma 25 (1999) HR 1313 1H, Patients Freedom from Restraint Act

Hunter R, Macalpine I. 1963 Three Hundred Years of Psychiatry 1535–1860: A History Presented in Selected English Texts. London: Oxford University Press

Hyde C, Harrower-Wilson C, Morris J. 1998 Violence, dissatisfaction and rapid tranquillisation in psychiatric intensive care. Psychiatr Bull 22: 477–480

Infantino J, Mustingo S. 1985 Assaults and injuries among staff with and without training in aggression control techniques. Hospital Community Psychiatry 36: 1312–1314

Jensen K. 1985 Comments on Dr. Stanley M. Soliday's comparison of patient and staff attitudes towards seclusion. J Nervous Mental Dis 173(5): 290–291

Jones R. 1999 Mental Health Act Manual, 6th edn. London: Sweet & Maxwell

Khan A, Cohen S, Chiles J, Stowell M, Hyde T, Robbins M, Bubble H. 1987 Therapeutic role of a psychiatric intensive care unit in acute psychosis. Comprehensive Psychiatry, 28: 264–269

Kingdon D, Bakewell E. 1988 Aggressive behaviour: evaluation of a non-seclusion policy of a district service. Br J Psychiatry 153: 631–634

Kinsella C, Brosman C. 1993 An alternative to seclusion? Nursing Times 89: 62–64

Klinge A. 1994 Staff opinions about seclusion and restraint at a State Forensic Hospital. Hospital and Community, Psychiatry 45: 138–141

Kumar A. 1997 Sudden unexplained death in a psychiatric patient – a case report: the role of the phenothiazines and physical restraint. Med Sci Law 37: 170–175.

Lanza M, Campbell R. 1991 Patient assault: a comparison of reporting measures. Quality Assurance 5: 60–68

Laposata A. 1988 Evaluation of sudden death in psychiatric patients with special reference to phenothiazine therapy: forensic pathology. J Forensic Science 33: 432–440

Lomax M 1922 The Experiences of an Asylum Doctor. London: George Allen & Unwin

Maier GJ. 1996 The role of talk down and talk up in managing threatening behaviour. J Psychosocial Nursing Mental Health Services 34(6): 25–30

Mason T. 1993 Seclusion theory reviewed: a benevolent or malevolent intervention? J Med Sci Law 33: 1–8

Mason T. 1994 Seclusion: an international comparison. J Med. Sci Law 34(1): 54–60

Mental Health Act 1983: Code of Practice 1990 London: Department of Health and Welsh Office

Merskey H 1991 Shell-shock. In: 150 Years of British Psychiatry, 1841–1991, eds: Berrios G, Freeman H. London: Gaskell, pp. 245–267

Mora G. 1967 History of psychiatry. In: Comprehensive Text Book of Psychiatry. eds: Freeman AM, Kaplan HI. Baltimore: Williams & Wilkins

Morales T. 1995 Least restrictive measures. J Psychosocial Nursing Mental Health Services 33: 42–43

Morrison P. 1990 A multi-dimensional scalogram analysis of the use of seclusion in acute psychiatric settings. J Adv Nursing 15: 59–66

Morrison P. 1995 Research in the effects of staffing levels on the use of seclusion. J Psychiatric Mental Health Nursing 2: 365–366

Morrison P, Lehane M. 1995 Staffing levels and seclusion use. J Adv Nursing 55: 1193–1202

Morrison P, Lehane M. 1996 A study of the official records of seclusion. Int J Nursing Studies 33(2): 223–235

Myers S. 1990 Seclusion: a last resort measure. Perspectives in Psychiatric Care, 26: 25–28

Nolan P. 1989 Face value. Nursing Times 85 (35): 62–65

Nolan P. 1993 A History of Mental Health Nursing. London: Chapman & Hall

Norris M, Kennedy W. 1992 The view from within: how patients perceive the seclusion process. J Psychosocial Nursing Mental Health Services 30: 7–13

Orr M, Morgan J. 1995 The medical management of violence In: Management of Violence and Aggression in Health Care, eds: Kidd B, Stark C. London: Gaskell

Outlaw FH, Lowery BJ. 1992 Seclusion: the nursing challenge. J Psycho-social Nursing Mental Health Services 30(4): 13–17

Palmstierna T, Wistedt B. 1995 Changes in the pattern of aggressive behaviour among inpatients with changed ward organisation. Acta Psychiatr Scand 91: 32–35

Parks J. 1996 Control and restraint training: a study of its effectiveness in a medium secure psychiatric unit. J Forensic Psychiatry, 7(3): 525–534

Paterson B, Leadbetter D, McComish A. 1998 Restraint and sudden death from asphyxia. Nursing Times 4: (44)

Pereira S, Beer D, Paton C. 1999 Good practice issues in psychiatric intensive care units. Psychiatr Bull 23: 397–404

Pilette PC. 1978 The tyranny of seclusion: a brief essay. J Psycho-social Nursing Mental Health Services 16 (10): 19–21

Pilowsky LS, Ring H, Shine PJ, Battersby M, Lader M. 1992 Rapid tranquillisation. A survey of emergency prescribing in a general psychiatric hospital. Br J Psychiatry 160: 831–835

Plutchik R, Karasu T, Conte H, Siegel B, Jerrett I. 1978 Toward a rationale for the seclusion process. J Nervous Mental Disease 166 (8): 571–579

Prins H 1994 Report of the Committee of Inquiry into the Death of Orville Blackwood and a Review of the Deaths of Two Other Afro-Caribbean Patients. London: Special Hospital Service Authority

Reed Committee. 1992 Review of Health and Social Services for Mentally Disordered Offenders and Others Requiring Similar Services. London: Department of Health/Social Services Office

Renvoize E. 1991 The Association of Medical Officers of Asylums and Hospitals for the Insane, the Medico-Psychological Association, and their Presidents. In: 150 Years of British Psychiatry, 1841–1991, eds: Berrios G, Freeman H. London: Gaskell

Richardson B. 1987 Psychiatric inpatients: Perceptions of the seclusion room experience. Nurs Res 36: 234–238

Rogers A, Pilgrim D 1996 Mental Health Policy in Britain: A Critical Introduction. London: Macmillan

Rosen H, DiGiacomo JN. 1978 The role of physical restraint in the treatment of mental illness. J Clin Psychiatry 39: 228–232

Shepherd M, Lavender T. 1999 Putting aggression into context: An investigation into contextual factors influencing the rate of aggressive incidents in a psychiatric hospital. J Mental Health 8(2): 159–170

Soliday SM. 1985 A comparison of patient and staff attitudes towards seclusion. J Nervous Mental Dis 173: 282–286

Soloff P, Gutheil T, Wexler J. 1985 Seclusion and restraint in 1985: A review and update. Hospital and Community Psychiatry 36: 652–657

Soloff P, Turner M. 1981 Patterns of seclusion. J Nervous Mental Dis 169: 1

Steele R. 1993 Staff attitudes toward seclusion and restraint, anything new? Perspectives in Psychiatric Care 29: (3)

Stevenson S. 1991 Heading of aggression with verbal de-escalation. J Psychosocial Nursing 29, 6–10

Swett C. 1994 Inpatient seclusion. Bull Am Acad Psychiatry Law 22(3)

Tooke S, Brown J. 1992 Perceptions of seclusion: Comparing patient and staff Reactions. J Psychosocial Nursing Mental Health Services 30: 23–26

Topping-Morris B. 1994 Seclusion: examining the nurse's role. Nursing Standard 8: 35–37

Torpy D, Hall M. 1994 Violent incidents in a secure unit. J Forensic Psychiatry 4(3): 519–544

Turnbull J, Aitken J, Black L. 1990 Turn it around: short term management of aggression and anger. J Psychosocial Nursing Mental Health Services 28: 6–12

Wells D. 1972 The use of seclusion on a university hospital floor. Arch Gen Psychiatry 26: 410–413

Whittington R, Mason T. 1995 A new look at seclusion: stress, coping and the perception of threat. J Forensic Psychiatry 6(2): 285–304

8

THE USE OF RESTRAINT

Mark Polczyk-Przybyla, Tom Morahan

INTRODUCTION

This chapter discusses the use of restraint in PICUs and aims to give the reader an overview of the development of current practice. The practice of physically restraining a patient in the context of psychiatric care may be accomplished in a variety of ways, using a range of methods. Therefore to be clear about the interventions that will be discussed the following definitions should be understood.

- Mechanical restraint: the use of inanimate devices to restrict the movement of an individual, e.g. body belts, hand cuffs etc.

- Manual restraint: physical contact between the individual being restrained and those providing the restraint designed to restrict the movement of the individual.

In this chapter we will be concentrating exclusively on manual restraint, as we do not advocate the use of mechanical methods under any circumstances when treating people in a PICU. The use of mechanical restraint is not sanctioned in any UK psychiatric setting. In some states of the USA and in other countries mechanical restraint can be practised. The use of seclusion (which may be seen as a form of restraint) is covered elsewhere (chapter 7).

Some of the use of sedative medications is also discussed elsewhere (Chapter 5) and so will not be mentioned here except to say that the use of manual restraint is often the precursor to the administration of such preparations.

HISTORICAL PERSPECTIVE

The first records of what might be termed as hospital provision for the mentally ill appear in the foundation deeds of Holy Trinity Hospital, Salisbury, in the 14th century. The deed states that beds will be provided where 'the sick are comforted, the dead are buried and the mad are kept safe until restored to reason . . .'. This would seem to identify madness as distinct from demonic possession and a condition best dealt with in a hospital environment.

Care in the community was also a method of dealing with the insane at this time, with the parish having a facility to provide funds so a relative of the unfortunate individual could stop work and provide supervision (? attendance allowance). It was also legal, according to manuals published for the guidance of justices, to use restraint in this community setting. An edition published in 1581 states that 'Every man may take his kinsman that is mad, and may put him in a house, and bind him and beat him with rods, without breach of the peace' (Allderidge 1979).

Throughout the 15th and 16th centuries the policy of confinement persisted although the mentally ill were treated alongside criminals and the poor. Workhouses and other such correctional facilities were considered to be appropriate repositories for the insane. The Vagrancy Act of 1744 empowered justices to order 'the confinement of persons of little or no estates who by lunacy or otherwise are furiously mad and dangerous to be permitted to go abroad, and to order that they be kept under lock and key and chained if necessary until cured'. This situation continued during the early 18th century until the mentally ill were confined in separate institutions from the criminal and other undesirables, the main reason for this apparently being the fear of contagion according to Foucault (1975).

The 18th century also saw the first moves towards what we now consider to be the humane treatment of the mentally ill. Through reformers such as Pinel in Paris and the Tuke family in England the philosophy of non-restraint evolved. This saw the advent of moral treatment in the York Retreat, which was founded in 1792 by the Tuke family. This small Quaker hospital had the philosophy that the mentally ill could be taught self restraint by kind example in an atmosphere modelled on the family with the patients in the role of errant children.

John Connolly tested the efficacy of this policy of non-restraint on a large scale in the Hanwell asylum in 1839 and found that it produced an improvement in the behaviour of the patients and as a result advocated the total abolition of mechanical restraint. Violent and dangerous patients were dealt with through a combination of manual restraint and seclusion. Solitary confinement cells were converted to padded seclusion rooms and emergency treatment units were used to deal with disruptive behaviour, the forerunners to today's PICUs (Soloff 1984).

So we arrive at the main method of managing violent and dangerous behaviour exhibited by acutely disturbed individuals today. Psychotropic medication, developed in the late 1950s, has played a significant role in reducing the incidence and duration of such acutely disturbed episodes but therein lies one of the most common uses of manual restraint, the forcible administration of parenteral medication. If this was not the initial aim of manually restraining an individual it is often the result.

INDICATIONS, CONTRAINDICATIONS AND ETHICS

In attempting to produce guidelines for the use of restraint in the modern PICU one soon realises that this is a complex issue beset with ethical and legal considerations. The act of laying hands on another without their consent is in some circumstances assault and is viewed as an infringement of civil liberties. The question is: under which circumstances, if any, is such an action acceptable or justifiable?

This question has been addressed by a number of authors (Stilling 1992, Tarbuck 1992, Hopton 1995) not only from the situational point of view but also examining the appropriateness of the various techniques or systems currently available. The consensus appears to be that manual restraint is justified in the following situations:

- To prevent imminent harm to the patient or others when all other options have proved ineffective.

- To allow the administration of compulsory treatment when clinically justified and legally sanctioned (derived from Hopton 1995).

In addition Guthiel and Tardiff (1984) also advocate the use of restraint and seclusion as a part of behavioural treatment or as contingent responses to certain behaviours. This is a controversial area as it opens the debate about aversive behavioural techniques and the effectiveness of negative reinforcers. An informal patient may be restrained as part of such a programme if they give their consent; however, if consent is to be valid it must be given freely and the patient must be able to withdraw it at any time. This would call the effectiveness of the programme into question as the patient is very likely to withdraw consent immediately after behaviour that prompts restraint. If agreement to this type of programme is a condition of admission, the validity of consent under these circumstances must be questioned (Crichton 1995). It is also under such circumstances that any physical restraint or seclusion may be experienced as purely punitive and therefore is ineffective in the long-term modification of behaviour.

Looking at the above it is clear that the majority of occasions when manual restraint is used will be in emergency situations, i.e. as a reaction to a potentially dangerous and acute incident. In this case it is the clinicians that are present at the time who will have to decide whether physical intervention is justified and necessary. This decision will be based on their knowledge of the individuals involved and an assessment of the level of risk the situation represents to those in the vicinity. As a general rule the decision will be made according to an assessment of the possible benefits the patient may gain balanced against the risks inherent in the procedure. Knowledge of any medical conditions or injuries that the patient has is essential in making this assessment as this may increase the risk of serious harm to the patient.

When restraint is used to administer medication as part of ongoing treatment, considerations such as the time and place in which the confrontation will occur and the number and mix of staff become more important. It is also vital that staff assess the potential risk to themselves as the act of manually restraining distressed and disturbed individuals is dangerous in itself. A study of assaults on staff in a psychiatric hospital found that 71% of injuries sustained by nursing staff were received in the act of restraining patients either in an attempt to seclude them or when trying to break up altercations between patients (Lion et al 1981).

According to Gillon (1986) the use of such intervention is ethically justified if the force used to carry out the restraint is less injurious to all than the behaviour it is meant to stop would be if allowed to go on. The issue of damage to property clouds the situation as the risk to others is harder to assess than in the case of a direct assault or a patient's deliberate attempts to harm him/herself.

The re-taking of absconding patients is another situation in which manual restraint may be indicated. However, just who and under what circumstances an individual may use force to detain or control another is not completely clear. The Criminal Law Act 1967 states that: 'A person may use such force that is reasonable in the circumstances, in the prevention of crime, or in effecting or assisting the lawful arrest of offenders or suspected offenders, or persons unlawfully at large' (Jones 1996 p. 38).

This part of the criminal law act gives hospital staff the authority to use 'reasonable force' to prevent a patient from committing some crime. It would also enable them to use manual restraint to return an absconded patient to lawful custody. This does not apply, however, if the patient is insane according to the McNaughton rules. In essence the McNaughton rules state that if a patient is deluded to the extent that they had no idea that what they were doing or were about to do was in any way wrong then no crime can be committed. In this situation Section 18 MHA (1983) provides the necessary powers. This section of the Mental Health Act details the circumstances in which a patient may be detained 'and returned to the hospital' by 'any approved social worker, by any officer on the staff of the hospital, by any constable, or by any person authorized in writing by the hospital managers'.

So, should a patient abscond or fail to return to hospital following leave under Section 17 MHA (1983) and provided that they are liable to detention under the Mental Health Act (1983), or if they are committing or suspected of committing an offence, anybody who works for the hospital or has written permission from the managers may use manual restraint to return them to that hospital. The time limits within which this may be done vary according to what section of the act the patient is liable to detention under; a detailed explanation of these limits can be found in Jones (1996).

Given these powers, any act of physical restraint, especially in a public place, needs serious consideration. As we have seen, restraining people in the relatively controlled environment is beset with dangers. These potential problems are magnified when outside the hospital grounds, as the reaction of members of the general public is not always predictable.

Another word of caution, these powers do not under any circumstances allow the forced entry into any premises in which the patient may be staying; only the police have this power under Section 135 MHA (1983).

Thus the manual restraint of an individual is a risky business; minor injuries to both the patient and staff are common. Therefore it is an intervention to be used only as a last resort when all other approaches have failed. The Joy Gardener case emphasises the seriousness of the risk. Joy Gardener was to be deported but died whilst being restrained by police officers trained in methods of restraining resistive individuals (Campaign against Racism and Fascism 1993). There have also been cases in hospital that have prompted examination of techniques used to restrain disturbed patients (Ritchie 1985) and the report of the Committee of Inquiry into Ashworth Hospital emphasises the need for nursing staff to attend 'Intensive courses in preventing violence' (Blom-Cooper 1992).

One thing that all of the literature is in agreement on is the need for a coherent approach or system that is known and used consistently by all staff. The recognition that an organized approach to restraint is necessary is no recent revelation. As long ago as 1794 Philippe Pinel wrote:

> If a madman suddenly experiences an unexpected attack and arms himself . . ., the director – always mindful of his maxim to control the insane without ever permitting that they be hurt – would present himself in the most determined and threatening manner but without carrying any kind of weapon. . . . At the same time the servants converge on him at a given signal, from behind or sideways, each seizing one of the madman's limbs. . . . Thus they carry him to his cell. . . . The employees are expressly forbidden to retaliate even if they are hit. (Fisher 1994)

Although the director's 'determined and threatening manner' may these days be seen as unlikely to encourage a non-violent outcome, the main point is that staff should adopt a co-ordinated method aimed at controlling the situation and causing no injury to the patient.

Training in the management of potentially and actually violent situations minimises the potential for injury to both staff and patients. There is evidence that the training alone plays a part in making the need to implement it less likely (Phillips and Rudestam 1995). It is possible that this is due either to an increased level of confidence in the staff dealing with a volatile situation or to elements of the training focused on 'talk down' techniques, or a mixture of the two. Either way the need for consistent training of all staff who may find themselves in such situations is reinforced.

In some areas a particular method of restraint is taught as a matter of policy and is therefore compulsory for all staff; others have a less rigid approach. The next part of this chapter will examine the systems that are currently in use and give an overview of their origin, basic principles and course structure. This is NOT a training manual. The intention is to give the reader a brief and objective critique of the methods and training that will at least promote an awareness of alternatives and at most aid in the choice of which system, if any, to pursue further. It is not the intention of the authors to advocate any one system above the others.

CONTROL AND RESTRAINT (C&R)

Origins

Control and restraint or C&R was developed in the 1970s as a method for restraining inmates in British penal establishments. This was a result of increased media attention and the inmates' growing awareness of their rights and entitlements. It therefore became necessary for the Prison Service to be seen to be acting in a professional and safe manner, using techniques that were legally sanctioned. The system also had to be consistent with Prison Rule 44(1) which states: 'An Officer in dealing with a prisoner should not use force unnecessarily and, when the application of force to a prisoner is necessary, no more force than is necessary shall be used'.

A further circular instruction explains: 'The use of force when it is not necessary, or the use of more force than is necessary to achieve the objective is both a criminal offence and a civil wrong'.

With this in mind the physical education branch of the Prison Service was tasked with devising a system that allowed the safe restraint and relocation of troublesome inmates (Brookes 1988).

A modified form of C&R found its way into the health service via the Special Hospital (High Secure) service (Ashworth, Broadmoor and Rampton Hospitals). Traditionally in these establishments staff were members of the POA (Prison Officers Association) and therefore had close connections with the prison service. Thus the migration of C&R to the high security hospitals was a natural step.

The advent of the building programme of Regional or Medium Secure Units (RSUs or MSUs) (Snowden 1985) meant that C&R spread outside high security establishments and found its way into general psychiatric hospitals as MSUs were initially either interim units converted from existing wards or purpose built units in the grounds of large psychiatric hospitals. From here it was but a small step to PICUs and then to general psychiatric services. At present C&R is taught and used in all types of adult psychiatric settings.

Basic principles

The C&R system relies on various holds or locks to immobilise the individual being restrained. The main type of hold is a variation on the theme of wrist locks. Central to the practice of C&R is the three person team; the minimum number of people that can safely carry out a restraint is three. Ideally five people are needed: the three person team, a leg person and a controller or coordinator. As with all of these methods it is stressed that the actual restraint of an individual is only to be attempted when all other less invasive techniques have been exhausted or when a potentially dangerous situation requires immediate intervention. Once this point has been reached the three person team approaches the patient in a wedge formation. The person at the apex of the wedge is designated 'No. 1' and is the only person to communicate with the patient. As the team approaches, 'No. 1' maintains the dialogue with the patient and continues to attempt to persuade him/her to stop the behaviour that is causing concern or to comply with the requests made by staff. If the required co-operation is not forthcoming, at a prearranged signal 'No. 1' takes hold of the patient's head and 'Nos 2

& 3' the arms and the patient is taken to the floor in a controlled manner. Once this has been achieved Nos 2 & 3 apply wrist locks. It is No. 1's role to protect the patient's head, maintain communication and ensure that the patient's airway remains clear. Incidentally the practice of referring to members of the team by number rather than name is as a result of C&R's origin in the Prison Service. The need to maintain the anonymity of the people restraining an individual is very serious because of possible reprisals from the individual or his associates. This does not apply to the same extent in hospital where it is likely that the patient will know the staff well and recognise them immediately.

The wrist locks are a controversial element in this system as, although the risk of injury to the wrist is minimal, with slight pressure it is possible to inflict considerable pain on the patient. These pain 'sanctions' are taught as part of the course as a method of encouraging the patient to co-operate with the requests made by No. 1 and to discourage protracted struggling by the patient. It is emphasised that the pressure on the locks that causes the pain is rarely necessary and should only be used when all attempts to gain the patient's compliance through verbal means have been exhausted; in effect it is a last resort in a last resort.

From this position on the floor the C&R system covers various procedures such as:

- Removal of clothing (if required for safety reasons).

- Relocation, e.g. to seclusion room.

- Climbing and descending stairs.

- Changing personnel in the event of fatigue or injury.

Breakaway techniques are covered by this system, as attempts at single-handed restraint are likely to result in injury to staff or patient or both. Breakaways are techniques that enable a member of staff to get free if grabbed by a patient; this covers holds from all angles on hair, clothing or other parts of the body.

A sample control and restraint policy can be found on p. 334.

Course structure

The C&R course is full time for five days, the first of which covers methods of de-escalation and verbal interventions aimed at avoiding the use of manual restraint. The remainder takes the students through the basic components of each technique and systematically builds on them. Each new item is introduced and demonstrated by the instructors, then practised by the students. This process of gradual addition of new material continues so that by the second half of the course the students are working in three person teams role-playing various scenarios.

The members of the group work with each other so that by the end of the course each student will not only be able to use C&R but will also be well acquainted with the experience of being restrained.

SCIP

Origins

The acronym SCIP stands for Strategies for Crisis Intervention and Prevention. This approach to physical restraint was developed in New York State and was imported to the UK in 1988. The first establishment to make use of the SCIP programme was the Loddon Unit in Basingstoke which caters for young people with learning disabilities. An important factor in the development of SCIP was the perception that with some of the other forms of physical restraint in use there were ethical issues especially in relation to causing physical pain to the person being restrained. There was also an idea that some of the existing techniques were open to abuse and therefore a safer method should be developed. The system's main objectives and techniques were adapted for adult psychiatry and a course developed in 1992 and since then a number of educational establishments and health service trusts have adopted the system and provide training. The system is also taught for use in other areas such as learning disabilities, schools, and facilities dealing with behavioural problems (Bond 1996).

Basic principles

SCIP's primary aim is the prevention of the crisis by the adjustment of the environment so that it discourages dangerous or aggressive behaviour. It also advocates the use of early intervention to prevent situations escalating to the point where physical restraint is necessary. The emphasis according to the programme is reassurance rather than control and all contact with the person causing concern is aimed at calming the situation without the need for physical intervention. If physical contact is deemed to be necessary the approach is graded in that the physical presence and amount of force are the minimum required to bring the situation back to one that is safe for all concerned. Any physical contact is terminated as soon as the patient is calm.

All of the holds that form the SCIP system focus on the long bones rather than joints and are therefore intended to be pain-free. The person being restrained should never be held face down so that they are always aware of what the restrainers are doing. This is intended to minimise the level of panic that the patient experiences and to maintain dignity. The holds are designed for one to four people depending on the level of control required, hence the gradient response. The first principle is always to attempt to gain the co-operation of the patient before applying more force.

Course structure

The SCIP course is full time for 5 days. The first day covers a number of theoretical topics such as the SCIP philosophy, statistics relevant to aggressive incidents, and precipitating factors for violence. This is followed by a demonstration of SCIP techniques. The remainder of the course is split between theoretical topics and the introduction and practice of the various physical techniques and methods that are used when restraining an individual. Table 8.1 shows the theoretical topics that are covered during the course.

In addition to the course work the students are asked to keep a reflective diary about their experiences and feelings whilst on the course, the salient points of which are discussed on day 5 as part of the overall discussion and evaluation of the course.

The instructors on these courses must attend an annual update session that is run by Master trainers from the UK and the USA. The instructor's certificates are reviewed every 2 years by Master trainers and all instructors must hold an up-to-date first aid certificate.

Table 8.1 – Topics covered by the SCIP course (Bond 1996)

Day	Topics covered
1	Individual aims and objectives Philosophy of SCIP Aggression, the statistics Why be violent? Precipitating factors What makes me angry?
2	Recognising aggression, the likely signs The environment Assessment of dangerousness Massage and aromatherapy
3	Communications Labelling Staff support and incident review
4	Assessment, action planning and management strategies
5	Discussion on the application of SCIP in various work settings

CONCLUSION

It is clear from the literature that an organised and standard approach to physical restraint is necessary both to increase the staff's confidence in managing potentially dangerous situations and in preventing injury to all concerned during the act of restraint.

The effectiveness of training in these techniques has been shown to reduce the incidence of violent situations and also reduce the likelihood of injury to both patient and staff. In their comparison of assaults and assault-related injuries between staff trained in aggression control techniques and untrained staff, Infantino and Musingo (1985) found significant benefits from training. The untrained group (n = 65) suffered 24 assaults of which 19 caused injury compared with only one assault on a member of the trained group (n = 31) that did not result in injury. In another study of the effectiveness of C&R, the authors found that, despite an increase in the number of staff injuries in the initial restraint phase, due mainly they felt to the practice of approaching the patient from the front, staff still had greater confidence in dealing with situations and found relocation and intervention easier (Parkes 1996).

The physical environment is also of vital importance although the potential for change may be limited.

Physical restraint should always be used as a last resort and training in non-physical methods of calming and managing potentially violent or destructive behaviours is vital for ALL staff who are likely to have contact with patients.

The two systems described above are the most used in the UK at present and although they have different origins and principles their aim is the same, to maintain safety in what is potentially an extremely hazardous area for all.

Any form of physical restraint is open to abuse by those practising it and having a standard system goes some way to minimising its likelihood. But in the final analysis it is the vigilance of all practitioners especially managers, and the training and retraining of staff, that will be most effective.

As stated at the beginning of the chapter, the authors do not advocate any one of the systems described above or others that may be in use above the rest, but we firmly believe that training in one of them is essential.

REFERENCES

Allderidge P. 1979 Hospitals, madhouses and asylums: cycles in the care of the insane. Br J Psych 134: 321–334

Blom-Cooper. 1992 Report of the Committee of Enquiry into Ashworth Hospital. London: HMSO

Bond K. 1996 Strategies for crisis intervention and prevention. Validation Document University of Hertfordshire

Brookes M. 1988 Control and Restraint Techniques: A Study into its Effectiveness at HMP Gartree. London: Home Office, Prison Department

Campaign Against Racism and Fascism. 1993 Defying the Repatriation Plan. London: CARF

Crichton J. 1995 Psychiatric inpatient violence: issues in English law and discipline within hospitals. Med Sci Law 35(1): 53–55

Fisher WA. 1994 Restraint and seclusion: A review of the literature. Am J Psychiat 151 (11): 1584–1591

Foucault M. 1975 Madness and Civilization: A History of Insanity in the Age of Reason. New York: Vintage Books

Gillon R. 1986 Philosophical Medical Ethics. London: John Wiley

Guthiel TG, Tardiff K. 1984 Indications and contraindications for seclusion and restraint. In: Tardiff K. (ed.) The Psychiatric Uses of Seclusion and Restraint Washington: American Psychiatric Press

Hopton J. 1995 Control and restraint in contemporary psychiatric nursing: some ethical considerations. J Adv Nursing 22: 110–115

Infantino J, Musingo S. 1985 Assaults and injuries amongst staff with and without training in aggression control techniques. Hosp Comm Psychiat 35(12): 1312–1314

Jones R. 1996 Mental Health Act Manual, 5th edn. London: Sweet & Maxwell

Lion JR, Snyder W, Merrill GL. 1981 Under reporting of assaults in a state hospital. Hosp Comm Psychiat 32: 497–498

Parkes J. 1996 Control and restraint training: A study of its effectiveness in a medium secure unit. J Forensic Psychiat 7(3): 525–534

Phillips D, Rudestam KE. 1995 Effect of nonviolent self-defense training on male psychiatric staff members' aggression and fear. Psychiatric Services 46(2): 164–168

Ritchie S. 1985 Report to the Secretary of State for Social Services Concerning the Death of Mr. Michael Martin. London: SHSA

Snowden P. 1985 A survey of the Regional Secure Unit Programme. Br J Psych 147: 499–507

Soloff PH. 1984 Historical notes on Seclusion and Restraint. In: Tardiff K (ed.) The Psychiatric Uses of Seclusion and Restraint. Washington: American Psychiatric Press

Stilling L. 1992 The pros and cons of physical restraints and behaviour controls. J Psychosocial Nursing 30 (3): 18–20

Tarbuck P. 1992 The use and abuse of control and restraint. Nursing Standard (6:) 52 30–2

9

THE COMPLEX NEEDS PATIENT

Zerrin Atakan

INTRODUCTION

In this chapter, we will deal with the kind of patient who has complex needs. More and more, especially in the inner city areas, mental health workers are encountering patients who not only suffer from a severe mental illness, but also have a number of additional problems, which further complicate their treatment and management. Very often, the treatment of the mental illness alone is not sufficient and the availability of resources catered specifically to their needs is scarce or non-existent.

Frequently, such patients are found at the psychiatric intensive care or acute in-patient units due to their disturbed behaviour. Their management, unless attention is paid to meet their specific needs, can be problematic and incomplete and the well-known 'revolving door' phenomenon is very likely to occur. At the intensive care units, patients with complex needs are often those who cannot be transferred out or discharged within four to eight weeks as their symptoms are resistant to treatment. They display frequent verbal or physical violence and find ingenious methods of abusing drugs, even in very carefully controlled ward environments.

Complex needs patients in PICUs:

- Symptoms resistant to treatment

- Frequent violent episodes

- Substance misuse

- Cannot be transferred/discharged in under 4 to 8 weeks

Box 9.1

We will attempt to define what the complex needs patient means and examine the most frequently seen categories of severe mental illness and additional problems with reference to their possible aetiological factors. Finally, we will examine how such patients can be treated and managed.

DEFINITION OF 'COMPLEX NEEDS PATIENT'

Over recent decades, with the development of Community Care philosophy and policies, the recognition of a 'new' group of mentally ill patients has emerged; the 'new long stay patient'. Other terms followed such as; 'young chronics', 'hard to treat', 'hard to place', 'treatment resistant', 'dual diagnosis' and 'challenging behaviour'. Most of these terms have overlapping meanings and are, to some extent, interchangeable.

Other terms used to describe complex needs patients:

- New long-stay patient
- Treatment resistant
- Young chronics
- Dual diagnosis
- Hard to treat
- Challenging behaviour

Box 9.2

Here we suggest the use of the term 'complex needs patient' to emphasise a needs based approach to their management and to steer away from negative and pessimistic terminology. The complex needs patient suffers from a severe mental illness, mainly in the form of schizophrenia or bipolar disorder, and in addition, has one or more additional problems such as another mental illness, substance abuse, medical problems, homelessness, history of abuse or lack of social support. More often than not, the same patient has a number of these problems at once as one problem tends to lead to another.

Characteristics of complex needs patients:

Severe mental illness *plus* one or more of the following:

- Another mental health problem
- Medical problems
- Substance abuse
- Homelessness
- Mild learning difficulty
- Lack of social support
- History of abuse
- Problems related to ethnicity

Box 9.3

BACKGROUND AND CHARACTERISTICS OF THE COMPLEX NEEDS PATIENT

Mann and Cree (1976) first developed the 'new long stay patient' concept. They defined this group as patients who had been in hospital continuously for more than one, but less than 5 years. Their national survey revealed this group to have multiple disabilities and problems. This group, apart from being resistant to treatment, were socially isolated, unskilled, had little family support and suffered from poor physical health. In addition, they presented with behavioural problems such as violence towards others, self-harm and extreme anti-social behaviour. Of these patients, 60% suffered from a psychotic disorder and 40% of these had been diagnosed as suffering from schizophrenia.

Characteristics of 'new long stay' patient*

- Psychotic illness
- Treatment resistant
- Poor physical health
- In hospital for more than 1, less than 5 years

- Behavioural problems
- Socially isolated
- Unskilled

Box 9.4

* Mann and Cree (1976)

A similar national audit carried out in the UK in more recent times (Lelliott *et al* 1994), examined a group of patients who had been in hospital continuously for more than 6 months but less than 3 years. This revealed similar findings to those found by Mann and Cree. Compared with earlier findings, the new long stay patients of the nineties were more likely to have more pronounced positive symptoms, exhibit more violence and abuse substances. In addition, they were more likely to be detained under the Mental Health Act.

Characteristics of 'new long stay' patient*

(in addition to Mann and Cree's findings):

- More positive symptoms
- Substance abuse
- In hospital for more than 6 months, but less than 3 years

- More violence
- Detained under the Mental Health Act

Box 9.5

* Lelliott *et al* (1994)

The terminology of 'treatment resistance', although more often conveying difficulties in response to medication, when studied closely, may reveal similar characteristics to the term 'new long stay'. Kane (1996) describes four main factors that can make patients difficult to treat: refractoriness to treatment, as the first factor, appears to have changed over time. In the 1960s about 70% of patients got better with antipsychotic treatments, whereas in the 1990s only about 50% of patients respond to conventional treatments. Kane lists other factors as:

- problems of adverse side-effects;
- non-compliance with treatment (as approximately 30% of patients become non-compliant within 1 year); and
- the problem of co-morbid conditions.

Anti-social and violent behaviours can also make patients difficult to treat. When we examine a typical non-compliant patient, very often we see that he does not perceive benefits in taking medication, has little or no daily supervision to ensure his medication intake, experiences side-effects, has little or no awareness of his illness and his symptoms make him suspicious, grandiose and anxious. These characteristics, coupled with substance abuse, further complicate the issue. Psychoactive substances can impair perception and interfere with judgement. Some drugs, especially alcohol, may act as chemical disinhibitors of aggressive impulses (Collins and Schlenger 1988). Behavioural disturbances and violence are further characteristics of the complex needs patient.

Factors leading to treatment resistance*

- Adverse side-effects
- Violence

- Non-compliance
- Co-morbidity

- Refractoriness to treatment (worse in 1990s compared with 1960s)

Box 9.6

* Kane (1996)

It is frequently observed that substances combined with a psychotic state can increase the risk of a patient wanting to act on his delusions and display violence. It is known that persons experiencing especially persecutory type delusions tend to act on them (Wessely *et al* 1993). Symptoms such as hostility, paranoid ideation and substance abuse are the most significant short-term predictors of violent behaviour. Link and Stueve (1994) studied the principle of 'rationality within irrationality' when the mentally ill patient feels threatened due to persecutory ideas and his internal control mechanisms are compromised. They argue that in these circumstances violence is more likely to occur. According to a detailed study they carried out they have found that symptoms such as; 'mind dominated by forces beyond your control', 'thoughts put into your head that were not your own' and 'that there were people who wished to do you harm', were significantly correlated with acts of violence.

It would be useful to examine some commonly seen subtypes of complex needs patients in more detail. These subtypes are categorised for purposes of examining each in more detail.

As mentioned previously, in reality a patient will have more than two problems and the nature of these problems are such that one problem can easily lead to another. For instance, a patient with a history of sexual abuse develops severe mental illness and with the loss of daily living skills, lacks social support and becomes homeless. He starts abusing substances to relieve his anxiety, and entering the subculture of the drug-dealing world, he develops serious physical problems and begins offending.

Severe mental illness and another mental health problem

Severe mental illness can lead to various disabilities, rendering the person suffering from it unable to function fully in society. Negative symptoms alone contribute enormously to psychosocial disability. As a result, the person can develop further mental health problems such as depression, anxiety, and hypochondriacal and obsessive symptomatology. With reduced self-esteem and hope, it is not uncommon for a patient to become suicidal, make repeated suicidal gestures or become involved in self-destructive behaviour.

Another commonly seen diagnostic category, especially found at the psychiatric intensive care units, is personality disorders. Antisocial, borderline and histrionic personality disorders or traits are among the most frequently encountered. In a study investigating the relationship between psychopathy and violence among patients with schizophrenia, it was found that co-morbidity of schizophrenia and psychopathy was higher in patients who displayed violence, compared with those who did not (Nolan et al 1999).

Patients with co-morbid borderline or antisocial personalities, by their tendency to violent acting out, poor impulse control, general insensitivity to others' feelings and demand for immediate satisfaction of their needs, may cause severe management problems within their environments. In certain instances, this may even lead to divisions among staff. Very often this may be at the expense of their severe mental illness where staff, overwhelmed by the negative feelings emanated by the patient, may review their beliefs about the sincerity of the patient's underlying psychosis.

Severe mental illness and substance abuse (dual diagnosis)

Although substance abuse is a type of mental health disorder, it constitutes a significant problem, which deserves to be examined under a separate heading. 'Dual' or 'double diagnosis' terms most often refer to this category and the number of such patients appear to be on the increase, despite the relative lack of services specifically tailored to their needs.

Over 90% of patients with schizophrenia are known to be using nicotine (Gritz et al 1985). About 50% of them are known to be abusing alcohol and/or illegal drugs ranging from cannabis to cocaine (Ziedonis et al 1994). According to one of the Epidemiological Catchment Area studies, 47% of patients with schizophrenia had a lifetime diagnosis of substance abuse (Pristach 1990). Although most of the studies on dual diagnosis originate from the USA, prevalence of substance abuse amongst the severely mentally ill is also known to be high in the UK. Young, male patients particularly appear to carry a higher risk and spend twice as many days in hospital as those without such problems (Menezes et al 1996). However, in practice it is believed that most patients with severe mental illness go undetected due to lack of regular drug or alcohol screening.

Patients with schizophrenia who abuse substances are also known to have worse outcomes compared to those who do not. This is shown to be true not only for patients with chronic conditions but also for those who are at the early stages of their illness (Kovasznay *et al* 1997). Interestingly, the outcome is not influenced by a lifetime use of substances in patients with affective disorder in the same longitudinal study carried out by Kovasznay *et al* (1997).

Such high rates of substance abuse amongst the severely mentally ill have many implications, ranging from genetic vulnerability to be a substance abuser, to 'normalising' the effects of negative symptoms and the side-effects of antipsychotic medication to psychosocial effects such as poor social status, involvement with criminal behaviour and exposure to chronic serious life events.

There are several hypotheses looking at the relationship between substance abuse and schizophrenia (rather than 'severe mental illness' as most research has been carried out with this diagnostic category):

- Causation model: states that substances cause or precipitate schizophrenia, especially in those individuals who are predisposed genetically or are vulnerable for environmental reasons.

- Self-medication model: suggests that patients take substances in order to counteract the effects of their antipsychotic medication, anxiety symptoms or negative symptoms of schizophrenia.

- Coincidental association model: the co-morbidity of schizophrenia and substance abuse is coincidental. Both disorders have similar age onset (late teens and early twenties) and male gender. However, if this model were true, one would expect similar substance abuse prevalence rates among patients with schizophrenia and in the general population of the same age and sex.

Suggested causal models between schizophrenia and substance abuse:*

- Substances cause or precipitate schizophrenia (Causal model)

- Substances are used to self-medicate (Self-medication model)

- Co-morbidity is coincidental (Coincidental association model)

Box 9.7

* Hambrecht and Häfner (1996)

Hambrecht and Häfner (1996) carried out a study of a representative first-episode sample of 232 schizophrenic patients and found that alcohol abuse, prior to first admission, was in 24% of the sample group, and drug abuse in 14%, which is twice the rates in the general population. They also revealed that in their group, alcohol abuse more often followed rather than preceded the first symptom of schizophrenia. On the other hand, drug abuse preceded the first symptom in 27.5%, followed it in about 40% and emerged within the same month in 34.6% of the cases. In other words, roughly 3 out of 10 co-morbid patients abused alcohol or illicit drugs before the first signs of schizophrenia emerged, and the rest started abusing around and after the onset. This study shows a remarkable association between substance abuse and first-onset schizophrenia. A similar study carried out in the UK confirms high rates of substance abuse at onset of psychosis, especially with young male patients carrying a higher risk of substance abuse compared to females (Cantwell *et al* 1999).

Although the association between substance abuse and first-onset schizophrenia appears to be clear, what is not yet so clear is which starts first. In another study where the severity of current substance abuse and onset of psychotic illness was examined, it was found that in almost all the cases categorised as moderate–severe substance abuse, the substance diagnosis predated the onset of psychosis (Rabinowitz *et al* 1998).

The association between criminal activity and substance abuse is well known. There also appears to be a relationship between schizophrenia and criminal activity. In the carefully controlled Camberwell study of crime and schizophrenia, the association between first-onset schizophrenia and convictions for violent and serious assaults were twice the amount in schizophrenic patients compared with the control group (Wessely *et al* 1994). In the same study, there was a small number of young African-Caribbean males with very long histories of both hospital admissions and criminal convictions. The reason why a particular group has such high rates is very complex and as Wessely later (1997) suggests, probably involves looking at the earlier age of onset, differential police response, social deprivation and drug abuse.

The question, therefore, would be: does the possibility of criminal behaviour increase further when a patient who suffers from schizophrenia also abuses substances? Using data from 3 sites of the National Institute of Mental Health (NIMH) Epidemiologic Catchment Area (ECA) surveys, Swanson *et al* (1996) found that after controlling for socio-demographic covariates, schizophrenia and major affective disorders were found to be associated with approximately fourfold increase in the odds of violence in one year (odds ratio = 3: 9) compared with normal controls. Furthermore, when substance abuse co-morbidity was the case, there was an even greater increase, approximately 17 times (odds ratio = 16.8) in the odds of violent behaviour.

To study the symptom profile of chronic patients with schizophrenia may also reveal information on the relationship between substance abuse and schizophrenia. There appears to be some evidence that it is especially patients who have predominantly positive and more affective symptomatology and display serious behavioural problems who also abuse substances. However, it is difficult to derive a causative association in between, without proper prospective studies.

It has been suggested that there is a shared genetic predisposition to alcoholism and schizophrenia (Kendler 1985). However, there needs to be further genetic linkage research to confirm such a link. The genetic links between substance abuse and schizophrenia are not known. However, there has been a long-established genetic link between manic-depressive illness and alcoholism. In a recent study, which examined this link, it was found that patients with bipolar illness not only had higher rates of abusing alcohol, but they also abused especially stimulant type drugs, compared to primary unipolar and control groups (Winokur *et al* 1998).

There is some data suggesting that anti-psychotic medications enhance the positive euphoric effects of certain substances, especially stimulants such as cocaine, whilst reducing paranoia-inducing aspects (Sherer *et al* 1989). In addition, anecdotal claims made by patients imply that cannabis and cocaine provide relief from negative symptoms of schizophrenia, anxiety and the side-effects of antipsychotic medication (Serper *et al* 1995).

Medication non-compliance appears to be significantly associated with substance abuse (Owen *et al* 1996). The reasons why a dual diagnosis patient may be poorly compliant with his medication can be varied. Very often he is advised not to combine his medication with substances. In addition, substance intoxication is very likely to affect his judgement and cause him to neglect to take medication. Thirdly, substances, by accentuating the side-effects of medications, contribute further to medication non-compliance.

Reasons for poor compliance among dual diagnosis patients:

* Following advice not to combine medication with substances

* Substance intoxication leading to neglect to take medication

* Substances accentuate the side-effects of medications

Box 9.8

It is important to find out which substance is being 'favoured' by the patient, although generally, it is known that most abusers take a number of drugs to 'regulate' their mood. Patients with schizophrenia are known to favour stimulants such as cocaine, amphetamine, caffeine, cannabis and alcohol. Cannabis is the most widely used substance around the world and some patients in certain areas may only be abusing cannabis. There is some evidence that cannabis can 'cause' or 'precipitate' a psychotic clinical picture or exacerbate symptoms in those who are predisposed to developing a psychotic illness (Mathers and Ghodse 1992). Cannabis abuse is the only lifetime substance use diagnosis that occurs more frequently in patients with schizophrenia than in those with affective psychosis (Kovasznay 1997). Patients who abuse cannabis on a long-term basis are also reported to have significantly more rehospitalizations, worse psychosocial functioning and more thought disturbance and hostility (Caspari 1999). Furthermore, even recreational use of cannabis or alcohol appears to increase the risk of tardive dyskinesia in patients with schizophrenia receiving neuroleptics (Olivera *et al* 1992, Zaretsky *et al* 1993). Further research is required to establish causal links between cannabis and other most frequently favoured substances and psychotic conditions.

Interestingly, it has been proposed that drug taking behaviour requires higher functioning level in patients with schizophrenia. This is based on studies showing that patients who also abuse drugs display less psychopathology, despite having a more complicated course of illness and worse outcomes (Dixon *et al* 1991). In other words, patients who are more severely disabled with their mental illness are at a lesser risk of abusing substances.

Although there is a strong link between severe mental illness and substance abuse, there is always a proportion of patients who do not abuse drugs. It may be important to find out what differentiates them from the group that does. So far, there has not been a clear answer given to this question. This merits attention and further research.

Severe mental illness, mild learning difficulty and challenging behaviour

Patients with mild learning difficulty usually fall between the generic adult and learning difficulty services and, more often than not, are provided with psychiatric care by the generic adult mental health services, without the benefit of specific training and services designed to cater for their needs.

To diagnose mental illness in patients with learning difficulty can at times be difficult as behavioural disturbances may have reasons other than mental illness. In addition, this problem increases as the severity of the learning difficulty becomes more profound. Symptoms in a patient with a more severe learning difficulty are difficult to recognise and not easily interpreted. Very often, the patient may not be able to express himself when being assessed for mental illness or not fully comprehend the assessment procedure.

Behavioural disturbances are not uncommon in patients with learning difficulties and they may have certain 'functions' or uses for the individual. It is very important to examine the dynamics of the disturbance when managing it. The behavioural disturbances displayed by patients with learning difficulty problems are also described as 'challenging behaviours'. Patients with severe mental illness and those with certain personality disorders can also display challenging behaviours.

Challenging behaviour is defined by Emerson (1995) as 'culturally abnormal behaviour(s) of such intensity, frequency or duration that the physical safety of the person or others is likely to be placed in serious jeopardy, or behaviour which is likely to seriously limit use of, or result in the person being denied access to, ordinary community facilities'. Aggression, destructiveness, self-injurious, non-aggressive problematic behaviours and streotypies are the types of behaviours, which are included here, and they may present harm to the individual and be challenging for carers and/or objectionable to the general public.

Challenging behaviours must be understood within their 'social context'. A behaviour, which may be acceptable within a certain cultural and social setting, may not be acceptable in another. Furthermore, it is important to understand the 'causes' or 'functions' of such behaviours. The management of disturbed behaviour should include finding out how a certain behavioural disturbance 'serves' the patient. It is not uncommon, for instance, that an aggressive outburst may help the patient to get the attention he needs, or in another instance, it may serve to help him escape from unwanted attention. Self-cutting behaviour may be to release anxiety. Finding other safe strategies to achieve the same goals can be a way to change these unacceptable behaviours.

According to a survey of self-injurious behaviour in people receiving services for learning disabilities, where 596 adults and children were screened, one-fifth (19%) of them displayed one or more self-injurious behaviour severe enough to cause tissue damage, at a rate of at least once per hour. A further 13% of these wore protective or restraining devices for all parts of the day and night (Oliver et al 1987). Emerson and Bromley (1995) studied the causes of such behaviours. They found that people with more severe disabilities showed more severe challenging behaviours. A significant minority (44%) of them showed more than one form of challenging behaviours. Cross-sectional analyses revealed specific clusters of problematic/aggressive and self-injurious behaviours. The most common functions of challenging behaviours appeared to be 'self-stimulation' for self-injurious behaviours, and 'securing the attention of carers' for aggressive behaviours.

It is crucial to have a better understanding of which behaviours are caused by what reasons. For instance, the behaviours of some learning disabilities patients may be due to neurological dysfunction (Reeves 1997). The inability to express oneself clearly can lead to frustration and formation of challenging behaviour. The patient learns to communicate with others in a dysfunctional way and staff, inadvertently, may further maintain this.

Severe mental illness and medical morbidity

Owing to exclusion from research studies, the real extent of medical co-morbidity in patients with severe mental illness is not generally acknowledged. Equally, mentally ill patients, especially those suffering from schizophrenia, are known not to report their physical complaints as much as others (Koranyi 1979). As a result, patients with severe mental illness very often receive less than adequate physical care.

Health professionals, especially mental health workers often do not recognise patients' physical health problems. In a study examining the physical health problems of mentally ill patients in California, it was found that mental health professionals only recognised 47% of patients' physical problems (Koran et al 1989). Furthermore, the more severe positive symptoms that a patient has, the more likely it is that both staff and the patient may underestimate or ignore a concurrent medical illness (Jeste et al 1996).

Unrecognised physical problems may exacerbate the symptoms of mental illness and severely affect the quality of life of patients. There is literature available which shows that patients with schizophrenia have a lower prevalence of some physical problems although they have a higher prevalence rate in others, compared to the general population and patients suffering from other mental disorders. For instance, rheumatoid arthritis is rarely seen in patients with schizophrenia (Eaton et al 1992), whilst they have an increased risk of developing cardiovascular disorders (Harris 1988) and non-insulin-dependant diabetes mellitus (McKee et al 1986). Although initially it was believed that patients with schizophrenia had a decreased incidence rate of cancer, more recently it has been shown that there is no significant difference in the overall prevalence of cancer between them and the general population (Tsuang 1983).

It has also been reported that in a subgroup of treatment-resistant patients with dual diagnosis, neurological dysfunction may be observed and such difficulties may further complicate their treatment (Levy et al 1996). Attending to co-morbid physical problems could have important implications for improving the patient's care and quality of life.

Severe mental illness and positive HIV status

With the growing concern of HIV infection and AIDS, there have been efforts to target certain at-risk groups to prevent further spread of the infection. Unfortunately, psychiatric populations do not appear to have been targeted, despite the evidence that they represent a vulnerable and disadvantaged segment of the population with a high risk of developing HIV infection. Large numbers of patients with severe mental illness may be living in the main drug-abusing neighbourhoods of inner-city areas and also have unprotected sex. According to a review article by Grassi (1996), several recent studies have shown that high-risk behaviour, especially intravenous drug abuse and non-protected sexual intercourse, is reported by 20–50% of psychiatric patients, particularly those affected by bipolar disorders and schizophrenia. Carey et al (1997) studied the risk behaviours of 60 severely mentally ill patients and found that 48% of men and 37% of women reported either having unprotected sex or sharing needles. Many participants were misinformed about HIV transmission and risk reduction. They tended to rate themselves at only slight risk for infection, undermining their motivation for condom use.

The prevalence of positive-HIV status in severely mentally ill patients is higher compared to the general population and nearly half of them are found to be unaware of their HIV status (Grassi 1996). About 50% of all patients with schizophrenia are also known to be abusing drugs and some of them may prefer substances such as cocaine due to its short 'high'. This creates a need for more frequent injections which in turn leads to an increasing likelihood of sharing syringes and HIV transmission (Davis 1998). In another study, the likelihood of injecting drugs was four times greater among psychiatric patients with a history of intranasal substance use compared with those without such use, three-and-a-half times greater among black patients than others, and five times greater among patients aged 36 or older (Horwath et al 1996). In addition, a 3-year longitudinal study shows a considerably higher risk of having more frequent future relapses for patients with manic depressive illness who are also intravenous drug users with HIV infection (Johnson et al 1999).

Although patients with a primary diagnosis of a severe mental illness are in the high-risk group of developing the infection, the prevalence of a first onset psychotic illness among HIV-positive patients is rare. According to a study where 1046 HIV-positive patients were screened, only 9 (0.9%) suffered from a psychotic illness. Seven of them were in late stages of the infection (Niederecker et al 1995). This data do not indicate a markedly elevated prevalence of psychosis in HIV-positive or AIDS patients.

The HIV status of a severely mentally ill patient should be of concern to the clinicians, especially when the patient has a history of drug abuse and unprotected sex. Establishing informed consent when carrying out an HIV test is crucial.

Severe mental illness and homelessness

Homelessness is one of the major problems a severely mentally ill patient is likely to have. Surveys of homeless persons carried out in different parts of the world show that a significant proportion of them suffer from serious mental and physical health problems. The reasons why a severely ill person becomes homeless may be varied and complex. However, according to a survey carried out in Munich, Germany, two thirds of the mentally ill homeless had become homeless after the onset of mental illness (Fichter et al 1996). In the same survey, amongst 146 homeless males, the lifetime prevalence rates were 12.4% for schizophrenia and 41.8% for affective disorders.

Presence of dual diagnosis such as schizophrenia and substance abuse constitutes a major risk to remain homeless or to become homeless again (Koegel 1988). According to a study carried out in New York, the combination of abusing drugs, persistent symptoms and impaired global functioning at the time of discharge increased the risk of being homeless again within 3 months of hospital discharge (Olfson et al 1999).

Furthermore, homelessness increases the risk of victimisation for the severely mentally ill. In one study, it was found that living in the city, abusing substances, having a secondary diagnosis of personality disorder and homelessness increased the risk of being a victim of a violent crime, at a rate two-and-a-half times greater than that of the general population (Hiday *et al* 1999). In another study, 44% of the subjects were the victim of at least one crime during the previous 2 months and the effect of the incident had a significant impact on their outcomes in terms of increased homelessness and decreased quality of life (Lam and Rosenheck 1998).

Severe mental illness and ethnicity

More and more societies have become multicultural environments, where people from different races, ethnic groups and cultures are living side-by-side. However, health services and other institutions do not yet appear to be 'in line' with the changes occurring within their immediate surroundings. British-born patients of West-Indian origins are especially known to be over-represented within the psychiatric services in the UK, and there are also services in various parts of the country populated by people from Asian origins. Although most may speak in English, the way in which the person expresses himself can often be a barrier between him and the staff members, if the cultural nuances are not understood. In addition, being unaware of certain cultural characteristics and needs can lead to misdiagnoses and mistreatments. In psychiatric intensive care units where the risk of behavioural disturbance is high, special attention should be given to cultural nuances and expressions. In such units, the ethnicity of staff should parallel its patients', as far as possible.

Studies in the UK show there is a higher prevalence of schizophrenia and higher levels of both voluntary and compulsory admissions among patients of West-Indian origin, even after more rigorous methods of detection are applied (Harrison *et al* 1997). A study, which measured the satisfaction with the mental health services, found that second-generation patients of West-Indian origin were significantly less satisfied with almost all aspects of the services that they received, than either older patients born in the West-Indies or white patients (Parkman *et al* 1997). It was also found in the same study that their dissatisfaction was highly related to the number of previous admissions, in that the more previous admissions they had, the more dissatisfied they were with the services.

It is crucial to acknowledge the ethnic characteristics and needs of the individual when assessing and treating him.

Severe mental illness and sexual or severe physical abuse

It is known that there is an established link between early sexual abuse and the development of mental health problems in adulthood. In a longitudinal prospective study, childhood sexual abuse and the development of major depressive illness, conduct disorder, suicidal behaviours and substance abuse at age 18, were significantly correlated (Fergusson *et al* 1998a). In the same study, it was found that most of the sexually abused children came from families with high levels of marital conflict, impaired parenting and parents who reported problems with alcohol. There appears to be a link especially between severe sexual abuse and an earlier onset of affective illness and personality disorder (Fergusson *et al* 1996b; Giese *et al* 1998; Cheasty 1998).

When assessing a patient with severe mental illness, special attention should be given to earlier traumatic experiences. Very often the patient may not volunteer information on emotionally sensitive issues such as sexual or severe physical abuse and yet, such traumatic events may have a severe impact on their later behaviour and conduct.

Severe physical abuse in early years may also lead to later mental health problems and it is not uncommon that physical and sexual abuse can go together. Growing up in an environment where physical violence is part of life, a child will develop various strategies to cope. Some may seek solace in abusing drugs or alcohol from very young ages while others may accept physical or verbal violence as a way to 'resolve' problems, thus repeating the dysfunctional interaction patterns which they have 'learnt' within their family settings. In fact, both physical and sexual abuses are associated with an increased likelihood of the use of alcohol, cannabis, and almost all other drugs for both males and females. Early onset of multiple drug abuse is especially common among those who have been both sexually and physically abused (Harrison *et al* 1997).

Until now, we have examined some of the most commonly seen types of complex needs patient. We will now look at how such patients can be treated and managed.

MANAGEMENT

The treatment and management of severely mentally ill patients with additional serious problems pose significant challenges for both in-patient and community psychiatric services. These patients are usually 'well known' within the service and their repeated re-admission often causes a sense of 'failure' among staff members. It is always disheartening to see previous good therapeutic work quickly being dissolved by the adversities a patient may encounter in the community. When the patient is re admitted, he will very often deny the severity of his problems and the existence of mental illness or substance abuse, despite the clear previous evidence for both. There may be some minimal co-operation whilst in hospital, especially in a locked environment such as an intensive care unit, where he makes 'promises' to keep away from substances or other problem behaviours. However, more often than not, these 'promises' are soon forgotten after discharge and there is a return to the previous cycle of events.

Our clinical experience suggests that most of the patients who cannot be transferred from the intensive care unit back to their catchment area wards within four to eight weeks, due to reasons other than resource problems, belong to this category. In places where there is no intensive care provision, such patients may be kept in acute wards where, due to low staff-patient ratios and at times lack of specialised training, patients may not receive the attention and care they require. Even in intensive care units, the management of such patients may be difficult due to lack of specialised training, appropriate acknowledgement of the additional problems or an appropriate treatment plan.

It is the experience of some psychiatric services in the UK that specialised units have been an essential addition to form a part of the comprehensive local mental health service. In the North West Region of England, a network of seven 'High Dependency Units' have been set up as a regional initiative. In South East London, there are two 'Challenging Behaviour Units' at the Bethlem Royal Hospital and at Bexley Hospital. These units offer a low secure service to the patients with complex needs who may require admissions of 3–24 months in order to address complex psychiatric, psychological, social and organic factors. A full multidisciplinary team is therefore essential when attempting to treat these patients. The types of therapeutic and psychological interventions are specified in the chapters on these subjects elsewhere in this book.

According to the experience of staff who work in such units some complex needs patients, following discharge, require a further period of highly staffed care. This may be in a hospital setting such as an open rehabilitation ward or in the community in a registered hospital hostel, possibly subject to the Mental Health Act or in a highly staffed community hostel. A small minority of patients may even require longer-term low secure care in a hospital setting if their needs and behaviour cannot be managed in a less secure setting.

Although there is a clear need to have more specialised services and treatment programmes tailored to the needs of patients with complex problems across the UK, employing certain strategies listed below may be beneficial when dealing with patients within existing services.

Assessing the complex need areas

It is not always the patient himself but the clinicians that need to acknowledge the existence of additional problems. The likelihood of failure of treatment in the long-term increases if the additional problems have not been adequately recognised and assessed. The emphasis can no longer be on the treatment of the mental illness alone. A needs-based approach will see the patient as an individual with individual needs and focus on all the problem areas.

The personality traits and additional mental health problems of a patient need to be elicited whilst assessing the mental state, bearing in mind that they are likely to be present in a 'difficult to treat' patient. It is crucial to recognise an underlying depression for instance, as the patient with a severe mental illness carries a higher risk of suicide. A detailed needs assessment will also reveal other problem areas such as homelessness, lack of social support and purposeful activities. A thorough medical examination and regular tests may also reveal unrecognised physical health problems in a patient who does not readily complain of poor health and is prone to develop serious illnesses.

At times some patients with mild learning difficulty may go unrecognised, especially if they have not been previously assessed for this. Atypical presentation of a psychotic illness should alert the assessor that there may be a mild learning difficulty. Furthermore, some repetitive problem behaviours can also be explained once this additional problem is acknowledged.

Again, it is well known that individuals who have been abused physically or sexually do not feel comfortable in disclosing their abuse. However, with thoughtful and tactful interviewing techniques, painful, traumatic experiences may be brought to the fore. In some cases, the abuse might still be going on, especially as patients with a severe mental illness can be open to exploitation.

Given that a considerable amount of patients with severe mental illness are also known to abuse substances, we will give special emphasis to the dual diagnosis cases. It should be borne in mind that such cases are known for having other co-existing problems, which are listed earlier. Their assessment requires more assertive methods of exploration than direct questioning. There are now techniques available, that enable clinicians to obtain rapid analysis of urine drug screening. For instance, methods such as, Triage 8, Sure Step and Frontline; these can give reliable results within minutes, showing whether the patient has recently abused drugs. Once a positive drug analysis is found, and provided that staff approach the problem with a non-judgemental manner, the patient is more likely to give information about his substance habit.

A detailed substance taking history is essential and should include:

- Length of abuse.

- Reasons for substance taking.

- Types of preferred substances.

- Method of use.

- Subjective experience.

- What the patient gains or loses from it.

- How it interacts with his medication and compliance.

Information on such aspects can significantly increase the clinician's insight into the patient's substance abuse problem and provide tools for imminent and future management. For instance, if the method of abuse is intravenous injection this may have important implications on HIV or other infections. Another patient may be 'self-medicating' due to unwanted dysphoria states, which may be overcome through more assertive treatment of the symptoms. It is important to remember that there is no such thing as a 'typical dual diagnosis patient'.

Most patients will initially deny they have problems with substances or that they suffer from a severe mental illness. Some centres advocate dealing with both problems at once because mental illness and substance abuse are seen as intrinsically connected and need to be treated concurrently (Brady et al 1996). In such a centre, they do not use different techniques and strategies to address each area separately. Following non-verbal, stress management techniques, such as relaxation and gentle movement exercises, with the reduction of dysphoria, patients appear to be more open to accepting that they may have problems in both areas. This phase is then followed by a 'classroom' approach when chalk and blackboard is used to increase awareness, with a special emphasis on maximising patient participation. Additional care is given to not overwhelming the patient with too much information. In later sessions, group confrontation, role-playing and peer-praise are used as important motivators to help individuals towards change.

Psycho-education

Patient empowerment plays an important part in the management of patients who have complex needs who may also feel that all control is being taken out of their hands, especially when they are receiving care at the intensive care units. Involving patients in decision making and taking responsibility for their actions requires on-going psycho-education. In addition to patients, carers also require information on aspects of mental illness and the impact of the additional problems and needs. This can be a daunting task, as very frequently it is seen that most patients cannot easily retain information. There is some evidence, however, that well-structured educational

Suggested topics for psycho-education:

- Mental health issues
- Medications and their side-effects
- Outcomes of unprotected sex
- Effects of substances

- Symptoms
- HIV infection
- Social skills
- Employment guidance

Box 9.9

sessions can have some impact on the patient's insight into their mental health problems, although not on their medication compliance (Macpherson *et al* 1996).

Patients with complex problems require information on a vast range of subjects. They will need to know about mental health issues, symptoms, the effects of substances, medications, their side-effects, employment guidance, the likely outcomes of unprotected sex, HIV infection and social skills training, to name only a few of the topics. Therefore, the timing and structure of the educational sessions are important. The language chosen has to be accessible. The information provided by the multidisciplinary team has to be consistent and well structured. Overwhelming the patient or the carer with too much information may lead to feelings of further alienation.

Pharmacotherapy of mild learning difficulty and challenging behaviour

Duggan and Brylewski (1998) carried out a systematic Cochrane review and searched for evidence for the efficacy of any antipsychotic medication when treating people with learning disability and schizophrenia. Unfortunately, the reviewers found no trial evidence to guide the use of antipsychotic medication in this group of people. They suggest following guidance from trials involving people with schizophrenia but without learning difficulty and call for an urgent need to carry out randomised trials. The same reviewers also searched antipsychotic medication for challenging behaviour and again found no evidence that antipsychotic medication helps or harms adults with learning disability and challenging behaviour. On the other hand, the use of Clozapine in a group of learning difficulty patients with challenging behaviour was shown to result in significant reduction in psychiatric symptoms and aggressive and self-injurious behaviour. The side-effects were also minimal (Cohen and Underwood 1994). In another study, Clozapine was again efficacious and well tolerated in 10 patients with learning difficulties who had either schizophrenia or bipolar disorder (Buzan *et al* 1998).

Pharmacotherapy of severe mental illness and substance abuse

The pharmacotherapy of dual diagnosis patients is a recently developing area. It studies both the pharmacokinetics of the substance and the psychotropics and their interactions. Animal studies show that cocaine seeking behaviour may be diminished by administering dopamine-1-like agonists to rats primed with cocaine previously (Self *et al* 1996). Deriving from this premise, Amantadine, a DA agonist, which is normally used to alleviate extrapyramidal side-effects, may therefore have a desired effect when used for prevention of a stimulant relapse. Some tricyclic anti-depressants, such as desipramine, a dopamine reuptake inhibitor, have also been suggested for prevention of cocaine relapse. In an open, double-blind, placebo controlled study, desipramine was given to cocaine-abusing patients with schizophrenia and the preliminary results suggest that cocaine-abusing schizophrenic patients who received desipramine for 12 weeks used less cocaine in a 15-month follow-up period than those who received the placebo (Wilkins 1997). Wilkins, in his review article, concludes that the treatment of cocaine abusing patients with schizophrenia may be enhanced with the addition of desipramine into the treatment regime and that cocaine-induced depression is alleviated with desipramine (1997). He also adds that cannabis, when taken concomitantly with cocaine, may also reduce the depressive symptomatology, whilst increasing hostility and suspiciousness.

It is suggested by research that one of the major reasons why patients with schizophrenia take substances is to 'self-treat' the negative symptoms or to reduce the side-effects of neuroleptics. For instance, cannabis has been shown to reduce negative symptoms, whilst increasing the positive symptoms of schizophrenia (Peralta and Cuesta 1995). Hence, targeting the treatment of negative and affective symptoms of schizophrenia may have beneficial effects on reducing the drive or the need to take substances.

As mentioned previously, an ideal medicine, for a stimulant abusing patient with schizophrenia, should target to reduce negative and positive symptoms and the drive to take stimulants. Clozapine has been shown to alleviate negative symptoms and, in principle, should have some effect on the drive to take drugs. In a study comparing substance-abusing patients with schizophrenia with non-abusing ones, Clozapine produced similar improvements in symptoms and psychosocial functioning levels. The history of substance abuse did not appear to negatively influence response to Clozapine (Buckley et al 1994). In a recent review article, Buckley advocates the use of Clozapine as the therapeutic option for patients with dual diagnosis as it has been shown to reduce alcohol, smoking and cocaine use (1998). Furthermore, it is suggested that Clozapine may also have antiaggressive effects (Buckley et al 1995). A retrospective analysis of 331 patients with schizophrenia showed that at baseline 31.4% displayed overt physical aggression and this rate fell to 1.1% after an average of a 47-week period on Clozapine (Volavka 1999). The author adds that this finding cannot be explained with sedation or antipsychotic effects alone, as the effect on aggression was more pronounced than that on other symptoms.

Other atypical neuroleptics may also have benefits for patients with dual diagnoses due to their less severe extrapyramidal side-effects. However, the efficacy of newer atypicals in reduction of substance abuse behaviour is not yet known. Flupenthixol, a typical neuroleptic, also known for its antidepressant properties, is suggested to reduce craving for cocaine (Gawin et al 1989).

Amidst newly emerging information regarding the reasons why patients with schizophrenia turn toward substances and that atypical neuroleptics may prove to be beneficial, it must be remembered that substance abuse behaviour cannot merely be explained with pharmacokinetics alone. Adding contingency management, psychoeducation and social skills training may enhance pharmacotherapy efficacy.

Specially designed services for dual diagnoses

Over the past decade, with increasing concern at the impact of dual diagnosis patients on existing resources, there has been a movement in creating specially designed services and treatment programmes. However, in the USA, the creation of such services integrating the substance misuse and adult mental health services has not been easy, due to separate funding sources or different administrative divisions. In the UK, although the substance misuse service is part of the mental health service, the day-to-day functioning of services and personnel are also known to be separate. There are some significant differences between these services especially in relation to their philosophies and treatment approaches. Mental health services have specially trained clinical staff and favour assertive efforts to maintain people on treatment, medication and psychosocial treatments. On the other hand, substance misuse staff can be people who have previously been drug abusers themselves (especially in the USA) and the patients are not treated in an assertive manner, but are expected to take responsibility and use voluntary organisations more often. These major differences need to be taken into consideration when a special programme to treat dually diagnosed patients is being planned.

One treatment model is that following the treatment of psychiatric illness, the substance abuse is treated. The other method involves concurrent but separate treatment of both psychiatric and substance misuse disorders, when different teams from both services treat patients. Both of these models can be applied when there are no integrated services available, but they require seamless planning and time management, with special care not to overload the patient. The third method, is the integrated model, where both disorders are treated concurrently by the same clinical team. This model requires the presence of well-integrated in-patient care and assertive community services with supportive living environments. Treatment methods vary within this model. Motivation-based treatments and engagement with services and psychosocial methods have both been advocated. This model can be costly and requires careful planning either of existing resources or the creation of new ones.

Although there are some studies showing that the third model with integrated case management services can lead to a better outcome in dually diagnosed patients (Rosenthal et al 1992, Ries and Comtois 1997), there does not appear to be any clear evidence that one model is superior to another, or that these models produce a better outcome compared with traditional services. A recent systematic Cochrane review, carried out by Ley et al (1999), aimed to evaluate the effectiveness of treatment programmes for people with dual diagnosis, and identified six studies which met their selection criteria. However, most of these studies were either small in size or did not report some important clinical outcome measures. The reviewers concluded that there is no clear evidence supporting an advantage of any one type of substance misuse programme over the value of standard care or another programme. They added that the current momentum for integrated services is not based on good evidence and suggest that the implementation of new specialist services should be within the context of simple, well designed controlled trials.

It can be suggested that within the intensive care unit settings, where there is a high staff to patient ratio, training staff in substance abuse issues may have beneficial effects on a proportion of dually diagnosed patients. Indeed, in our clinical experience, providing regular information on the adverse effects of substances, rewarding abstinence by outings away from the unit and other tokens along with use of atypical neuroleptics have been beneficial in increasing the motivation to stop abusing drugs in a number of patients.

Motivation to stop abusing substances can be very low in dually diagnosed patients and may vary according to the substance abused. In a study of outpatients, the percentage of low motivational level (precontemplation and contemplation) was 41% for opiates and 60% for cocaine (Ziedonis and Trudeau 1997). The same authors used a motivation-based treatment to increase the level of motivation for change. In addition, they advocate the use of community reinforcement approaches, treatments focusing on engagement with treatment, finding external and internal levers to increase motivation, case management and blending traditional substance abuse psychotherapy approaches with mental health treatment with atypical neuroleptics, in order to achieve extended abstinence.

Staff-related issues and staff burnout

One of the most important aspects of good practice within the intensive care unit setting involves cohesive multidisciplinary teamwork. A humane approach to all kinds of adversity as the adopted philosophy, a good mix of various complementary skills among the members of the team, availability of training and further staff empowerment, a well structured ward programme and decent physical surroundings are among the essential elements to create a harmonious and cohesive intensive care unit. However, it is also very easy for things to go terribly wrong in an emotionally charged environment.

One of the main problems in dealing with complex needs patients in psychiatric intensive care units or acute wards is staff 'burnout'. Being exposed to violence on a daily basis can change an individual's reaction to them over time. It is known that some may become emotionally exhausted and lose patience and tolerance, whilst others may feel demoralised and alienated from their patients and begin avoiding contact with them. Emotions experienced can vary, even within the same day, from anger and resentment to sadness, fear and anxiety. Staff may feel exhausted with such a strongly felt range of emotions experienced within a short period. Such emotions, if they are left unexplored and not briefed on an on-going basis, may even lead to psychological disturbances. In a study carried out to measure and compare 'burnout' between staff who worked with patients displaying challenging behaviour in hospital-based bungalows and a community unit, it was found that hospital-based staff were less satisfied with their salaries, enjoyed their contact with their patients less, were more emotionally exhausted and found their training to be less adequate, compared with community based staff (Chung and Corbett 1998).

It is important that staff understand the causes of challenging behaviours. If they do not, staff may inadvertently ensure the long-term maintenance of unwanted behaviour. In a study examining staff's beliefs about the causes of challenging behaviour and their responses to them, the belief systems of experienced and inexperienced staff were compared (Hastings *et al* 1995). Experienced staff held beliefs that were consistent with present knowledge on challenging behaviours and distinguished between the behaviours in terms of their causes, whilst the inexperienced staff did not. This data is interpreted as emphasising the importance of a 'needs-based' approach and staff training, when managing challenging behaviour.

There are numerous ways of avoiding staff 'burnout'. It is crucial that management of psychiatric intensive care units and acute in-patient units take into account that 'burnout' is a strong possibility. Management should arrange regular staff support groups in addition to regular and relevant staff training to furnish staff with ways of coping and delivering appropriate and humane care to those most likely to have the most complex problems.

SUMMARY

In this chapter, we have attempted to define the type of patient who has complex needs and examined them under several subheadings. Many of these patients are found in intensive care units where they may require care for longer periods compared to patients with less complicated conditions. These patients not only suffer from a severe mental illness, but also have additional diagnoses or problems, which complicate and worsen their clinical outcome. Very often one problem can lead to another and there is an accumulation of adverse factors. Patients with schizophrenia appear especially prone to substance abuse and create serious management problems for the services. This chapter also includes information on management strategies for the complex needs patient and discusses the preferred choice of treatments.

ACKNOWLEDGEMENTS

The author thanks Catherine Ebenezer, Senior Librarian at Lambeth AMH Library, who helped with the literature search, Tim Foster who helped in editing this chapter, and her daughter Sanem Atakan who made the much needed coffee and tea whilst working.

REFERENCES

Brady S, Hiam CM, Saemann R, Humbert L, Fleming MZ, Dawkins-Brickhouse K. 1996 Dual diagnosis: A treatment model for substance abuse and major mental illness. Com Men Health J 32(6): 573–578

Buckley PF, Thompson P, Way L, Meltzer HY. 1994 Substance abuse among patients with treatment-resistant schizophrenia: characteristics and implications for clozapine therapy. Am J Psychiatry 151(3): 385–389

Buckley PF, Bartell J, Donenwirth K, Lee S. Torigoe F, Schulz SC. 1995 Violence and schizophrenia: clozapine as a specific antiaggressive agent. Bull Am Acad Psychiatry Law 23(4): 607–611

Buckley PF. 1998 Substance abuse in schizophrenia: a review. J Clin Psychiatry (suppl. 59)3: 26–30

Buzan RD, Dubovsky SL, Firestone D, Dal Pozzo E. 1998 Use of Clozapine in 10 mentally retarded adults. J Neuropsychiatry Clin Neurosciences 10(1): 93–95

Cantwell R, Brewin J, Glazebrook C, Dalkin T, Fox R, Medley I, Harrison G. 1999 Prevalence of substance misuse in first-episode psychosis. Br J Psychiatry 174: 150–153

Carey MP, Carey KB, Weinhardt LS, Gordon CM. 1997 Behavioural risk for HIV infection among adults with a severe and persistent mental illness: patterns and psychological antecedents. Comm Ment Health J 33(2): 133–142

Caspari D. 1999 Cannabis and schizophrenia: results of a follow up study. Eur Arch Psychiatry Clin Neurosci 249(1): 45–49

Cheasty M, Clare AW, Collins C. 1998 Relation between sexual abuse in childhood and adult depression: case-control study. BMJ 316(7126): 198–201

Chung MC, Corbett J. 1998 The burnout of nursing staff working with challenging behaviour clients in hospital-based bungalows and a community unit. Int J Nurs Stud 35(1–2): 56–64

Cohen SA, Underwood MT. 1994 The use of Clozapine in a mentally retarded and aggressive population. J Clin Psychiatry 55(10): 440–444

Collins J, Schlenger W. 1988 Acute and chronic effects of alcohol use on violence. J Studies on Alcohol 4(6): 516–521

Davis S. 1998 Injection drug use and HIV infection among the seriously mentally ill: a report from Vancouver. Can J Common Ment Health 17(1): 121–127

Dixon L, Haas G, Weiden PJ, Sweeney J.1991 Drug abuse in schizophrenic patients: Clinical correlates and reasons for use. Am J Psychiatry 148: 224–230

Eaton WW, Hayward C, Ram R. 1992 Schizophrenia and rheumatoid arthritis: a review. Schiz Res 6: 181–192

Emerson C. 1995 In: Challenging behaviour. Analysis and intervention in people with learning difficulties. Cambridge: Cambridge University Press

Emerson E and Bromley J. 1995 The form and function of challenging behaviours. J intellect Disabil Res 39(5): 388–398

Fergusson DM, Lynskey MT, Horwood LJ. 1996a Childhood sexual abuse and psychiatric disorder in young adulthood: I. Prevalence of sexual abuse and factors associated with sexual abuse. J Am Acad Child Adoles Psychiatry 35(10): 1355–1364

Fergusson DM, Horwood LJ, Lynskey MT. 1996b Childhood sexual abuse and psychiatric disorder in young adulthood: II. Psychiatric outcomes of childhood sexual abuse. J Am Acad Child Adoles Psychiatry 35(10): 1365–1374

Fichter MM, Koniarczyk M, Greifenhagen A, Koegel P, Quadflieg N, Wittchen HU, Wölz J. 1996 Mental illness in a representative sample of homeless men in Munich, Germany. Euro Arch Psychiatry and Clin Neurosciences 246: 185–196

Gawin FH, Allen D, Humblestone B. 1989 Outpatient treatment of 'crack' cocaine smoking with flupenthixol decanoate. Arch Gen Psychiatry 46. 322 325

Giese AA, Thomas MR, Dubovsky SL, Hilty S. 1998 The impact of a history of childhood abuse on hospital outcome of affective episodes. Psychiatr Serv 49(1): 77–81

Grassi L. 1996 Risk of HIV infection in psychiatrically ill patients. AIDS Care 8(1): 103–116

Gritz ER, Stapleton JM, Hill MA, Jarvik ME. 1985 Prevalence of cigarette smoking in medical and psychiatric hospitals. Bulletin of Society of Psychologists in Addictive Behaviours 4(3): 151–165

Hambrecht M, Häfner H. 1996 Substance abuse and the onset of schizophrenia. Biol Psychiatry 40: 1155–1163

Harris AE. 1988 Physical disease and schizophrenia. Schiz Bulletin 14(1): 85–96

Harrison G, Glazebrook C, Brewin J, Cantwell R, Dalkin T, Fox R, Medley I. 1997 Increased incidence of psychotic disorders in migrants from the Caribbean to the United Kingdom. Psychol Med 27(4): 799–806

Harrison PA, Fulkerson JA, Beebe TJ. 1997 Multiple substance use among adolescent physical and sexual abuse victims. Child Abuse Negl 21(6): 529–539

Hastings RP, Remington B, Hopper GM. 1995 Experienced and inexperienced health care workers' beliefs about challenging behaviours. J Intellect Disabil Res 39(6): 474–483

Hiday VA, Swartz MS, Swanson JW, Borum R, Wagner HR. 1999 Criminal victimisation of persons with severe mental illness. Psychiatr Serv 50(1): 62–68

Horwath E, Cournas F, McKinnon K, Guido JR, Herman R. 1996 Illicit-drug injection among psychiatric patients without a primary substance use disorder. Psychiatry Serv 47(2): 181–185

Jeste DV, Galdsjo JA, Lindamer LA, Lacro JP. 1996 Medical co-morbidity in schizophrenia. Schiz Bulletin 22(3): 413–430

Johnson JG, Rabkin JG, Lipsitz JD, Williams JB, Remien RH. 1999 Recurrent major depressive disorder among human immunodeficiency virus (HIV)-positive and HIV-negative intravenous drug users: findings of a 3-year longitudinal study. Compr Psychiatry 40(1): 31–34

Kane JM. 1996 Factors which can make patients difficult to treat. Br J Psychiatry 169 (suppl. 31) 10–14

Kendler KS. 1985 A twin study of individuals with both schizophrenia and alcoholism. Br J Psychiatry 147: 48–53

Koegel P, Burnam MA, Farr RK. 1988 The prevalence of specific psychiatric disorders among homeless individuals in the inner city of Los Angeles. Arch Gen Psychiatry 45: 1085–1092

Koran LM, Sox HC, Marton KI, Moltzen S, Sox CH, Kraemer HC, Imai K, Kelsey TG, Rose TG, Levin LC, Chandra S. 1989 Medical evaluation of psychiatric patients. Arch Gen Psychiatry 46: 733–740

Koranyi EK. 1979 Morbidity and rate of undiagnosed physical illnesses in a psychiatric clinic population. Arch Gen Psychiatry 36: 414–419

Kovasznay B, Fleischer J, Tanenberg-Karant M, Jandorf L, Miller AD, Bromet E. 1997 Substance use disorder and the early course of illness in schizophrenia and affective psychosis. Schiz Bulletin 23(2): 195–201

Lam JA, Rosenheck R. 1998 The effect of victimisation on clinical outcomes of homeless persons with serious mental illness. Psychiatr Ser 49(5): 678–683

Lelliott P, Wing JK, Clifford P. 1994 A national audit of new long-stay psychiatric patients I: Method and description of the cohort. Br J Psychiatry 164: 160–169

Levy M, Saemann R, Oepen G. 1996 Neurological co-morbidity in treatment-resistant dual diagnosis patients. J Psychoact Drugs 28(2): 103–110

Link B, Stueve C. 1994 Psychotic symptoms and the violent/illegal behaviour of mental patients compared to community controls. In: Monahan and Steadman (Eds) Violence and Mental Disorder. 137–159. Chicago: University of Chicago Press

Macpherson R, Jerrom B, Hughes A. 1996 A controlled study of education about drug treatment in schizophrenia. Br J Psychiatry 168: 709–717

Mann S, Cree W. 1976 'New' long stay psychiatric patients: a national sample survey of fifteen mental hospitals in England and Wales 1972/73. Psychol Med 6: 603–616

Mathers DC and Ghodse AH. 1992 Cannabis and psychotic illness. Br J Psychiatry 161: 648–653

McKee HA, D'Arcy PF, Wilson PJK. 1986 Diabetes and schizophrenia–a preliminary study. J Clin Hosp Pharmacy 11: 297–299

Menezes PR, Johnson S, Thornicroft G, Marshall J, Prosser D, Ebbington P, Kuipers E. 1996 Br J Psychiatry 168(5): 612–619

Niederecker M, Naber D, Riedel R, Perro C, Goebel FD. 1995 Incidence and aetiology of psychotic disorders in HIV infected patients. Nervenartz 66(5): 367–371

Nolan KA, Volavka J, Mohr P, Czobor P. 1999 Psychopathy and violent behaviour among patients with schizophrenia or schizoaffective disorder. Psychiatr Serv 50(6): 787–792

Olfson M, Mechanic D, Hansell S, Boyer CA, Walkup J. 1999 Prediction of homelessness within three months of discharge among inpatients with schizophrenia. Psychiatr Serv 50(5): 667–63

Oliver C, Murphy GH, Corbett JA. 1987 Self-injurious behaviour in people with mental handicap: a total population study. J Ment Def Res 31: 147–162

Olivera AA, Kiefer MW, Manley NK. 1990 Tardive dyskinesia in psychiatric patients with substance abuse disorders. Am J Drug Alc Abuse 16: 57–66

Owen RR, Fischer EP, Booth BM, Cuffel DJ. 1996 Medication noncompliance and substance abuse among patients with schizophrenia. Psychiatr Serv 46(8): 853–858

Parkman S, Davies S, Leese M, Phelan M, Thornicroft G. 1997 Ethnic differences in satisfaction with mental health services among representative people with psychosis in south London: PRISM study 4. Br J Psychiatry 171: 260–264

Peralta V, Cuesta MJ. 1995 Negative symptoms in schizophrenia: a confirmatory factor analysis of competing models. Am J Psychiatry 152 (10): 1450–1457

Pristach CA, Smith CM. 1990 Medication compliance and substance abuse among patients with schizophrenia. Hosp Community Psychiatry 41: 1345–1348

Rabinowitz J, Bromet EJ, Lavelle J, Carlson G, Kovasznay B, Schwartz JE. 1998 Prevalence and severity of substance use disorders and onset of psychosis in first-admission psychotic patients. Psychol Med 28(6): 1411–1419

Reeves S. 1997 Behavioural misdiagnosis. Nurs Times 93(19): 44–45

Ries RK, Comtois KA. 1997 Illness severity and treatment services for dually diagnosed severely mentally ill outpatients. Schiz Bulletin 23(2): 239–246

Rosenthal RN, Hellerstein DJ, Miner CR. 1992 A model of integrated services for outpatient treatment of patients with co-morbid schizophrenia and addictive disorders. Am J Addictions 1(4): 339–348

Self DW, Barnhart WJ, Lehman DA, Nestler EJ. 1996 Opposite modulation of cocaine-seeking behaviour by D_1- and D_2-like dopamine receptor agonists. Science 271(5255): 1586–1589

Serper MR, Albert M, Richardson NA, Dickson S, Allen MH, Werner A. 1995 Clinical effects of recent cocaine use on patients with acute schizophrenia. Am J Psychiatry 152: 1464–1469

Sherer MA, Kumor KM, Jaffe JM. 1989 Effects of cocaine are partially attenuated by haloperidol. Psychiatry Res 27: 117–125

Swanson JW, Borum R, Swartz MS, Monahan J. 1996 Psychotic symptoms and disorders and the risk of violent behaviour in the community. Criminal Behaviour and Mental Health 6: 309–329

Tsuang MT, Perkins K, Simpson JC. 1983 Physical diseases in schizophrenia and affective disorder. J Clin Psychiatry 44: 42–46

Volavka J. 1999 The effects of clozapine on aggression and substance abuse in schizophrenic patients. J Clin Psychiatry 60 (suppl.) 12: 43–46

Wessely S, Buchanan A, Reed A, Cutting J, Everitt, Garety P, Taylor P. 1993 Acting on delusions I: Prevalence. Br J Psychiatry 163: 69–76

Wessely S, Castle D, Douglas A, Taylor PJ. 1994 The criminal careers of incident cases of schizophrenia. Psychol Med 24, 483–502

Wessely S. 1997 The epidemiology of crime, violence and schizophrenia. Br J Psychiatry (suppl. 32) 170: 8–11

Wilkins JN. 1997 Pharmacotherapy of schizophrenia patients with co-morbid substance abuse. Schiz Bulletin 23(2): 215–228

Winokur G, Turvey C, Akiskal H, Coryell W, Solomon D, Leaon A, Mueller T, Endicott J, Maser J, Keller M. 1998 Alcoholism and drug abuse in three groups–bipolar I, unipolars and their acquaintances. J Affect Disord 50(2–3): 81–89

Zaretsky A, Rector NA, Seeman MV, Fornazzari X. 1993 Current cannabis use and tardive dyskinesia. Schiz Res 11: 3–8

Ziedonis DM, Kosten TR, Glazer WM, Frances RJ. 1994 Nicotine Dependence and schizophrenia. Hosp Community Psychiatry 45: 204–206

Ziedonis DM, Trudeau K. 1997 Motivation to quit using substances among individuals with schizophrenia: Implications for a motivation-based treatment model. Schiz Bulletin 23(2): 229–238

10

THERAPEUTIC ACTIVITIES WITHIN PSYCHIATRIC INTENSIVE CARE UNITS

Brenda Flood, Sarah Hooton

INTRODUCTION

Treatment within psychiatric intensive care units (PICUs) has traditionally concentrated on medical interventions and the containment of acutely disturbed individuals, with previously little emphasis on the use of therapeutic activities. In a recent survey of PICUs in the UK, Best (1997) identified that over 90% of staff felt that management of problematic behaviour, intensive nursing, the safety of the patient and others were the main functions of the unit; 79% identified therapeutic activities as a function of PICUs but, as noted by Moore (1998), the provision of intensive individualised therapy programmes is difficult when patients are only on the ward for a short period of time. The ability of staff to offer therapeutic activities has been limited further as there has been a shift towards a custodial rather than a therapeutic model of care. This has been forced upon many units because of large numbers of detained patients, an increase in paper work and a decrease in multidisciplinary team working (Nuffield Institute 1998). The Sainsbury Centre (1998) believed that 'Organised activity is important, not only therapeutically or to maintain interest and engagement, but also because of research showing that activities which are disorganised and unpredictable lead to increased rates of violence on psychiatric wards'. The literature suggests that activities can not only enhance an individual's development, but also assist in the management of problematic behaviour and maintenance of a safe environment.

The type of activities that can be offered within a PICU require careful consideration in order to meet the acute, complex and challenging needs of the patient population. Clinicians are faced with the task of identifying appropriate strategies and ensuring the necessary structures and systems are in place in order for therapeutic activities to be safely and consistently provided.

This chapter aims to provide clinicians with an introduction to the relevant literature supporting therapeutic activities and presents a practical approach towards developing and maintaining a therapeutic programme within a PICU. It will explore the benefits and limitations of providing a therapeutic programme and describe how these activities can be effectively implemented within this specialised environment.

ACTIVITY

Activity incorporates self-maintenance tasks, productive activity/work and leisure pursuits. All of these activities are fundamental to meeting basic human needs.

'The healthy individual has his daily life activities organised into a satisfying pattern which is important to health and life satisfaction' (Kielhofner 1980).

Patients with mental illness may have a diminished ability to perform these tasks successfully which affects their ability to fulfil life roles and routines. Using activities therapeutically can enable patients to develop and maintain the skills required for social functioning. The programme can incorporate both diversional and treatment specific activities, which should be valued by and have meaning for the patient.

Activities can be used purely to occupy the mind, distracting the individual's attention from disturbing symptoms (e.g. listening to music, going for a walk, board games), or be specifically selected and identified in the individual's care plan to develop and maintain the patient's functioning (e.g. relaxation, anger management techniques, cooking, art therapy). (Figure 10.1). Whether an activity is diversional or treatment-specific is determined not by what the activity is but how it is used.

The use of activities as a therapeutic tool has long been recognised. As early as 2600 BC 'The Chinese taught that disease resulted from organic inactivity and used physical training for the promotion of health' (Creek 1990). In Ancient Greece music was used to soothe delirium, and many Greek philosophers linked mind with body and recommended the use of activity to maintain health. They also recognised the diversional value of activity and its value in the treatment of mental diseases (Hopkins and Smith 1988). In 1786 in Paris, Pinel introduced work treatment. It was also at this time that William Tuke founded the Retreat in York, England. He also used work or 'occupation therapy' but encouraged treating patients in a humane and rational manner, which he called 'Moral Treatment'. Clinicians who employed the principles of moral treatment 'used normal daily routines of activity to bring patients back into productive satisfying participation in the social group' (Kielhofner and Nicol 1989).

Activities can be a valuable therapeutic tool when they are specifically selected and aim to meet identified patient needs, but they can also be beneficial when they occur

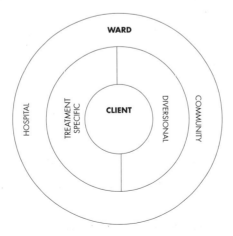

Figure 10.1 – Therapeutic activities

spontaneously and are diversional in nature. Some of the benefits patients with mental illness can experience from engaging in specific activities are outlined below. The benefits of activities can be enhanced when provided within the framework of a wider structured programme.

Benefits of engaging in activities

- Enhance feelings of self worth.
- Maintain present level of functioning.
- Provide opportunities for meaningful communication and appropriate socialisation.
- Increase ability to solve life stresses.
- Increase insight and understanding of mental illness.
- Enable orientation to surroundings and reality.
- Focus concentration on to productive pursuits.
- Facilitate self expression.
- Encourage patients to take personal responsibility.
- Promote choice.
- Maintain a routine and provide a structure.
- Provide patients with a purpose and focus to their day and their admission.
- Increase levels of confidence.
- Replace lost roles.
- Enable the assessment of a patient's functional performance and mental state over a period of time.
- Provide opportunities for developing life skills.
- Provide pleasurable experiences.

THE THERAPEUTIC PROGRAMME

The therapeutic programme can be considered to be the overall structure within which activities are provided. It is a combination of planned, structured as well as spontaneous activities which can be both diversional or treatment specific. It includes activities related to self care, leisure, education and work, which reflect a balanced lifestyle and can occur on a group or individual basis. These are facilitated by the multidisciplinary team and can occur within the immediate environment, the wider hospital or involve accessing community facilities. Figure 10.2 provides an example of a unit-wide therapeutic programme within which individual activities such as self-care tasks can be incorporated.

Shepherd and Lavender (1999) stated that planned, structured activities and the prioritisation of individual time with patients can reduce social isolation and levels of boredom. They also provided opportunities for the reinforcement of socially appropriate behaviour. The role activities play in developing individual skills and abilities is well documented. As well as this many studies indicate or directly link engagement in activities to reduced levels of violence within inpatient psychiatric units. Howells and Hollin (1989) found support for the view that lack of planned activities could actually contribute to violence. In particular, they cited a study by Drinkwater (1988), who showed that during periods without planned activities, violent behaviour was likely to be four times higher than during more structured times. In another study Shepherd and Lavender (1999) noted that no incidents were reported to have taken place in therapeutic contexts. This is supported by Torpy and Hall's (1993) study of aggressive incidents in a medium secure unit over a 3-year period, in which they found that no violent assaults occurred when patients were in occupational therapy areas, the gym or outdoor spaces. Similarly Fottrell (1980) found that violence and frustration is more prevalent during periods of little therapeutic activity. Nelson et al (1995) obtained the views of patients within a psychiatric unit, who identified therapeutic and environmental factors which contributed to their levels of aggression. These included: lack of attention from staff, not enough to do and boredom, lack of access to the outdoors and insufficient explanation of the rules.

These findings confirm the need for patients to have access to activities within inpatient psychiatric units. These activities should be specifically planned and an appropriate environment created in order for them to be effectively implemented. The results of a study undertaken by Palmstierna et al (1991) in a Swedish PICU suggest that ward environment and treatment approaches which are less punitive

Monday	Tuesday	Wednesday	Thursday	Friday	Saturday	Sunday
Community Meeting	Craft group	Cooking group	Social skills	Education		
Relaxation	Quiz/Games	Life skills group	Computer sessions	Art therapy	Trip out	Communal meal
Multi gym	Badminton	Multi gym	Art/Craft activities	Pool competition	Video night	

Figure 10.2 – A therapeutic programme

and not solely focused on containment, but still consider the patients' illness, safety and legal restrictions, are more likely to reduce levels of aggressive behaviour. These findings are supported by Canastey and Roper (1997) who found that by providing a less controlled environment, levels of frustration and aggression can be reduced.

All these studies indicate that structured activities within a ward environment, whilst at the same time allowing patients a degree of choice and control, can directly reduce levels of frustration and aggression.

THE PATIENT GROUP AND THE ENVIRONMENT

The needs of these patients differ from those in open wards due to the consistently greater risk in the behaviour they exhibit, such as violence toward self and others. Best (1996) showed that these patients are characterised by affective extremes and rapid fluctuation in mood, delusional beliefs, hallucinations, poor interpersonal skills, limited concentration, limited cognition and are often disoriented in time and place. Damage to property is another feature, which was noted by Musisi et al (1989), as is the risk of absconding, highlighted in research completed by Gentle (1996). Other behaviours closely associated with intensive care patients include: impaired impulse control resulting in physical and verbal aggression, decreased tolerance, increased frustration and irritability due to limited ability to express themselves fully, chaotic thoughts and routine, as well as disturbed sleep patterns.

Hospitals are unfamiliar environments, where there is often limited personal space and privacy, and few opportunities for patients to make choices or have control over their situation. In addition, PICU patients have other factors to contend with, e.g. a high staff to patient ratio, often decreased access to facilities as security and safety is a priority; a concentration of other highly disturbed individuals resident on the units, with overcrowding and rapid turnover. This can result in the patients presenting negative behaviour in response to the environmental constraints and structures. They may have difficulty establishing rapport, be unable to trust staff, feel disempowered, choose to isolate themselves and may demonstrate increased levels of verbal and physical aggression. This in turn may have an adverse effect on their motivation and level of self worth.

If patients are encouraged to channel their energies into productive pursuits, which have been carefully considered, not only would this lead to increased feelings of self worth and empowerment, but also may have the positive effect of reducing problematic behaviour. The incorporation of therapeutic activities into the ward routine and culture, may create an environment which plays a significant part in the management of difficult behaviour and levels of safety may be created, whilst at the same time addressing individual needs.

Case history

Simon is a 29-year-old man on his first admission to a PICU. He presented with manic features including pressure of speech, increased activity levels, irritability and sexual disinhibition. The team felt that appropriately to channel his excess energy, a dual approach to treatment had to be adopted. Simon had an interest in sporting activities so this, as well as medication was introduced into his treatment plan. He attended the gym daily, which was facilitated on a one-to-one basis initially. This provided him with an enjoyable and safe outlet in which he could expend his excess energy and alleviate his distressing symptoms.

DEVELOPING A THERAPEUTIC PROGRAMME

In order to provide a relevant and effective therapeutic programme staff should aim to meet the needs of the patients and consider the risk factors presented by the acute nature of the patients' illness and the environmental constraints. This next section will identify and discuss the practical considerations necessary for successful implementation of activities on the ward. This is divided into two interrelated parts, one being the factors required to establish a ward routine, programme or culture and the other focusing on the implementation of specific activities.

Establishing a ward therapeutic programme

The therapeutic programme needs to be an integral part of the overall service provided on the ward, the success of which is significantly affected by the multidisciplinary team's understanding, commitment and facilitation of this fundamental form of treatment. The following points should be considered in order to ensure the successful implementation of a unit programme.

- All staff need to have an understanding of the rationale for engaging in activities to ensure effective support and implementation for this structure. The adoption of a shared philosophy requires leadership and support from the multidisciplinary team, which can be aided by having a clear statement of purpose in the ward operational policy. An identified individual(s) with appropriate skills and experience should be responsible for the overall coordination of the programme.

- Patients should receive information upon admission, which clearly outlines the principles of the therapeutic programme, and the expectation that they will be required to engage in these activities as part of their treatment during their admission. This can be in the form of a leaflet, which describes the types of activities available or verbally from the team or named nurse.

- The multidisciplinary team, in conjunction with the patient, should decide on the appropriate activities for the individual based on the assessment findings. This should be discussed in the team clinical meeting and agreed with the patient, where possible.

- Activity programmes should combine diversional and treatment specific activities. Each individual should have a specific programme to address areas of need which takes into consideration their current mental state and behaviour, interests, level of functional performance, cultural background and future plans following discharge. This should be documented in the individual's care plan, with a copy of the programme given to the patient.

- The patient's performance within the activities should be regularly reviewed and progress/changes reported with regard to the individual's mental state, behaviour and level of functioning. This may result in the need to adapt their programme accordingly.

- The daily structure within the unit should be based on the common needs of patients, with specific treatment activities incorporated into this overall approach (Table 10.1).

- Sufficient support at both management level and amongst staff is essential. Adequate staffing levels to ensure that an activity can be facilitated is a basic requirement if the therapeutic programme is to remain consistent. Staff should have dedicated time to provide this activity which includes time to plan, implement and evaluate its effectiveness and not be expected to undertake other responsibilities for the duration of the activity. Staff not actively engaged in a specific activity can provide valuable support, by ensuring appropriate patients attend, that noise levels are kept to a minimum and respecting the need not to disturb patients whilst engaged in an activity.

- There should be adequate opportunity for staff to receive the appropriate training to enable them competently and confidently to provide relevant

Table 10.1 – Proposed basic ward structure

9–10 am	Self care tasks:	Washing, dressing, making bed, breakfast
10–12 pm	45 min activity:	Quiz, badminton, art, community meeting, indoor gardening
12–2 pm		Lunch and rest period
2–4 pm	45 min activity:	Life skills group, relaxation, self awareness, social skills, cooking session
4–6 pm		Dinner and rest period
6–8 pm	Leisure:	Football, pool competition, bingo, board games

individual and group activities. Staff should also receive supervision from an appropriately qualified member of the team in order to offer continued support and guidance.

- During the planning process resource implications should be identified with sufficient provision made for ongoing funds and materials/equipment.

- In order to maintain a high profile and promote the programme, systems should be developed to support it. A weekly programme of unit activities should be displayed in a prominent position as well as patients having their own specific programme. Staff should know what activities are planned and when. This could be built into shift handovers in which the allocation of staff to certain unit activities occurs if not already preplanned.

- Mechanisms should be in place for the multidisciplinary team to plan, evaluate and adapt the overall programme regularly, e.g. a monthly programme planning and review meeting.

This overall framework will enable patients to develop and maintain a routine, which will also assess changes in mental state and behaviour over a period of time. Such a framework will maximise the benefits of both individual and group activities related to self care, activities of daily living, productive and social/leisure pursuits. This not only provides staff with a focus for treatment, but also clearly demonstrates what is expected of patients.

Case history

Bob is a 38–year–old man with a long history of mental health and behavioural problems. During his admission to the PICU, he was frequently prone to violent outbursts directed towards staff and would press panic alarm buttons, much of which the team considered to be attention seeking behaviour. The occupational therapist chose to use an activity (painting) to engage him in a purposeful, non-confrontational way, therefore meeting his immediate need for individual attention and directing his energy towards a task. This demonstrated to the team that Bob was willing and able to engage in a practical activity, during which time no incidents occurred. Whilst the occupational therapist was working with the patient in the communal area the team was aware of the rationale for the activity and maintained an unobtrusive presence to support the activity. The benefits of engaging Bob were acknowledged including the monitoring of his mental state, enabling self-expression and reinforcing socially appropriate behaviour. This approach was continued by other members of the team to assist in his overall management and treatment.

Implementation of therapeutic activities

In order to prepare for activities within the PICU it is important to take into account the needs of the patient, establish treatment aims with the patient and consider how to adapt an activity to meet individual needs. Preparation for an activity session needs to consider the following five areas:

Environment

- The environment plays a significant part in meeting each patient's treatment goals. It should be organised in such a way as to enable patients to function and engage effectively. In many units the environmental design and space available is less than adequate and therefore requires innovative techniques to ensure the setting can be made appropriate for that particular activity.

- The overall management of the environment and organisation of the space, including the layout of furniture should reflect the group aims, patient group and the type of activity. This will have a significant effect on the level of interaction, the patient's sense of inclusion in the activity and the patient's ability to access resources. For example, a room should be at an appropriate temperature and have suitable light to enhance a patient's performance.

- The type of activity and the number of patients will dictate the most suitable location. This is often limited by the availability of space and safety issues. For example an activity requiring patient concentration and quiet should be within an area where there are few interruptions or noise from the ward, whereas those activities which are social in nature could take place in a communal area.

- Depending on the aims of the activity the facilitator can create a certain type of atmosphere. If a relaxed and welcoming environment is wanted, tea and biscuits could be provided; on the other hand an activity could be presented in a structured way in order to promote a work atmosphere allowing the patients to focus on a specific task.

- Wherever practicable, following appropriate risk assessment, patients should be encouraged to access other environments, within the hospital or local community to promote community living skills and reintegration. For example, utilising local leisure and sports centres, shops and cafés.

Resources

- It is important to identify what activities are required prior to the purchase of equipment. The investment in a sufficient range of resources should support the programmed activities and provide choice for patients engaging in diversional activities.

- An allocated budget will be required to maintain the range and availability of resource materials. This should be accessible to the activity facilitators.

- Prior to patients accessing a particular activity it is the clinical team's responsibility to assess their suitability to use resources required in the activity. The team assessing the patient's level of risk based on their current presentation and previous history could achieve this, e.g. assessing the patient's level of safety before attending a craft group in which scissors will be available. Staff facilitating the activity should have made the team aware of the equipment used within it; this will assist the team to make an informed decision.

- Patients involved in an activity using equipment such as glue, clay, tools, can be closely supervised, the equipment can be locked away before and directly after use, or adapted equipment could be used which minimises the level of risk.

Staffing

- In order to maximise the effectiveness and ensure consistency in the provision of therapeutic activities a designated person, responsible for progamme coordination and implementation of activities would be most appropriate.

- Staff on shift need to be aware of activities planned and enough people should be made available to directly facilitate or support the activity in terms of calling residents and motivating them to attend. This can be best achieved during staff handovers.

- Continuity and consistency in the provision of activities is important for individuals who have experienced chaotic and disruptive lifestyles prior to admission. Therefore activities should occur when they have been planned and at the time designated, wherever possible.

- Staff require sufficient time to plan the activity on the day, ensuring the room has been prepared, the equipment is available and the patients have been reminded of the activity.

- Recording of observations made during the activity should be incorporated into the time allocated to the activity.

Relaxation group

Case history

A relaxation group was held on the ward each Monday afternoon. It took place in a group room a small distance away from the ward communal area. Most chairs were moved out of the room, with some left around the edge for those who preferred to sit. Mats were laid on the floor, curtains were drawn and signs informing others that the group was in session placed strategically to ensure minimum disturbance. Staff were aware that the group was occurring and made sure that the ward remained relatively quiet and prevented unnecessary interruptions.

Activity

- The activity selected, should be based upon the identified needs of the patient(s). Each activity should have a specific aim, which may be to meet the individual's recognised treatment needs or for recreational purposes. These aims should be documented in order to ensure staff and patients are aware of why they are engaged in a particular activity. A file could be held centrally with current activity rationales accessible for staff (Figure 10.3).

- In order to monitor a patient's progress throughout their participation in an activity, records must be kept and contain sufficient as well as relevant information on a patient's behaviour, skills and interactions. An example of

---

Aim
To assist patients to cope more appropriately with stress and tension. To increase patient's level of awareness of the effect stress has on their feelings and behaviours.

Objectives
To provide a safe non-threatening environment for patients to utilise, learn and practice a range of relaxation techniques. To provide opportunities for patients to discuss the effect of stress and the techniques used. To assist patients to generalise relaxation techniques into their everyday lives.

Practical details
Location – Quiet, group room
Time – Monday 2.00–2.30
Facilitator – OT & Nurse
Equipment required – Cassette player and cassettes, relaxation mats
Criteria for group attendance – Open to patients on ward
  Patients should have an interest and/or desire to learn techniques
  Patients should be able to attend/concentrate for 30 minutes
  Patients' behaviour should not be disruptive to others

Figure 10.3 – Activity rationale

a form, which could be utilised to gather relevant information about a patient's performance, is given in Figure 10.4.

- The use of individual and group activities is dependent on the needs of the patient, which should be monitored on an ongoing basis. In some circumstances it may be appropriate for a patient to commence interacting on an individual basis, either because their behaviour is too disruptive or they are not yet able to cope within a group setting. It may be appropriate for some patients to initially undertake individual activities within a group setting to encourage socialisation and normalisation.

- It is important that activities are both achievable and challenging. If they are too easy or too difficult the patient can experience frustration. This could be perceived as a negative experience for the patient who may be less likely to engage in the future. It is therefore necessary to grade activities in order that the patient can experience success.

Preparing lasagne

This can be graded at different levels:

1. Purchase a ready-made lasagne, where all the patient has to do is place it in oven, time the meal and serve.
2. Prepare a lasagne using ready-made pasta and cheese sauces.
3. Prepare a cheese sauce using raw ingredients and ready-made pasta sauce.
4. Use all raw ingredients and provide a salad to accompany the meal.

The level of support given by staff would vary throughout this process. Initially this may be more practical and hands on, but gradually become less direct and more supportive in nature.

Date of activity:___/___/___Name of client:_____Name of activity:_____

Content: *(Brief details of format & activity completed.)*

Motivation: *(Willingness to attend, participation in activity, observed level of interest)*

Behaviour/Social Skills: *(Level & type of interaction, changes in mood/mental state, inappropriate or unsafe behaviour, non verbal communication)*

Cognition: *(Level of understanding, ability to follow verbal/written instructions, concentration, memory, problem solving, decision making, literacy & numeracy)*

Task Performance: *(Assistance required, accuracy, speed/impulsivity, gross motor control, planning, organising and sequencing tasks.)*

Facilitator: _____ Signature:_____Date: __/__/__

Figure 10.4 – Activity progress notes

Patient

- The patient should wherever possible be fully involved in deciding what activities they will participate in and the reasons why. This should be based on the patient's interests and needs and relate to their cultural beliefs.

- Patients should be informed of what is expected of them in terms of participation in the unit programme upon admission. Initially their involvement in the programme may be minimal or observational in nature. In some circumstances it may be necessary for the team initially to provide external structure/guidelines encouraging the patient to engage. The ultimate aim is to enable the patient to internalise this structure and make informed decisions about attendance at activities.

- A number of methods can be employed to increase the patient's motivation to participate in the therapeutic programme. If the patient is fully involved in determining their activity timetable, aware of benefits and given an individual, personalised copy of this, it is likely to improve their levels of motivation. It may be necessary to remind patients when they are due to attend activities on their timetable. It can be difficult to maintain the balance between enforcing attendance at an activity staff know will be of benefit and giving up after one refusal by the patient. This is best achieved through negotiation and maintaining respect for the patient's choice.

- The patient's ability to participate in a certain amount and type of activity is affected by their mental state. This should be considered and staff need to maintain realistic expectations of what the patient can practically achieve.

SUMMARY

This chapter has discussed a practical and achievable approach to treatment that can improve the overall quality of care received by the patient. It has outlined how activities used within a PICU can positively affect the patient's functioning, the ward atmosphere and the quality of staff interactions.

Some key factors have been highlighted which could assist a PICU in establishing, implementing and maintaining a ward therapeutic programme. Fundamental to this process is a multidisciplinary team commitment to this approach to care. The team should have realistic expectations as to what can be achieved, a clear, staged process of change and a recognition that this process will be gradual and may not always run smoothly. Each service should identify those factors, which may preclude the effectiveness of a programme and develop practical solutions to address them.

There are clearly documented benefits of providing therapeutic activities for patients who are admitted to psychiatric intensive care units, but these are not always easy to initiate and maintain. It is important to be aware of and to address the potential constraints and limitations within a PICU. The main difficulties appear to be associated with the environment, the patient group and staff practices/attitudes. Environmental constraints such as the lack of space, poor decor, inadequate resources, and lack of support and availability of staff can all contribute to the difficulties of implementing an activities programme. This requires staff to be flexible and innovative in order to maximise the potential of the service. The acute nature of the patients' illness and the intense level of input required poses a challenge for staff, which may lead to staff becoming de-motivated or burnt-out. A supportive therapeutic programme structure may assist staff to cope with these challenging needs, by focusing their energies on productive pursuits. It is recognised that considerable time and energy is often employed to maintain control, levels of safety and security. It has been demonstrated in the literature that the provision of activities can have a positive effect on an individual's progress and levels of aggression. Review of current practices could allow for an increased emphasis on the provision of activities programmes and therefore contribute to the creation of a more therapeutic and safe environment.

REFERENCES

Best D. 1996 The developing role of occupational therapy in psychiatric intensive care. Br J Occupat Therapy 59 (4): 161–164

Best D. 1997 Unpublished work

Canastey K, Roper J. 1997 Removal from stimuli for crisis intervention: using least restrictive methods to improve the quality of patient care. Issues Mental Health Nursing 18: 35–44

Christiansen C, Baum C. 1991 Occupational therapy overcoming human performance deficits. Slack Inc, New Jersey

Creek J. 1990 Occupational Therapy Practice and Mental Health. Edinburgh: Churchill Livingstone

Finlay L. 1998 Occupational Therapy Practice in Psychiatry. London: Croom Helm

Finlay L. 1994 Groupwork in Occupational Therapy. London: Chapman & Hall

Fottrell E. 1980 A study of violent behaviour among patients in psychiatric hospitals. Br J Psych 136: 216–221

Gentle J. 1996 Mental health intensive care: the nurses' experiences and perceptions of a new unit. J Adv Nurs 24: 1194–1200

Hopkins H, Smith H. 1988 In: Willard, Spackman Occupational Therapy, 7th edn. Lippincott, Philadelphia

Howells K, Hollin C. 1993 Clinical Approaches to Violence. Chichester: Wiley

Hume C, Pullen I. 1994 Rehabilitation for Mental Health Problems – An Introductory Handbook, 2nd edn. Edinburgh: Churchill Livingstone

Kielhofner G. 1980 A Model of Human Occupation Part 2: Ontogenesis from the perspective of temporal adaptation. AJOT 34: 657–663

Kielhofner G, Nicol M. 1989 The Model of Human Occupation: A Developing Conceptual Tool for Clinicians. BJOT 9: 210–214

Moore C. 1998 Acute inpatient care could do better. Survey Nursing Times 94 (3)

Muir-Cochrane E, Harrison B. 1996 Therapeutic interventions associated with seclusion of acutely disturbed individuals. J Psych Mental Health Nurs 3 (5): 319–325

Musisi S, Wasylenki D, Morton R. 1989 A psychiatric intensive care unit in a psychiatric hospital. Canadian J Psychiatry 34 (4): 200–204

Nelson N, Kaufman J, Silverstein B, Shields J. 1995 Patient and staff views on factors influencing assaults on psychiatric hospital staff. Issues Mental Health Nursing 16 No 5: 433–446

Nuffield Institute For Health. 1998 The mental health nursing care provided for acute psychiatric patients. Research Bulletin June

Palmstierna T, Huitfeldt B, Wistedt B. 1991 The relationship of overcrowding and aggressive behaviour on a psychiatric intensive care unit. Hospital and Community Psychiatry 42 (12): 1237–1240

Shepherd M, Lavender T. 1999 Putting aggression into context: an investigation in contextual factors influencing the rate of aggressive incidents in psychiatric hospitals. J Mental Health 8: 159–169

Sainsbury Centre. 1998 Acute Problems: A Survey of the Quality of Acute Psychiatric Wards. London Sainsbury Centre

Torpy D, Hall M. 1993 Violent incidents in a secure unit. J Forensic Psychiatry (3) 517–544

FURTHER READING

Allan E, Brown R, Laury G. 1988 Planning a psychiatric intensive care unit. Hospital and Community Psychiatry 39 (1): 81–83

Carpenter W, McGlashan T, Strauss J. 1997 The treatment of acute schizophrenia without drugs: An investigation of some assumptions Am J Psychiatry 134: 1 14–20

Cohen S, Khan A. 1980 Antipsychotic effect of milieu on the acute treatment of schizophrenia. Gen Hosp Psychiatry 12: 248–251

Felthons A. 1984 Preventing assaults on a psychiatric inpatient ward. Hospital and Community Psychiatry 35 (12)

Friis S. 1986 Characteristics of a good ward atmosphere. Acta Psychiatr Scand 74: 469–473

Goldney R *et al.* 1985 The psychiatric intensive care unit. Br J Psychiatry 146: 50–54

Gunderson J. 1980 A re-evaluation of milieu therapy for non-chronic schizophrenic patients. Schizophrenia Bulletin 6 (1): 64–69

Jeffry A, Goldney R. 1982 An innovation: the psychiatric intensive care unit. Australian Nurses' Journal 12 (5): 42–43, 49

Mitchell G. 1992 A survey of psychiatric intensive care units in Scotland. Health Bulletin May 50 (3): 228–32

Zigmond A. 1995 Special care wards: are they special? Psychiatric Bulletin (19): 310–312

SECTION 2:
FORENSIC AND
RISK ISSUES

11

RISK ASSESSMENT AND MANAGEMENT

Stephen M Pereira, Maurice Lipsedge

Part One: The violent patient

INTRODUCTION

Many view risk assessment as being firmly within the realm of forensic mental health practitioners. In everyday practice, however, all mental health practitioners knowingly or unknowingly pay attention to those factors that give rise to concern, either in the patient's history or at presentation. Indeed, the Care Programme Approach (Department of Health 1992) requires the assessment of need including risk. Mention of a formal risk assessment often arouses anxieties in staff carrying out the assessment. 'Risk assessment is surrounded by an aura of mystique, which it does not deserve. The basis for risk management is a thorough clinical assessment, which any multi-disciplinary team should be able to undertake' (Maden 1996).

This chapter focuses on those issues relevant to everyday practice encountered by PICU multidisciplinary teams. De-institutionalisation has lead to a larger number of potentially high risk patients living in the community, some not in receipt of adequately resourced care. Owing to a shortage of inpatient beds, especially in inner cities, largely those who are seriously at risk to others or themselves are usually admitted to these beds. Thus, there has been increased preoccupation with risk identification of patients. It is important to get this right as often as possible, not least because at least half of reported incidents of assault are thought by victims to be avoidable (Aiken 1984).

Various inquiries into homicides and serious incidents comment on the inability of services to manage seriously disturbed individuals with difficult behaviour and the lack of appropriate facilities for this group, e.g. the Clunis Inquiry (1994). Various other shortcomings have been identified: poor or absent consultant supervision; poor communication of important information within the team and other relevant people (including relatives); lack of opportunities for training in risk assessment and inadequate resources of space and of trained staff (Birley 1996). It is impossible to conclude whether there is a real or apparent increase in violence. Increased awareness, fear of litigation and better methods of recording and reporting may account for higher figures in recent times. However, a review by Taylor and Gunn (1999) concluded that, over a 38-year period, there was little fluctuation in the numbers of people with a mental illness committing criminal homicide. In the UK, the Confidential Inquiry into Suicide and Homicide (1999) found that people convicted of homicide have substantial rates of mental disorder (44%) but most do not have severe mental illness or a history of contact with mental health services (Shaw et al 1999). Shaw et al's data correspond to around 40 homicides per year by people who have been in contact with mental health services in the previous 12 months. Shaw et al's was from a total of 718 homicides reported to the inquiry. Discussion of risk assessment invariably involves risk to self, although risk to others is a larger public preoccupation.

Maden (1996) in his excellent review advocates the importance of distinguishing between the assessment of dangerousness and that of risk. Violence researchers (e.g. Steadman *et al* 1993) also urge mental health professionals to be concerned with risk, rather than dangerousness for the following reasons. Firstly, risk can be objectively assessed, secondly, the context in which the risk behaviour occurs can be considered, thirdly, risk can be subdivided into further manageable components and finally risk is not static and therefore lends itself to be managed over time.

The PICU clinician is often asked to make an assessment of risk at various stages.

- At the community interface, e.g. police stations, A&E departments, Section 136 rooms, prisons, courts.

- At the inpatient interface, e.g. acute and other inpatient facilities.

- Within the PICU, e.g. at admission, ongoing assessments, considering leave arrangements.

- At the point of discharge from the PICU.

The ability to carry out a comprehensive risk assessment is often compromised by the urgency of the request for admission to the PICU and acuteness of the patient's behavioural disturbance. Some other factors that can influence a thorough risk assessment and the subsequent decision to admit or not are:

- Training and experience of the assessor.

- Availability of clinical information.

- Knowledge of local service, e.g. training, experience of staff managing the situation.

- Availability of local resources.

It is important to consider the factors that are available from research whilst assessing patients at the community interface. These are listed in Table 11.1.

Swanson *et al* (1990), in a massive survey of the general population, the Epidemiologic Catchment Area (ECA) study in the USA, found that delusional symptoms, independent of diagnosis, appear to have a significant association with violence. Patients with a combination of delusions and alcohol abuse had a high risk of violence. Other community surveys (e.g. Link and Stueve 1994) showed similar findings. The delusions that were particularly relevant included delusions of influence and control, e.g. that one's mind was dominated by forces beyond one's control, thoughts were being inserted into one's mind and there were people who wished to do one harm. Particular mental disorders with high rates of violence include schizophrenia, major affective disorder and substance abuse.

Table 11.1 – Risk factors associated with violence (Clinical Practice Guidelines, The Royal College of Psychiatrists 1998)

Demographic or personal history
- A history of violence
- Youth, male gender
- Stated threat of violence
- Association with a subculture prone to violence

Clinical variables
- Alcohol or other substance misuse, irrespective of diagnosis
- Active symptoms of schizophrenia or mania, in particular if:
  - delusions or hallucinations are focused on a particular person
  - there is specific preoccupation with violence
  - there are delusions of control, particularly with a violent theme
  - there is agitation, excitement, overt hostility or suspiciousness
- Poor collaboration with suggested treatments
- Antisocial, explosive or impulsive personality traits

Situational factors
- Extent of social support
- Immediate availability of a weapon
- Relationship to potential victim

Whilst it is clear that violent people are more likely to demonstrate symptoms of mental disorder and that those mentally disordered are more likely to be violent, it is important to put these findings into perspective. Swanson's ECA study shows that 4–5% of violent acts are committed by persons with major mental illness. When linked with co-morbid substance abuse the figure rises by another 5–6%. Substance abusers without mental illness contributed to 27% of violent acts. The Confidential Inquiry (1999) found that of 500 homicides for whom psychiatric reports were available (out of a total of 718 reported homicides, 1996–1997), 102 were in contact with mental health services at some time. However, only 71 had a mental disorder. The commonest diagnosis was personality disorder (20 cases). Alcohol and drug misuse was common.

Table 11.2 – DSM-IV categories which include violence and aggression

1. Alcohol-related disorders
2. Amphetamine intoxication
3. Inhalant intoxication
4. Phencyclidine intoxication
5. Antisocial personality disorder
6. Borderline personality disorder
7. Dementia
8. Delirium
9. Intermittent explosive disorder
10. Mental retardation
11. Conduct disorder
12. Oppositional defiant disorder
13. Post-traumatic stress disorder
14. Personality change due to a general medical condition, aggressive type
15. Sexual sadism
16. Schizophrenia, paranoid type

A UK study of violence and verbal abuse in 233 accident and emergency departments found that alcohol, waiting times, recreational drug use and patient expectations were perceived as the main causes of violence (Jenkins *et al* 1998). Table 11.2 lists some mental disorders which include violence.

When assessing risk, it is important to enquire not only into the harm being threatened, but also about a variety of other factors, as outlined below:

SOME QUESTIONS TO ASSIST A RISK ASSESSMENT FRAMEWORK

Harm factors

Harm that has occurred, or that is being threatened.

- Description and frequency of the threat or act or thought or fantasy (is this provoked or spontaneous)?
- What risk is being considered, e.g. harm to self or others?
- How serious is the potential harm?
- How serious was the act/s (or if committed did the patient express remorse)?
- Why is the harm being considered or, if committed, reason for the act?
- What is the intent?
- Who or what is at risk?
- Is there a concrete plan, e.g. when, where?
- Does the patient have access to instruments of harm?
- What is the likelihood of harm occurring?

Diagnostic factors

- Does the patient suffer from a mental illness?
- How active are the features of the patient's illness?
- Does the patient have an associated substance abuse and/or personality disorder, e.g. antisocial, borderline, sadistic?
- Does the patient suffer from a developmental or acquired brain damage or disorder?

Predispositional/historical factors

- Does the patient have a previous history of violence?

- Are there any relevant childhood or familial factors?

- Does the patient suffer from chronic anger, hostility, resentment, low tolerance for frustration, have difficulty in delaying gratification, a sadistic orientation?

- Does the patient have a history of loss of control?

- Is the patient impulsive?

- Has the patient exhibited remorse for his/her past acts?

Contextual factors

- Does the patient have stress factors, e.g. loss, frustration, provocation?

- What are the patient's usual coping strategies?

- Does the patient feel well supported by family and/or professional carers?

- In an inpatient ward:

  - is the ward overcrowded?

  - is there a high number of temporary staff?

  - does it lack clear leadership, training, experience and morale?

- Is the patient frank and cooperative or guarded, irritable, defensive?

- Is the patient over aroused, agitated and excited?

- Is the patient compliant with prescribed treatments?

  - is the patient on the appropriate medication, taking an appropriate dose?

  - is the patient engaging with nursing, OT, psychological interventions?

- How disruptive/dangerous is the patient's current behaviour?

N.B. Obtaining collateral information, carrying out a detailed mental state examination and reviewing past case notes are important for a good risk assessment.

Prediction of violence is very difficult. A reasonable degree of success can be achieved in short-term prediction, i.e. the near future, but not so for longer-term violence prediction. Published research so far does not provide any clear consensus on criteria that would be clinically useful, across the different varieties of clinical settings. In addition these difficulties arise due to variations in the period covered, choice of predictor items, patient sampling, level of detail provided in the studies, methods of analysis and the way in which available actuarial scales are used.

Thus, various actuarial measures have been used in risk assessment. These are fraught with methodological difficulties, e.g. inter-rater reliability; conceptual difficulties, e.g. definition of violence; and measure different target behaviours, e.g. internally, externally directed violence. Some actuarial measures assess risk factors, e.g. Novaco Anger Scale, Barratt's Impulsivity Scale, Hare Psychopathy Checklist, Maudsley Assessment Delusions Schedule. Various other aggression scales are also in use, e.g. Staff Observation Aggression Scale, Overt Aggression Scale, Global Aggression Scale. Self rating, e.g. Hostility and Direction of Hostility Questionnaire and general questionnaires, e.g. Buss Durkee Hostility Inventory, have also been used. For a review of some of these measures, see Mak and Koning (1995) and Monahan and Steadman (1994). It must be emphasised that none of these measures are a substitute for a comprehensive history and clinical examination of a patient.

EVENTS THAT INDICATE IMMINENT VIOLENCE IN PSYCHIATRIC SETTINGS

The rate of violence towards mental health workers is much higher than in any other occupation. Psychiatric nurses are particularly at risk. A review by Whittington (1994) indicated that 90% of assaults by psychiatric patients are directed at nurses. This figure is not surprising given their role as direct, round-the-clock caregivers and is a significant occupational risk. Rates of violence against psychiatrists range from 32 to 42%. Jones (1985) found that of assaults in psychiatric facilities, 65% were against staff and 32% were directed at other patients or property. Various attempts have been made to examine the accuracy of patient behaviour as a predictor of imminent violence. Powell *et al* (1994) examined antecedents for 1000 incidents in three psychiatric hospitals over a 13-month period. They allocated incidents to 15 categories of antecedents. The most common antecedents were:

- Patient agitation or disturbance

- Restrictions being placed on patients associated with routine hospital regime

- Provocation by other patients, relatives, visitors.

Interestingly, they found that incidents arising from staff members initiating contact with patients was very rare. The study also confirmed the experience of most PICU clinicians that a small number of largely detained patients were involved in a high number of incidents. These patients were more likely to commit assaults after certain incidents, e.g. self-harm, absconding and arson. Whittington and Patterson (1996) studied verbal and non-verbal behaviour immediately prior to assault. These included: verbal abuse, high overall activity, standing uncomfortably close, etc. However, a large number of these behaviours were also exhibited by patients who did not assault staff members. There is, on the other hand, general agreement amongst researchers that only a small number of assaults occur in the absence of any behavioural predictors (3% of the sample in the Whittington Study). The clinical practice guidelines (CPG) also identified possible antecedents of violence. Some other researches (e.g. Aiken 1984, Lanza 1988) believe that the highest predictor for assault is what has been variously described as the 'pre-assaultative tension state' or the 'acute excitement phase'. These cues may seem obvious, but go unheeded on many occasions. Taken together with the experience of many clinicians, it may be suggested that the above factors in younger male patients who are more acutely ill, e.g. floridly psychotic and under-medicated, may lead them to present with higher rates of violence.

SOME FACTORS LEADING TO VIOLENCE IN PICU

Sheridan *et al* (1990) identified some of these factors in inpatient settings that apply equally to PICUs. These include:

- Patient–staff conflict (e.g. limit setting, denial of privileges)

- Conflict with other patients

- Patient's personal problems (e.g. money, family, social problems)

- Events internal to patients (e.g. delusions, hallucinations, confusion).

McNeil and Binder (1994), in their study of 330 patients admitted to a locked short stay unit, explored the relationship between acute psychiatric symptoms, diagnosis and short-term risk of violence. The proportions of violence by diagnosis were: schizophrenia 36%, mania 28%, organic psychosis 27%, the rest 12%. A complex analysis of BPRS (Brief Psychiatric Rating Score) and the OAS (Overt Aggression Scale) showed three summary scores significantly associated with violence. These were hostile-suspiciousness, agitation-excitement and thinking disturbance. Palmstierna and Wistedt (1990) found that risk factors for aggressive behaviour are of limited value in predicting the violent behaviour of acute involuntarily admitted patients. The only predictors of some value in the immediate future (first 8 days) was previous damage to property or person, and in the near future (first 28 days) was use of drugs other than alcohol.

Derived from available literature and clinical experience, some of the features are summarised below.

Cues suggestive of imminent violence

Physical cues

These are largely features of motor overactivity and include:

- Agitation, arousal, restlessness, pacing

- Physical tension, rigid posture, erratic movements
- Threatening gestures or stance
- Glaring, breathlessness, aggressive to objects (e.g. thumping tables, walls) or self (e.g. banging head).

Mood cues
- 'Irritable', 'upset', angry, 'high' or elated, lability of mood.

Speech cues
- Verbal threats, abuse, swearing
- Complaining, demanding or refusal to communicate
- Loud and pressured speech.

Thought and perceptual cues
- Inability to concentrate or register information
- Unclear or disordered thought processes
- Bizarre, paranoid, persecutory, violent thoughts and delusions
- Active hallucinations, usually auditory, sometimes visual
- Preoccupation with violent themes in thinking
- Confusion, disorientation.

Boundary cues
- Perception by patient that his/her own space/boundaries, privacy is being violated
- Persistent intrusion by patient of others' personal space, e.g. standing very close.
- Insistence that demands be met immediately, however unrealistic.

Contextual and past cues
- Early warning signs elicited from previous episodes of violence
- Current reports from carers, other patients or self of angry feelings, unmet demands
- Current use of illicit substances or alcohol
- Poor frustration tolerance and other coping strategies.

Therapeutic cues

- Breakdown in rapport

- Uncooperativeness, lack of encouragement

- Usually worsening mental state

- Failure to respond to reassurance, de-escalation, time out or other previously successful, agreed strategies.

RISK MANAGEMENT

There is acknowledgement from various inquiry panels that, even in the best run service, the possibility remains that something may go wrong. The UK National Confidential Inquiry into Homicides (Shaw *et al* 1999) recognised that mentally ill patients committed only a small proportion of homicides annually and that these patients were only a small fraction of the total number of psychiatric patients. It also called for recognition of the limitations to what treatment of mental illness alone could achieve in preventing homicides.

The key issue, however, remains that, whilst one may not be able to eliminate the risk of a serious untoward incident, various systems can be put into place to reduce the risk of these occurring. 'Inquiries into homicides by psychiatric patients suggest that, when things do go wrong, it is usually because of basic failures in procedure. If services are based on good clinical practice, most risk can be safely managed' (Maden 1996). Some of the systems referred to above have been further discussed in the chapters on Management of the Acutely Disturbed patient (Chapter 2) and Good Practice Issues in PICUs (Chapter 17).

Reith (1998) identified four major themes that were consistently lacking in care provided to violent patients:

1. Thoroughness (detailed and accurate recording of information)

2. Communication and liaison (proper inter-agency cooperation and real team working)

3. Listening to all members of the clinical team (recognising and valuing the contribution of all staff, especially junior members, who are in contact with the patient)

4. Listening to those closest to the patient (careful attention being paid to the experience and understanding of relatives and carers).

Some of these issues have been also highlighted by the Department of Health, UK in Building Bridges (1995): 'The key principle of risk assessment is to use all available sources of information . . .' and the Blom-Cooper Inquiry (1995): 'Professionals need to be trained to trust the experienced judgement of close family rather than rely on their own impressions made at one isolated assessment', to name a few.

The National Confidential Inquiry in its full report, Safer Services, make 31 recommendations for changes in clinical practice. These include: training in risk assessment, documentation, use of specific drug and psychological treatments, changes in the Mental Health Act to allow compulsory treatment, e.g. in the community, etc.

In the PICU setting, risk management should be considered in multiple domains.

The patient domain

With a view towards adequately managing risk on the PICU, as much information as possible should be obtained via referral forms, and full discussion with the referring service prior to admission. Very urgent clinical need takes priority over this requirement but this should very much be the exception rather than the rule.

Standardised assessment forms, incorporating a clinical risk assessment framework and some objective measures help contribute towards obtaining a fuller picture. This also reduces the risk of idiosyncratic PICU assessments based on personality, judgmental attitudes, level of training on part of the assessor. Response times to requests for admission to PICU should be derived by local discussion with contracted referrers. This gives a clear idea as to the type of risk being managed and over a defined period of time. Clinical experience shows that disturbance is moderated over a period of time by initiated treatment strategies including appropriate nursing interventions, adequate medication regimens, appropriate placements. This is especially true for disturbance due to mental illness, but not necessarily so for those with personality disorders, co-morbid substance misuse, acquired or developmental brain disorders and treatment resistant conditions.

Those patients considered unsuitable for admission to the PICU should be discussed further in detail with the referring teams. This would serve the purpose of providing a second multidisciplinary team opinion and advice regarding management of the patient. These opinions should be accepted in the spirit in which they are given rather than 'we don't require them to tell us what to do', or viewed as being undermining of the care plan in place. Feedback should be provided to referrers as soon as possible for those who are accepted or not, to the PICU. Clinical situations can change rapidly. All PICU assessments should be flexible to acknowledge this.

Once admitted to the PICU, multidisciplinary protocols derived from the most up-to-date guidance from peer bodies, research, audit, code of practice, should govern all clinical practice. Some of the areas thus regulated are outlined below. Risk assessment should occur as often as is required in the PICU, clearly documented, with at least one or two full multidisciplinary team risk reviews involving referrers and all involved carers.

The discharge from the PICU should contain clear guidance regarding identified risk factors, the context in which risk behaviours occur, and suggested multidisciplinary strategies to manage them. It is essential that referrers at the very least attend predischarge reviews of their patients. This ensures a smooth transition of care back to the catchment area wards. Unless PICUs are adequately resourced with community or assertive outreach services, discharge should always occur back to the catchment area wards to enable full planning and delivery of previously identified care needs by the referring catchment area teams.

Every service should identify the small group of mentally ill patients who are most at risk, especially to others, when relapsing, in the community. Doing so enables the service to fast track admissions to the appropriate secure facility or environment. However, good practice would suggest this should be to the acute open inpatient ward in the first instance, with appropriate safeguards, e.g. predetermined medication, nursing strategies, to prevent labelling and thus stigmatisation of this group of patients as being always violent. In a significant number of cases, even such patients usually settle down on admission to the open ward.

The staff domain

PICUs can be particularly effective in safely modifying the outcome of violent, destructive acts, once they have started. However, the real expertise of PICU clinicians should be in the area of early identification of violent, aggressive thoughts, feelings and behaviour, thereby preventing their occurrence at best, or reducing their frequency at the very least.

All staff in the PICU should be trained to recognise the early warning signs predisposing to violence. This entails drawing up individual risk assessment profiles. In order to do this crucial information should be gleaned from past notes, discussion with referrers, other professional carers and relatives. This should be as detailed and accurate as possible. Particular attention is paid to psychopathology, personality factors, coping strategies, past violence (see risk assessment framework). This should be incorporated in multidisciplinary team care plans.

Ability to identify risk factors in itself is insufficient to manage it, within the PICU. Staff should be able to respond to the many crises that develop in an effective and professional manner. For example, there is evidence to show that training in the methods of control and restraint (C&R) can lead to a reduction in violent behaviour and injury to both staff and patients. Reasons suggested include greater confidence engendered in staff by such training, enabling them to defuse situations before they escalate (Gold Award 1976, Lion 1977). Before employing C&R, other strategies such as time out, talking down and de-escalation techniques (see Chapter 3) should be considered. This presumes that staff teams possess skills in verbal and behavioural interventions and are able to react to patients in a non-provocative manner (Tardiff and Sweillam 1982).

Thus a balance is required between professional, confident management and rigid judgmental authoritarian attitudes that may develop. This in itself may predispose to further violence. Over-controlling, authoritarian staff rarely socialise with patients and have little person to person contact with them, unless the interaction involves limit setting or confrontation (Sanson-Fisher *et al* 1979, Hodges *et al* 1986). Being able to identify issues relevant to counter-transference e.g. a professional's negative feelings towards a patient, especially with chronically disturbed and personality disordered or dual diagnosis patients can play an important role in provocation and therefore prevention of patient violence.

Although, seclusion rooms are used as part of a risk management plan, a significant number of PICUs do not have these. No strong evidence-based conclusions can be derived from the literature advocating or diminishing the usefulness of this practice. If employed, staff should have rigorous training in avoiding the situation escalating to a level requiring seclusion and in the monitoring standards expected once a patient is in seclusion.

Clear evidence-based protocols are required in the use of rapid tranquilisation and emergency medication (see Chapter 4) as part of an effective risk management plan. Distinctions need to be drawn between short-term and long-term usage of medication in risk management, e.g. administration of benzodiazepines as required in schizophrenic patients is significantly high. It is possible that staff resort to medication too easily and increasing non-medication techniques may reduce the need for such prescriptions (Paton *et al* 2000).

The multidisciplinary domain

Psychological therapies are effective in reducing levels of violence. For example, cognitive behavioural therapy is effective for anger problems (Beck and Fernandez 1998). Some patients respond to a primarily behavioural programme. Talking and listening must be regarded as active interventions, as they are greatly valued by patients (The Royal College of Psychiatrists 1998). All PICUs should have dedicated input from a psychologist, not only to help develop effective interventions for patients, but also to provide regular support and supervision to staff working in this high risk subspecialty. The role of an occupational therapist in the PICU is discussed elsewhere in the book (see Chapter 10). The role of the pharmacist in advising medication strategies and planning medication reviews is a very important one. Dedicated input from social workers or support workers is crucial in helping to understand family dynamics, social stresses and supports and in providing practical help. This goes a long way in allaying short-term anxiety, irritability, reduces provocation and helps long-term planning of care at an early stage. The important contributions made by other professional carers and relatives in risk assessment and management cannot be over-emphasised. Their involvement is mandatory in planning care.

The environmental domain

Several factors affect how the therapeutic milieu can influence effective management of risk. These include design, quality, comfort of accommodation, as well as staff support, patient participation in decision making, e.g. community meetings and patient autonomy. It may be suggested that the milieu is one of the most important factors influencing the outcome of treatment. Psychotic patients (e.g. in PICUs) seem to benefit primarily from a milieu with a high level of support, practical orientation, order and organisation (Frilis 1986). This may help to maintain a low level of anger and aggression.

Drinkwater and Gudjonsson (1989) found that for the majority of patients observed on the ward, 89% of their day consisted of no planned activities. She reported that the frequency of violent incidents was, on average, four times higher during periods without planned activities, in addition to other prohibited behaviours, e.g. being verbally abusive, breaking ward rules. It has been suggested that wards with low levels of planned activities and staff–patient interaction appear to foster violence.

Ensuring an appropriate mix of skills and staff gender has a role in risk management. Reports from both psychiatric and forensic hospitals show that employing female staff on male wards (Levy and Hartocollis 1976) or male staff in a female-only PICU at Rampton High Security Hospital (Carton and Larkin 1991) led to a reduction in violent incidents.

The organisational domain

The main features are summarised in the risk management framework below. This includes clear management support of clinical staff in ensuring a safe and clinically effective environment for patients. Firm backing from managers leads to a high morale amongst staff. Organisational responsibilities include training, specification of responsibilities, appraisal of performance and job stability (The Royal College of Psychiatrists 1998).

Developing policies, e.g. prosecution of violent patients, should be carefully considered by organisations. With the growing number of violent patients being admitted to hospital, a principled, uniform, rational deterrent response needs to be in place to protect other patients and staff. Most carers find this very difficult to do for ethical, legal and professional considerations.

Drinkwater and Gudjonsson (1989) suggest the following advantages in reporting serious assaults on staff:

• It highlights the seriousness of the offence to the patient.

- It ensures that the offence is properly recorded and investigated by an independent authority.

- It is the court who decides the appropriate outcome for criminal offences, not the clinical team.

- It enables staff to apply for compensation for personal injuries, e.g. to the Criminal Injuries Compensation Board.

- It helps maintain staff morale, which tends to be poor in settings where physical assaults are common.

There are some arguments against having such a policy. Some would consider such policies as being radical, open to abuse, affecting patient confidentiality and that violent attacks are an occupational hazard that staff members should learn to accept. Although, some contend that prosecuting a patient is never justified, this position is unwarranted (Appelbaum and Appelbaum 1991). Having such a policy regarding persecution of patients prevents inconsistent, idiosyncratic decision making and sends a clear message to habitually violent patients.

Table 11.3 – Important PICU multidisciplinary team skills to assist risk management

1. Initiate, communicate, develop rapport and a caring professional relationship with patients.
2. Listen effectively, communicate clearly.
3. Learn to identify verbal and non-verbal cues.
4. Write concise, easily understood, legible case notes.
5. Validate perceptions.
6. Create a therapeutic milieu by individual and collective participation in programmes.
7. Develop easily available and clearly understood risk management plans.
8. Watch for signs of negative attitudes to patients, environmental stresses and examine own coping strategies.
9. Pay attention to personal and professional development.
10. Ask for help in managing difficult situations.

It is important that PICU teams develop a culture of change and learning. Mason and Chandley (1999) suggest that units which have such cultures not only quickly develop strategies that keep them abreast of recent advances in their field but also 'become places in which it is pleasurable to work and morale is high. They offer job opportunities and experience and there is a feeling of worth in the establishment'.

A FRAMEWORK FOR RISK MANAGEMENT

Harm factors

Well rehearsed, clearly understood

- Management of acute disturbance protocols, displayed/easily available

- Experienced, trained staff delivering well rehearsed interventions, e.g. de-escalation

- Regular reviews by keyworker and the multidisciplinary team of the risk assessment and management plan

- Clear action plan, communicated to all appropriate individuals, within and outside teams, organisations

- Critical incident analysis after all events.

Diagnostic factors

- Review of diagnosis and associated conditions

- Comprehensive and thorough case notes review of past history, adverse incidents, response to interventions etc.

- Highlighted risk factors, early warning signs of relapse with patients

- Easy accessibility of such information involving high risk individuals especially when seen in emergency settings, e.g. community, Accident and Emergency.

Predispositional/historical factors

- Past history of violence (descriptions of act/s, intent, remorse, weapons used if any, severity of injury, outcome), expression of remorse

- Childhood factors (brutality or deprivation, decreased warmth, affection in the home, early loss of parent, fire setting, bed wetting, cruelty to animals)

- Psychological profiles of high risk individuals, e.g. anger, self view as a victim, resentful of authority, recklessness, impulsivity.

Contextual factors

Particular attention is paid to

- Ward design and safety issues (e.g. lines of observation), suitability of placement and secure areas on wards

- Alarm systems and rehearsed contingency plans

- A well-structured therapeutic milieu

- Careful assessment of immediate and longer-term social supports

- Accessibility to named and experienced link workers to fast-track known violent patients to appropriate care

- Accessibility to longer-term risk minimisation strategies, e.g. short- and long-term psychotherapies.

Organisational and management factors

- Well-developed policies, procedures, protocols covering all areas of clinical practice

- Well-defined, regularly updated management policies and leadership in areas of risk strategy

- Collaboration with service users in planning clinical environments, policies, monitoring practices

- Regular availability and monitoring of staff training, e.g. risk assessment and management, morale, multidisciplinary working

- Policies sensitive to patient care in relation to overcrowding, individuality and choice, privacy, gender and ethnic mix, ward layout, safe activity areas, etc.

- Central recording and regular clinical audit, e.g. seclusion, control and restraint, adverse incidents

- Well-developed liaison with local services, e.g. police, forensic.

Part Two: The suicidal patient

INTRODUCTION

Violent and self-destructive behaviour can, of course, co-exist and, as with predictions of violence, forecasts of deliberate self-harm can be safely made only for fairly short periods. By the same token, risk must be reviewed in the light of changes and symptoms and alterations in the personal, domestic, social and legal circumstances of the patient. As with predictions of violence, a realistic short time-frame and ongoing reviews are essential.

A rolling in-house training programme on suicide awareness and prevention will reduce the frequency of false-negative predictions. It is salutary to recall that many of the suicides reported to the Confidential Inquiry (1996) were totally unexpected by medical and nursing staff.

However, completed suicide is a relatively rare event and many patients on the PICU will have identifiable risk factors such as co-morbidity, personality disorders or a past history of deliberate self-harm. The high rate of false-positive predictions might demotivate staff by creating a sense of complacency or of frustration at ostensibly unnecessary restrictions on patients and the imposition of a regime of intrusive surveillance. It is hoped that specific guidelines will reduce the risk of a counter-productively excessive caution on the one hand and a casual recklessness on the other. Reduction of the risk of suicide in the PICU requires vigilant awareness of the various factors which might increase the frequency of deliberate self-harm. Recognised risk factors include:

- Declared intent

- A previous history of deliberate self-harm

- Clinical risk factors

- 'Malignant alienation'

- Demographic and social factors

- Physical features of the unit.

Declared suicidal intentions

A threat to harm oneself should never be disregarded. Even the most transparently 'manipulative' threat has to be assessed in the context of the patient's current mental state, preoccupations, frustrations and personal and social circumstances. Conversely, the absence of any declared suicidal intention does not mean that the risk is negligible.

For example, patients with persecutory delusions and threatening auditory hallucinations sometimes kill themselves as a way of escaping from imaginary torturers and executioners, even in the absence of a frank depressive illness.

Previous history of deliberate self-harm

It is dangerous to assume that there is little risk just because a particular patient has survived numerous previous episodes of deliberate self-harm (DSH). One per cent of patients who harm themselves will go on to commit suicide within one year, while the risk of subsequent suicide during the 10 years after an episode of deliberate self-harm is 30 times higher than in the general population.

Clinical risk factors

Fifteen per cent of patients with bipolar-affective disorder and 10% of people with schizophrenia kill themselves. In schizophrenia, the risk of suicide is often associated in young people (especially men) with a fear of deterioration, and also after a recent discharge and development of insight. Alcohol and drug addiction also have a well-known association with suicide (King 1984).

'Malignant alienation' (Watts and Morgan 1994)

Just as the quality of the relationship between patients and staff can be a strong predictor of violence (Beauford et al 1997), and the initial therapeutic alliance helps in evaluating psychiatric patients' risk of violence, so the lack of a therapeutic alliance also correlates with a higher risk of suicide. 'Malignant alienation' describes a potentially lethal distancing of the patient from staff, from other patients and from relatives. This is particularly likely to happen with patients who are regarded as manipulative or attention-seeking.

Demographic and social risk factors

Although suicide is commonest in the elderly, there has been a significant increase in suicide in young men over the past 15 years (Hawton et al 1997). Other risk factors include divorce, unemployment and recent bereavement. Further demographic and social factors that are worth noting are that suicide is more common in men, in those aged over 45, divorced, single or widowed and is associated with unemployment and retirement. Highest rates are in social classes I and V. Other associations have been made with broken homes in childhood, loss of role, mental and physical illness, and social disorganisation, including criminality, drug and alcohol misuse.

Physical safety features of the unit

Structures such as brackets or curtain rails should not be weight-bearing whilst false ceilings should not provide easy access to electric wiring. Windows must be made of unbreakable glass and stairwells have to be made safe. Obviously exit from the unit has to be controlled.

Search procedures have to be implemented according to clear guidelines to remove potentially dangerous objects such as scissors, lighters, etc.

EVALUATION AND MANAGEMENT OF SHORT-TERM SUICIDE RISK

- Evaluate past and recent deliberate self-harm and declared intention and preparations

- Assess mental state and look for despair, pessimism, anhedonia, morbid guilt, severe insomnia, self-neglect, agitation and panic attacks

- Consider recent adverse life events

- Assess the quality of relationships with staff and others. Has the patient established a working alliance with the key worker or any other member of the team?

- The patient should be explicitly encouraged to approach staff when distressed and to discuss suicidal ideas openly.

Caution (Morgan and Stanton 1997)

- The period shortly after admission carries a high risk of deliberate self-harm

- Extra vigilance is also required during shift handovers

- With a misleading clinical improvement and temporary amelioration of distress, but without resolution of stress factors, be aware of the possibility of a reluctance to talk specifically about suicide (the patient's level of distress might fluctuate markedly throughout the day).

Observation

Intensive, supportive observation allows close monitoring of behaviour and mental state. The level of supportive observation has to be agreed jointly by the patient's key worker together with medical and other members of the team. It must be recorded and passed on to all the unit staff as well as to the patient. The level of observation can be intensified unilaterally by the nursing staff and reviewed at every change of nursing shift as well and regularly by senior nursing and medical staff.

Repeatedly asking patients the same questions with each change of staff can have an obvious alienating effect. On the other hand, one-to-one, special or continuous care observation provides an opportunity for staff to work intensively with the suicidal patient using a cognitive approach to suicidal preoccupations. See helpful guidelines on cognitive therapy for suicidal behaviour (Weishaar and Beck 1990).

The Good Practice Statement of the CRAG/SCOTMEG Working Group with Mental Illness (1995) provides clear guidelines on nursing observation.

REFERENCES

Aiken GJM. 1984 Assaults on staff in a locked ward: Predictions and consequences. Med Sci Law 24: 199–207

Appelbaum KL, Appelbaum PS. 1991 A model hospital policy on prosecuting patients for presumptively criminal acts. Hosp and Community Psychiatry, 42: 1233–1237

Beauford JE, McNiel DE, Binder RL. 1997 Utility of the initial therapeutic alliance in evaluating psychiatric patients' risk of violence Am J Psychiatry 154: 1272–1276

Beck R, Fernandez E. 1998 Cognitive behaviour therapy in the treatment of anger: a meta-analysis. Congitive Therapy and Research, 22: 63–74

Birley J. 1996 Homicide and suicide by the mentally ill. J Forensic Psychiatry 7: 234–237

Blom-Cooper L. 1995 The Falling shadow – One Patient's Mental Health Care 1978–1993. Report of the Committee of Inquiry into the Events Leading up to and Surrounding the Fatal Incident at the Edith Morgan Centre, Torbay on 1 September 1993 (Chair: Louis Blom-Cooper). London: Duckworth

Carton G, Larkin E. 1991 Reducing violence in a Special Hospital. Nursing Standard, 5(17): 29–31

Clunis Inquiry. 1994 The Report of the Inquiry into the Care and Treatment of Christopher Clunis (Chair: Jean Ritchie QC). London: HMSO

Confidential Inquiry into Homicides and Suicides. 1996 Report of the Confidential Inquiry into Homicides and Suicides by Mentally Ill People. London: Royal College of Psychiatrists

CRAG/SCOTMEG Working Group on Mental Illness, May 1995. Final Report. Nursing Observation of Acutely Ill Psychiatric Patients in Hospital: A Good Practice Statement

Department of Health. 1992 The Health of the Nation. Strategy for Health in England. London: HMSO

Department of Health. 1995 Building Bridges – A Guide to Arrangements for Inter-agency Working for the Care and Protection of Severely Mentally Ill People. London: HMSO, p. 88

Drinkwater J, Gudjonsson GH. 1989 The nature of violence in psychiatric hosptials. In: Clinical Approaches to Violence. K. Howell, C.R. Hollin (eds). Chichester: John Wiley

Frilis S. 1986 Characteristics of a good ward atmosphere. Acta Psychiatr Scand 74: 469–473

Gold Award. 1976 A program for the prevention and management of disturbed behaviour. Hospital and Community Psychiatry 25: 725–727

Hawton K, Fagg J, Simkin S, Bale E, Bond A. 1997 Trends in deliberate self-harm in Oxford, 1985–1995. Br J Psychiatr 171: 556–560

Hodges V, Sanford D, Elzinga R. 1986 The role of ward structure on nursing staffing behaviours: an observational study of three psychiatric wards. Acta Psychiatr Scand 73: 6–11

Jenkins MG, Rocke LG, McNicholl BP, Hughes DM. 1998 Violence and verbal abuse against staff in accident and emergency departments: a survey of consultants in the UK and the Republic of Ireland. J Accid Emerg Med 15: 262–265

Jones MK. 1985 Patient violence: report of 200 incidents. J Psychosocial Nurs Ment Health Serv 23: 12–17

King E. 1994 Suicide in the mentally ill: an epidemiological sample and implications for clinicians. Br J Psychiatr 165: 658–663

Lanza ML.1988 Factors relevant to patient assault. Issues in Mental Health Nursing 9: 239–257

Levy P, Hartocollis P. 1976 Nursing aides and patient violence. Am J Psychiatr 133: 429–431

Link BG, Stueve A. 1994 Psychotic symptoms and the violent/illegal behaviour of mental patients compared to community controls. In: Monahan J, Steadman H J (eds) Violence and Mental Disorder: Developments in Risk Assessment. Chicago: University of Chicago Press, 137–160

Lion JR. 1977 Training for battle: thoughts on managing aggressive patients. Hosp Community Psychiatr 38: 875–882

Lipsedge M. 2000 Clinical risk management in psychiatry. In: Vincent C (ed) Clinical Risk Management, 2nd edn BMJ

McNeil DE, Binder RL. 1994 The relationship between acute psychiatric symptoms, diagnosis and short term risk of violence. Hosp and Comm Publishers Psychiatry 45: 133–137

Maden A. 1996 Risk assessment in psychiatry. Br J Hosp Med 56: 78–82

Mak M, Koning PD. 1995 Clinical research in aggressive patients, pitfalls in study design and measurement of aggression. Prog Neuro-Psychopharmacol and Biol Psychiatr 19: 993–1017

Mason T, Chandley M. 1999 Managing Violence and Aggression. A Manual for Nurses and Health Care Workers. Edinburgh: Churchill Livingstone

Monahan J, Steadman HJ. 1994 Violence and Mental Disorder: Developments in Risk Assessment. Chicago: University of Chicago Press

Morgan HG, Stanton R. 1997 Suicide among psychiatric inpatients in a changing clinical scene. Br J Psychiatr 171: 561–563

Palmstierna T, Wistedt B. 1990 Risk factors for aggressive behaviour are of limited value in predicting the violent behaviour of acute involuntarily admitted patients. Acta Psychiatr Scand 81: 152–155

Paton C, Banham S, Whitmore J. 2000 Benzodiazepines in schizophrenia. Psychiatric Bulletin 24: 113–115

Powell G, Caan W, Crowe M. 1994 What events precede violent incidents in psychiatric hospitals? Br J Psychiatr 165: 107–112

Reith M. 1998 Risk assessment and management: lessons from mental health inquiry reports. Med Sci Law 38. 09 93

The Royal College of Psychiatrists. 1998 Management of Imminent Violence: Clinical Practice Guidelines to Support Mental Health Services: OP 41, March 1998

Sanson-Fisher RW, Poole D, Thompson V. 1979 Behavioural patterns within a general hospital psychiatric unit: an observational study. Behv Res Ther 17: 317–332

Shaw J, Appleby L et al. 1999 Mental disorder and clinical care in people convicted of homicide: national clinical survey Br Med J 318: 1240–1244

Sheridan M, Henrion R, Robinson L, Baxter V. 1990 Precipitants of violence in a psychiatric inpatient setting. Hosp Community Psychiatr 41: 776–780

Steadman HJ, Monahan J, Robbins P, et al. 1993 From dangerousness to risk assessment: implications for appropriate research strategies. In: Hodgins S (ed) Crime and Mental Disorder. Sage, 39–62

Swanson JW, Holzer CE, Ganju VM, Jono RT. 1990 Violence and psychiatric disorder in the community: evidence from the Epidemiologic Catchment Area Surveys. Hosp Community Psychiatry 41: 761–770

Tardiff K, Sweillam A. 1982 Assaultative behaviour among chronic patients. Am J Psychiatry 139: 212–215

Taylor P, Gunn J. 1999 Homicides by people with mental illness: myths and reality. Br J Psychiatr 174: 9–14

Watts D, Morgan HG. 1994 Malignant alienation. Br J Psychiatr 164: 11–15

Weishaar ME, Beck AT. 1990 The suicidal patient: how should the therapist respond? Hawton K, Cowen P (eds) In: Dilemmas and Difficulties in the Management of Psychiatric Patients. Oxford Medical Publications

Whittington R. 1994 Violence in psychiatric hospitals. In: Wykes T (ed) Violence and Healthcare Professionals. London: Chapman & Hall, 23–43

Whittington R, Patterson P. 1996 Verbal and non-verbal behaviour immediately prior to aggression by mentally disordered people: enhancing the assessment of risk. J Psychiatr Mental Health Nursing 3: 47–54

12

THE INTERFACE WITH FORENSIC SERVICES

James Anderson

INTRODUCTION

Psychiatric intensive care is at the interface with forensic psychiatric services because both share a common clinical problem – violence. This is the behavioural disability which characterises the majority of patients within the forensic psychiatric service. Knowing how to evaluate violence, and quantify the risk of future violence, is the essence of risk assessment. Knowing when to refer a particular patient to forensic psychiatric services is an important part of effective risk management. Understanding what services are offered by forensic psychiatry is a necessary precondition to using that service effectively.

The aim of this chapter is to provide guidelines to those working outside forensic psychiatry on what is and what is not available within that service. The assessment of dangerousness is discussed elsewhere, but dangerousness in terms of risk to others is pivotal to an evaluation of a patient's need for secure care. It is therefore pivotal to know whether that patient warrants referral to forensic psychiatric services.

It is unrealistic, given existing resources, to imagine that forensic psychiatric services could, or should, manage all those patients who are violent. But knowing which patient should be managed in a more secure setting, whether that be intensive care or the local medium secure unit, is our current concern. However, there are no absolute rules or fixed access criteria; local services vary and are in a state of flux, developing new services for old problems. Many facilities at one time provided within the old asylums are being re-invented and re-named.

The Butler Committee Report (1975), which was particularly influential and which provoked the modern development of regional secure units, recognised that there was 'a yawning gap' between the special hospitals (maximum secure) and the increasingly liberal asylums. The latter were shutting beds and could offer less in terms of secure facilities than they had hitherto. Twenty-five years later we still have that gap and despite the continuing fall in total psychiatric bed numbers there are now more people aged 15 to 44 in psychiatric hospitals than there were 10 years ago. This increase is most pronounced among young men who account for over 40% more hospital episodes than they did 10 years ago (Department of Health 1995). It is young men, both in the community at large and amongst the mentally ill, who account for most violence (Walmsley 1986.) It is also this group that are associated with drug and alcohol abuse – a factor which, in conjunction with serious mental illness, significantly increases the risk of violent behaviour (Monahan and Steadman 1994).

Community care of the mentally ill is a policy which has been welcomed by patients and their families alike. Nonetheless, as time goes by, it is evident that in many parts of the country, most notably in the inner cities, there are inadequate facilities for acute psychiatric admissions and for the 'new long stay' (Milmis Project Group 1995). Recognition of these deficiencies in the service has prompted the development of specialised secure facilities which include: medium secure units, low secure units, challenging behaviour, psychiatric intensive care, etc. These are all expensive resources, and generally over-subscribed, so establishing the clinical criteria for admission for each type of facility is an important priority for purchasers and providers alike.

THE MEDIUM SECURE UNIT – FORENSIC PSYCHIATRIC SERVICES AT THE INTERFACE WITH GENERAL PSYCHIATRY

The medium secure unit is the hub of forensic psychiatric services in most districts. It is the inpatient facility, the academic base and the home base for most community forensic psychiatric services. In response to the Butler Report medium secure units were developed to take patients who were persistent absconders, who represented a risk to the public, were seriously disruptive to hospital regimes or who exhibited persistent and impulsive violence – these being the criteria originally considered in a working party set up by the UK Ministry of Health in 1961 (cited in Eastman 1993). Since the first medium secure units were built there has been increasing awareness of the psychiatric needs of the mentally disordered offender (Reed Committee 1992) and increased public concern about community care of the mentally ill. Whether justified or not, there is a perception of increasing risk to the public from the mentally ill in the community. This has provoked a flurry of legislation ostensibly to tighten professional procedure in community care. There has been a corresponding increase in the awareness and concern about risk in the general psychiatric patient population (Milmis Project Group 1995). The Milmis Project has demonstrated increasing bed occupancy, falling bed numbers, a high level of assaults and sexual harassment by patients on other patients or staff, premature discharges and a dependence on secure facilities in the private sector. The current composition of patients within the medium secure unit reflects these various demands. Although there is some regional variation, by far the majority of inpatients come from prison or the courts. Less than 25% come from general psychiatric services, and less than 10% from Special Hospital (Gunn and Taylor 1993).

Forensic psychiatric services are developing to meet these differing demands. They include:

- *Inpatient facilities.* Bed numbers are increasing and services becoming more specialised. There is an awareness of the need for long-term medium security (a provision which at the moment is virtually non-existent). There is recognition of a need for low secure beds, challenging behaviour and intensive care facilities. Some UK National Health Service Trusts are developing these latter facilities within the forensic directorate; others are separate. However, they are developed, it is important that clear clinical boundaries are established to ensure that patients are appropriately placed.

- *Community forensic psychiatric services* are developing in recognition of the commonality of many patients in general and forensic psychiatric services, particularly those patients who are recognised as potentially dangerous but may not have offended. These community-based services can offer advice and expertise in risk assessment and management. Adopting a strategy of assertive outreach for patients who are recognised as potentially dangerous if untreated, will hopefully ameliorate the risk of violent behaviour to others – whether such patients are being rehabilitated following previous admission to the medium secure unit, or identified as potentially dangerous by the general service. However, local experience suggests (Buchanan, personal communication) the weight of numbers means that community forensic services must be developed as an integrated service with general psychiatry, involving joint clinical management as opposed to a completely separate parallel service.

- *Court diversion schemes* have developed in recognition of the frequency with which the mentally ill become involved in the Criminal Justice System. Once involved, they often experience unacceptable delay before they receive hospital treatment while languishing in prison. Court diversion schemes have significantly reduced these delays and are now established in many parts of the country (James and Hamilton 1991).

- *Forensic psychiatry in prison.* Most forensic psychiatric services attempt to provide regular liaison with their local prisons. This is in recognition of the level of psychiatric morbidity in both the remand and sentenced prisoner populations (Gunn *et al* 1991, Brooke *et al* 1996). Unfortunately for many schizophrenic patients in the inner city, prison is an established part of their itinerary. If such patients are to be well managed, it is important that general and forensic psychiatrists alike acknowledge this reality. Trying to provide an integrated service that monitors the psychiatric population in the community, psychiatric hospitals, the courts and prison can reduce the distress that results when the seriously mentally ill are committed to prison. Nonetheless there is evidence that much psychiatric morbidity in prison remains undetected. Where it is detected, the nature of the prison regime and actions of the courts can make effective delivery of care difficult, many patients being discharged from court before psychiatric contact is established (Birmingham *et al* 1998).

The forensic psychiatric service has a wide constituency ranging from patients in Special Hospital, patients in prison and attending court, outpatients and patients within the general psychiatric service. The latter include those considered a serious enough risk to warrant forensic psychiatric management, or having special treatment needs particular to forensic, psychiatry, e.g. sexual offending, morbid jealousy, etc. Obviously the service can offer advice on the suitability of referral of a particular patient and clearly, if indicated, offer a bed for patient admission. If the clinical criteria are suitable, but no bed is available locally, the patient may be admitted to a private medium secure unit. What the service cannot do is manage all patients who exhibit violent behaviour.

GUIDELINES ON ACCESS TO IN-PATIENT FORENSIC CARE

With the burgeoning of costs for the treatment of mentally disordered offenders, a need has arisen to identify more rigorously the factors that characterise those requiring forensic secure services. In some parts of the UK this has led to the formalisation of access criteria to forensic services (Eastman and Bellamy 1998). Whilst still at the evaluation stage, it is hoped that these criteria will provide guidelines which will not only encourage a consistent approach within the service, but also provide referral guidelines to external agencies. However, there are limitations to such an approach. Admission policies must to some extent reflect the local context, although there is a need to establish clearly delineated clinical boundaries between different types and levels of secure facilities.

The most common reasons for the general psychiatric services to request forensic psychiatric advice are:

- To obtain a risk assessment.

- To transfer a patient to the medium secure unit.

The approach to risk assessment is described in a number of excellent reviews (Gunn and Taylor 1993, Royal College of Psychiatrists 1996) and I commend these. The latter is published as a pocket-sized booklet and is an invaluable companion. The protocol for risk assessment is described as follows:

The standard psychiatric assessment including the following:

History

- *Previous violence and/or suicidal behaviour.*

- *Evidence of rootlessness or 'social restlessness', e.g. few relationships, frequent changes of address or employment.*

- *Evidence of poor compliance with treatment or disengagement from psychiatric aftercare.*

- *Presence of substance misuse or other potential disinhibiting factors, e.g. a social background promoting violence.*

- *Identification of any precipitants and any changes in mental state or behaviour that have occurred prior to violence and/or relapse.*

Are the risk factors stable or have any changed recently?

- *Evidence of recent severe stress, particularly of loss events or the threat of loss.*

- *Evidence of recent discontinuation of medication.*

Environment

- *Does the patient have access to potential victims, particularly victims identified in mental state abnormalities?*

Mental state

- *Evidence of any threat/control override symptoms: firmly held beliefs or persecution by others (persecutory delusions), or of mind or body being controlled or interfered with by external forces (delusions of passivity).*

- *Emotions related to violence, e.g. irritability, anger, hostility, suspiciousness.*

- *Specific threats made by the patient.*

Conclusion

A formulation should be made based on these and all other items of history and mental state. The formulation should, as far as possible, specify factors likely to increase the risk of dangerous behaviour and those likely to decrease it. The formulation should aim to answer the following questions:

- *How serious is the risk?*

- *Is the risk specific or general?*

- *How immediate is the risk?*

- *How volatile is the risk?*

- *What specific treatment, and which management plan, can best reduce the risk?*

I would elaborate one aspect of this protocol and that is the evaluation of potential violence because this dictates where in the hierarchy of supervision and security the patient should be managed.

By and large, it is violence and the risk of further serious violence that determines the patient's admission to forensic psychiatric facilities. This is true of the offender and non-offender population alike. It is true that on occasions the courts or the Mental Health Unit at the British Home Office will dictate the level of security a patient requires, regardless of clinical need, but that is relatively unusual. It remains the case that the seriousness of a patient's violent behaviour will dictate the level of security that patient requires.

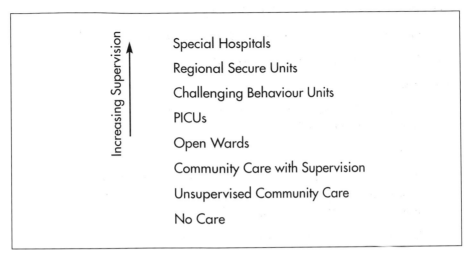

Figure 12.1 – A hierarchy of supervision and security within the English Hospital System (from Gunn and Taylor 1993)

Admission assessment therefore focuses on violence in the context of a full risk assessment. In evaluating previous violence (and by implication risk of future violence) it is important to obtain as much information as possible about previous behaviour including: previous criminal record, witness statements, arresting officers' statements, etc. However, a significant minority of patients show highly dangerous behaviour not 'officially recognised' or processed through the Criminal Justice System, prior to their admission. It is then necessary to establish the gravity of the patient's current violent behaviour. This is relatively easy if they are subject to criminal proceedings because it will be stated as the charge. However it is important to attempt to re-create the details of the offence as accurately as possible. This is not only because the charge may underestimate (or less commonly overestimate) the seriousness of what took place, but also because a charge as such gives little information about motivation for the offence. For instance, 'attempted murder' gives little information about motivation: the stabbing of a young man by another outside a pub at 11.30 pm on Saturday night in the context of an alcohol-inflamed argument has very different implications to the near strangling of a young woman by a young man in the context of a sadistic sexual assault.

If the patient has not offended but has been violent in the community or in hospital, it is important to obtain as much detail of that violence as possible: from the patient, family and friends, GP, social workers, nursing staff, etc.

To assess violence, therefore:

- Obtain the arresting officer's statement (by ringing the police station in which he was charged).

- Read witness statements (sometimes these are difficult to obtain, but should be provided by the Crown Prosecution Service or solicitors, if you are providing a psychiatric report).

- Speak to witnesses.

- Speak to family or friends, GP, social worker, nursing staff.

The index offence, or the 'equivalent' behaviour associated with the patient's admission to hospital, can be ranked in severity. It can also be quantified by its frequency. Behaviour should be evaluated in the patient's life-span of violent behaviour and conclusions drawn about whether there is a changing pattern of offending or violence.

Secure care admission criteria (from Eastman and Bellamy 1998)

Behaviour Category 1

- Murder

- Manslaughter

- Attempted murder

- Infanticide

- Arson with intent to endanger life

- Rape (against men or women)

- Causing death by reckless driving

Behaviour Category 2

- Aiding or abetting suicide

- Administering poison

- Arson with recklessness towards life

- Concealment of birth

- Contact sexual offending (not rape but including attempted rape)

- False imprisonment (e.g. kidnapping)

- Grevious bodily harm (GBH)

- Possession of a firearm

- Reckless driving

- Robbery

- Threats to kill
- Wounding with intent to cause GBH

Behaviour Category 3

- ABH (Actual Bodily Harm)
- Affray
- Aggravated burglary
- Arson (no recklessness or intention to endanger life)
- Attempted assault
- Blackmail
- Breaking and entering
- Burglary
- Common assault
- Criminal damage
- Deception
- Forgery
- Fraud
- Going equipped to steal
- Handling stolen property
- Non-contact sexual offences
- Possession of an offensive weapon
- Public nuisance offences
- Public order offences
- Theft
- Trespass

Offences can be categorised according to seriousness (as above) and this schema can be adopted to provide guidelines to access different levels of security (Eastman and Bellamy 1998). The major determinant of acceptance to admission in the non-offender population is also violence. Offen and Taylor (1985) found violence was the precipitant to referral in all but 13 (18%) of their series of referrals to an interim secure unit. The more serious the violence, the more likely it was that a bed would be made available. Treasaden (1985) found in a review of four Interim Secure Units (ISUs) that violence was the behavioural indication for admission in the majority (67–83%) with fire raising (19–24%) and sexual behaviour (3–10%). Violent behaviour in the non-offender population can be ranked in terms of its equivalent to the offence categories described above. As a rule of thumb, offences of violence equivalent to category one, will require admission to medium or maximum secure care. The major factor determining which of the two is the level of continuing risk. Offences or violence equivalent to offence Category 2 can generally be managed in medium secure care. Offences of Category 3 can generally be managed in low secure care. In all cases the major additional factor to the level of security they require being their continuing risk of such behaviour.

This approach is summarised in Figure 12.2.

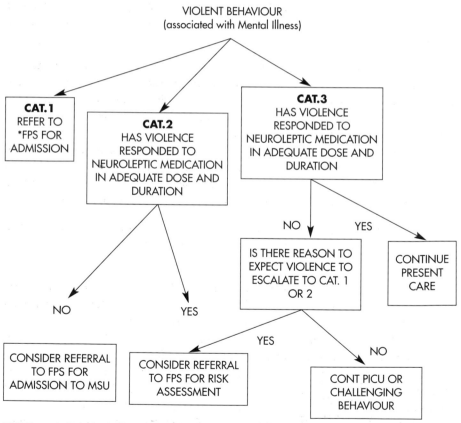

*FPS Forensic Psychiatric Services

Figure 12.2 – Guidelines on access to different levels of secure care

So violence is categorised in terms of <u>severity</u> and quantified in terms of <u>frequency</u>. Risk of repeated violence in the short and longer term, is also assessed. Furthermore if there is <u>specific pathology</u> that predicts serious violence (whether or not that has taken place to date), this may indicate the need for secure care, e.g. morbid jealousy. The risk of violence taking place on the unit itself should be considered, i.e. what level of continuing risk does that patient pose and to whom.

If the patient should <u>abscond</u> from hospital, it must be decided if he or she represents a <u>serious, immediate risk</u> to the general public, or only to named individuals. If it is named individuals only, do those individuals live nearby or not?

Another major consideration in assessing a patient's need for specialist forensic involvement is the <u>psychopathology</u> they exhibit. Forensic psychiatry has developed specialised interest and skill in the management of particular disorders. Sexual pathology, for instance, is almost exclusively dealt with by forensic psychiatry. Other pathologies are also more commonly encountered by forensic psychiatrists, because of their association with offending and dangerous behaviour, e.g. morbid jealousy, erotomania, sadistic fantasies, etc.

<u>Personality disorder</u>, which will often preclude a patient's admission to general psychiatric services, will not necessarily do so from forensic psychiatric care. It is often the presence of personality disorder in conjunction with serious mental illness that perpetuates the risk of violence. This conjunction of mental illness and personality disorder may be an indication for admission to medium secure care. However, it is notable that very few patients are detained in medium secure care under the legal category of psychopathic disorder, the majority being designated as mentally ill. This contrasts with Special Hospital where approximately 25% of patients are detained under the legal category psychopathic disorder (Dell and Robertson 1988).

Other <u>co-morbid factors</u> include drug and alcohol abuse; those with diagnosed drug and alcohol misuse are much more likely to be violent than those with mental illness alone.

The majority of patients in medium secure care are detained under criminal sections of the Mental Health Act, and many of them under <u>restriction orders</u>. The increasing number of patients subject to restriction orders has had significant impact on the ability to discharge patients. Unfortunately there is some evidence that this has increased the average duration of admission, the net result being that, despite increasing numbers of medium secure beds, it remains as difficult to admit a patient as it was ten years ago (Brown 1998). The influence of the Mental Health Unit, Home Office in determining where a patient is admitted from prison can override clinical decisions on the patient's security needs. In other words the Home Office can dictate that a patient be admitted to medium secure care even if the clinicians involved feel that his risk to others does not warrant this. Certainly in maximum secure hospitals there are patients who are considered too high a <u>political profile</u>, to allow their care in lower levels of security. Furthermore it is not just the patient's risk to others if they should abscond that should be considered, but also whether they have <u>dangerous friends</u> who might execute an escape attempt, possibly exposing staff and other patients to risk.

Although an attempt should be made to determine the patient's security needs on current clinical grounds, this judgement may be influenced by previous experience of that patient in other settings. It is surprising how many extremely disturbed patients settle rapidly, without any change in medication, when they move into a more secure environment.

HOW TO MAKE A REFERRAL

First and foremost, know what you want: advice, moral support, a risk assessment or a transfer? Advice can be enormously reassuring, and as a matter of principle good liaison between general and forensic psychiatric services helps to establish a culture of dialogue which itself tends to facilitate good working relationships and discourages entrenched protectionist attitudes and policies. Nonetheless it has its drawbacks: advice is informal and inevitably does not represent a formal risk assessment. Forensic psychiatrists can be hesitant about making judgements without undertaking a formal assessment if a potentially violent patient is released on the basis of such a judgement.

If you feel the patient is inappropriately placed in psychiatric intensive care and warrants admission to medium secure care, make the case persuasively.

1. Provide a full history with as much supportive information as possible, e.g. informant history, arresting officer's statement, previous criminal record, witness statements.

2. Provide a multiaxial diagnostic formulation.

3. Detail treatment to date and indications for referral including:

    • violence category of index offence or equivalent behaviour.

    • Perceived risk of continued violence including seriousness of risk, whether risk is specific or general, whether risk is immediate, how volatile the risk is.

It is very unusual for forensic psychiatric services to admit a patient without undertaking a multidisciplinary assessment themselves. It is important therefore that the referrer can treat the patient safely while awaiting the outcome of that assessment. Patients detained in psychiatric intensive care are often an unknown quantity in terms of their previous history of violence so the unit should have the structural capacity and personnel to contain potentially serious violent behaviour.

THE WAY AHEAD

Forensic psychiatry is a relatively young speciality that many general psychiatrists see as the cuckoo in the nest, monopolising resources that might otherwise have been enjoyed by all. Sadly there is some truth in all this. The public and political preoccupation with what is seen as 'the failure of community care' has shifted the focus and resources of much of psychiatric practice towards the severely mentally ill. Many psychiatrists resent the preoccupation with risk and the fact that much of their practice is dictated by statutory expectation rather than patient need.

On the other hand, forensic psychiatry can be seen as having developed in response to real need. Its separation from general psychiatry was a necessary part of its development. Perhaps now is the time to see its reintegration. To do so requires good liaison, and acknowledgement of shared interests and responsibilities. So while there must be adequate numbers of medium secure beds, there must also be adequate beds and resources provided for general psychiatry in psychiatric intensive care units, rehabilitation, and in the community. It is only then that forensic psychiatric patients can be fully reintegrated with the community, and general psychiatric patients receive the level of secure care appropriate to their needs.

ACKNOWLEDGEMENT

I am grateful to Dr Nigel Eastman for permission to reproduce the Behaviour Gravity Categories from Admission Criteria to Secure Services Schedule (ACSeSS) (Eastman and Bellamy 1998). Other aspects of the evaluation of violence risk are also derived from ACSeSS and from discussion with Dr Eastman.

REFERENCES

Birmingham L, Mason D, Grubin D. 1998 A Follow-up Study of disordered men remanded to prison. Criminal Behaviour and Mental Health 8: 202–213

Brooke D, Taylor C, Gunn J, Maden A. 1996 Point prevalence of mental disorder in unconvicted male prisoners in England and Wales. Br Med J 313: 1524–1527

Brown C. 1998 Trends in Admissions to a Regional Secure Unit 1983–1996. London: R Coll Psychiatrist, Winter Meeting

Butler Committee Report. 1975 Better Services for the Mentally Ill. London: Home Office/DHSS

Dell S, Robertson G. 1988 Sentenced to Hospital. Maudsley Monograph No. 32. Oxford: Oxford University Press

Department of Health. 1995 Mental Health in England. London: Department of Health

Eastman NLG. 1993 Forensic psychiatric services in Britain. Intern J Law Psychiatry 16: 1–26

Eastman NLG, Bellamy S. 1998 Admission criteria to secure services and service definitions. Unpublished

Gunn J, Maden A, Swinton M. 1991 Treatment needs of prisoners with psychiatric disorders. Br Med J 300: 338–341

Gunn J, Taylor PJ. 1993 Forensic Psychiatry Clinical Legal and Ethical Issues. London: pp. 624–640, 716. Butterworth-Heinemann

James DV, Hamilton LW. 1991 Assessing efficacy and cost of a psychiatric liaison service to a magistrates' court. Br Med J 303: 282–285

Milmis Project Group. 1995 Monitoring Inner London mental illness services. Psychiatr Bull 19: 276–280

Monahan, Steadman HJ. 1994 Violence and Mental Illness. Chicago. University of Chicago Press

Offen L, Taylor PJ. 1985 Violence and resources: factors determining admission to an interim secure unit. Med, Sci and the Law 25: 165–171

Reed Committee. 1992 Review of Health and Social Services for Mentally Disordered Offenders and Others Requiring Similar Services. London: DOH/Home Office

Royal College of Psychiatrists. 1996 Assessment and Clinical Management of Risk of Harm to Other People. Council Report CR53. London: R Coll Psychiatrists

Treasaden IH. 1985 Current practice in Interim Secure Units. In: L. Goslin (ed.) Secure Provision. London: Tavistock

Walmesley R. 1986 Personal Violence. Home Office Research Study No. 89. London: HMSO

13

THE PROVISION OF INTENSIVE CARE IN FORENSIC PSYCHIATRY

Harvey Gordon

In some countries, the practice of forensic psychiatry is confined to providing psychiatric evaluation to the court (Harding 1993). In England and Wales, forensic psychiatrists are involved in the assessment and treatment of patients who have been charged with an offence or convicted by a court and, since the 1959 Mental Health Act, patients may be transferred to forensic psychiatric units without being charged with any offence. Most of these patients would now be detained on Section 3 of the 1983 Mental Health Act, though a few may be subject to Section 2 of the same Act. Consequently, when the Reed Committee reported (Department of Health and Home Office 1992), it covered not only mentally abnormal offenders, but also 'those requiring similar services'.

In reality, therefore, there is an overlap between general and forensic psychiatry rather than any sharp demarcation. It can indeed be arbitrary whether or not a patient in the community or a psychiatric hospital is charged with a criminal offence (James and Hamilton 1991, Cripps et al 1995). Most patients admitted to regional secure units or Special Hospitals have previously received treatment in general psychiatric hospitals (Parker 1973, Cope and Ndegwa 1990, Murray 1996).

Considerable tension may exist between general and forensic psychiatrists, and related health professionals, as to which patients are accepted for transfer into forensic psychiatric units, and then subsequently back to the general psychiatric sector, though liaison is better in some areas compared to others. Such professional border disputes must contribute little benefit to patients who may find themselves caught between differences of perspective between clinicians. The issue was indeed identified at the time of the genesis of medium secure units by the Butler Committee (Home Office and Department of Health and Social Security 1975). That report reflected a contemporaneous one by the Department of Health and Social Security (1974) on security in psychiatric hospitals, which concluded that medium secure units were needed for patients presenting with severely disruptive behaviour, with a diagnosis of mental illness, mental handicap or psychopathic or severe personality disorder. Admission to a medium secure unit would be decided by multidisciplinary assessment, taking account of the potential risk to others and risk of self injury, and the prospects of response to treatment.

In practice, patients on Section 3 of the 1983 Mental Health Act, if psychotically disturbed may be located in intensive care units in general psychiatric hospitals (Mortimer 1995), medium secure units (Kennedy et al 1995a, b) and in Special Hospitals (Grounds et al 1993a).

Violence by patients in psychiatric hospitals is common (Crighton 1995) though its severity tends to rise with the level of security provided (Larkin et al 1988). Most psychiatric hospitals have found it necessary to provide intensive care facilities in order to separate the more violent and disturbed group from the more behaviourally stable majority (Ford and Whiffin 1991, Beer et al 1997, Allan et al 1998). Risk of harm to fellow patients and staff, potential for self harm, absconding behaviour, and the tendency for any unit's functioning to be adversely affected by the degree of restrictions or resources needed for the most disturbed patients have led to the provision of locked facilities in general psychiatry.

Intensive care units in general psychiatric hospitals have their counterparts in intensive or special care areas or units in medium secure facilities and in Special Hospitals. Whilst the literature on intensive care units in general psychiatry is extensive, that pertaining to intensive or special care in forensic psychiatry is sparse. A history of violence to some degree is characteristic of virtually all patients admitted to forensic psychiatric units, the ethos of which is the assessment and treatment of the mental disorder and its associated violence and antisocial behaviour.

Studies of regional secure units in England and Wales have described a broad range of patient variables (Higgins 1981, Faulk and Taylor 1984, Bullard and Bond 1988, Rix and Seymour 1988, Cope and Ndegwa 1990, Higgo and Shetty 1991, Sugarman and Collins 1992, Torpy and Hall 1993, Kaul 1994, Cripps *et al* 1995, James 1996, Murray 1996, Mohan *et al* 1997). However, none of these have, as yet, provided data on which patients within them have tended to be more violent or in need of intensive care, though one such study is currently in progress in North West London (Broughton – personal communication). Studies reflecting the use of intensive or special care facilities in Special Hospitals are also relatively few in number (Larkin *et al* 1988, Coldwell and Naismith 1989, Carton and Larkin 1991, Mason and Chandley 1995, Brook and Coorey 1996, Gordon *et al* 1998).

Many medium secure units have provided an intensive care area, e.g. the Denis Hill Unit in the Bethlem Royal Hospital, which can be brought into effect with extra nursing staff when required. Other medium secure units have more permanent intensive care wards, such as the Shaftesbury Clinic, the Reaside Clinic and the Three Bridges Unit. Patients may be transferred into the intensive care unit from elsewhere in the medium secure unit or directly, if appropriate when admitted. It is assumed that placement in the intensive care facility can be harmoniously negotiated but at present this is not known. Health professionals, especially nursing staff in intensive care units, in general psychiatry are known to often feel professionally isolated (Zigmond 1995), but in the hitherto relatively small medium secure units perhaps more mutual understanding regarding patient location has been developed. Clearly an intensive care facility, whether in general or forensic psychiatry, should provide an effective service to its feeder units, with the understanding that patients should stay no longer in intensive care than is necessary.

The majority of patients admitted to medium secure units suffer from schizophrenia or a related psychosis (Higgins 1981, Faulk and Taylor 1984, Bullard and Bond 1988, James 1996, Murray 1996). Although it was originally felt that some patients with personality disorder would be suitable for medium secure units, most are disinclined to admit such patients other than by transfer from Special Hospitals and then only after extra careful assessment (Faulk and Taylor 1984, Bullard and Bond 1988), though one partial exception is the Trent regional secure unit which is disposed towards admission of offender patients with a diagnosis of personality disorder on assessment sections under Part III of the 1983 Mental Health Act (Kaul 1994). The avoidance by medium secure units of many patients with personality disorder is not necessarily inappropriate, however, as the more severe group of personality disordered patients can be highly disruptive unless in a well-contained therapeutic environment providing an extended length of stay. On the other hand, blanket rejection of patients on the basis of diagnosis alone is of doubtful ethical soundness.

The limitations of general psychiatric facilities and medium secure units have been outlined in regard to the types of patients they find too difficult to manage successfully. Coid (1991), in a survey of the private sector, found that the group of patients most difficult to place in the public sector were those presenting with persistently challenging behaviour, on Section 3 of the 1983 Mental Health Act, suffering from severe schizophrenia, mild or moderate mental handicap or brain damage. Murray (1996), in a review of all the medium secure units in England, found that these units had proved unable to provide adequately for those offender patients requiring medium security over a long period of time, i.e. several years, and separately the problematic non-forensic patients on Section 3 of the 1983 Mental Health Act, most of whom had schizophrenic illnesses which were more resistant to treatment than usual. More than 20 years after the Butler Report the issue of the provision of facilities for the persistently disturbed psychotic outside the Special Hospitals remains unresolved, and one of the parameters always provided by Special Hospitals, namely extended length of stay, is found to be necessary. However the provision of long-term medium security may prove far more complex in practice than in theory (Taylor et al 1996).

Whether patients located for periods in intensive care areas in medium security resemble those difficult to place patients described by Coid (1991) or are those referred to by Murray (1996) is not currently known. Neither is it known whether these are the same group who find themselves transferred from medium to maximum security, though clinical impression suggests it might be. Bullard and Bond (1988), in their study of a precursor to the Reaside Clinic, found that 10% (seven cases) of their patient group required transfer to a Special Hospital, four of the seven being young female patients with a diagnosis of personality disorder, two of whom also had a degree of mental impairment. Higgo and Shetty (1991), in a study of the Scott Clinic in Liverpool, found that, over a 6-year period, about 10% of patients leaving the unit were transferred to a Special Hospital. Cope and Ward (1993), in the Reaside Clinic, found that almost one-third of patients transferred there from a Special Hospital required transfer back to the Special Hospital, noting a special concern about the risks associated with patients legally categorised as psychopaths with a propensity towards sexual violence. However the overt dangerousness of that group would be more likely to manifest itself in the community than in hospital, and indeed the violence perpetrated by a patient in the community may not in all cases correlate with that in hospital (Gordon *et al* 1998).

Broughton's ongoing study in the Three Bridges Unit will be the first to throw some light on the use of an intensive care facility in a medium secure unit. A clear picture of the use of such provision has not yet revealed itself, except that replication within medium security of an intensive facility as in general psychiatry has emerged.

The Special Hospitals have been the subject of extensive professional and public review and criticism over the last two decades (Department of Health and Social Security 1980, Bluglass 1992, Department of Health 1992, Department of Health and Home Office 1992, Special Hospitals Service Authority 1993). However they continue to provide sizeable proportions of patients who could be safely managed elsewhere in lesser degrees of security if such were available (Maden *et al* 1995). Around the time of the Butler Report, Tidmarsh (1974) referred to the impression that the Special Hospitals were having to accept patients who previously would have been treated in general psychiatric hospitals. The Special Hospitals have continued to provide humane asylum in some cases, a concept which became unpopular but has stood the test of time even if its optimum modern characteristics may take a different form, at least for the group who are not a serious danger to the public (Munetz *et al* 1996). The role of the therapeutic environment is also a concept still adhered to theoretically but not always fully appreciated in practice in general and forensic psychiatry (Cohen and Khan 1990).

Larkin *et al* (1988), in a study in Rampton, found that the rate of serious violence within the hospital was significantly higher than in general psychiatry. He found the highest rates were in Rampton's female intensive care unit, though reasons for that were unclear. A follow-up study by Carton and Larkin (1991) found that the acquisition of skills in the use of control and restraint techniques had led to reduction in the levels of serious violence.

Larkin *et al*'s study pointedly illustrates that most units in Special Hospitals are segregated by gender, compared to the widespread integration available elsewhere in psychiatry (Special Hospitals Service Authority 1991, Taylor and Swann 1999).

Coldwell and Naismith (1989), in what was then Park Lane Hospital for male patients only (subsequently Ashworth Hospital), found an excess of patients in their male special care ward who were detained on Section 3 of the 1983 Mental Health Act, albeit that did not reach statistical significance. A similar finding is reported by Gordon *et al* 1998 in a study at Broadmoor Hospital, where it applied both to male and female patients in their respective special care units. It therefore seems that patients on Section 3 who are behaviourally disturbed in general psychiatric hospitals or regional secure units who require transfer to Special Hospitals tend to remain disturbed at least for a period of time. The clinical state of such patients seems to be somewhat independent of the environment in which they receive treatment, though in due course improvement does occur. The absence of unrealistic expectations on length of stay for these patients may here be a positive benefit, allowing the patient to improve at his or her own pace. However, this need not preclude the construction of appropriate alternative long-term secure facilities for such patients elsewhere (Taylor et al 1996). Such facilities need to provide not only a lengthy placement, but also a flexibility and a range of therapeutic facilities within a secure perimeter.

The special care units in Special Hospitals are the buffer zones of psychiatry, the outer limits of the therapeutic stratosphere. It is of considerable note that the study in Broadmoor Hospital showed that the special care units were used mainly by patients with chronic schizophrenia or a related psychosis, the proportion of transfers into them of psychopathic patients being uncommon, especially for males. Within a secure psychiatric hospital, most of the violent incidents are perpetrated by the acutely or chronic mentally ill. This is, however, more true for male patients than for female patients for whom borderline personality disorder also accounts for sizeable numbers of transfers into special care and is reminiscent of Bullard and Bond's study (1988), in which several female borderline patients required transfer to a Special Hospital.

The operational problems in the special care units in Special Hospitals have focused around two different groups with differing lengths of stay. The average length of stay in special care in the Broadmoor study was about four months for females and about 6 months for males. A significant minority continued to show protracted challenging behaviour in excess of two years, with a few cases even beyond 5 or more years. Mason and Chandley (1995) in Ashworth Hospital have described these persistently challenging cases. Most of these patients suffer from a chronic schizophrenic illness, though there may be an occasional case of exceptional difficulty where there is superadded brain damage. The proposal to reduce seclusion for these patients is helpful (Special Hospitals Service Authority 1995), but the notion that seclusion could be abolished for this group is based on ideological and clinical naivety. In two particularly rare cases known to the author, seclusion has been reduced only by the controversial use of mechanical restraint to allow the patient to get up safely (Gordon et al 1999). However these are unusual cases and most patients in special care units in Special Hospitals can usually be transferred back to an ordinary ward in the hospital within a reasonable time. A length of stay of 4–6 months in most cases may seem rather long in comparison to length of stay in general psychiatry, but it is not unduly long when considered in the context of the average length of stay in a Special Hospital which is about 8 years (Grounds et al 1993b).

Some advantages accrue by separating the more chronic group from those requiring only shorter periods in special care. Brook and Coorey (1996) described the opening in Ashworth Hospital of such an acute intensive care unit in September 1994 in an attempt to have a more consistent environment for the separate more chronically disturbed group. Similar changes were made at Broadmoor Hospital in January 1997, although in practice blending of the two groups still tends to occur.

A major issue for special care units in Special Hospitals is their reputation as 'punishment wards'. Similar concerns have been expressed in regard to intensive care units in general psychiatric hospitals (Ford and Whiffin 1991, Zigmond 1995). Whether such punitive impressions can be entirely avoided may be doubtful, even if the clinicians working in such units do not employ such a philosophy of care. Regular liaison with the units from which the patient has been transferred to special care, close sharing of relevant information with managers, and encouragement of visiting by legal and other legitimate agencies with an interest in mental health is helpful.

Although forensic psychiatry's focus is that of the violent patient, some patients in forensic psychiatric units of medium or maximum security pose a greater threat than others either in the short term or on a more protracted basis. The provision of an intensive or special care facility allows the more stable group within the hospital to undertake their treatment and rehabilitation without undue excessive restrictions. Additionally the more disturbed and dangerous patient may be located in a unit more appropriate to his or her needs and that of others. It is vital, however, that, once sufficient progress has been achieved, the patient returns to a more liberal area of the hospital. In the author's experience, achieving that requires close cooperation with medical colleagues as well as a degree of patience but also firmness and determination, without which an intensive or special care facility can become an injustice in some cases.

REFERENCES

Allan ER, Brown RC, Laury G. 1998 Planning a psychiatric intensive care unit. Hosp Community Psychiatry 39(1): 81–83

Beer MD, Paton C, Pereira S. 1997 Hot beds of general psychiatry: a national survey of psychiatric intensive care units. Psychiatr Bull 21: 142–144

Bluglass R. 1992 The Special Hospitals should be closed. Br Med J 305: 323–324

Brook R, Coorey PR. 1996 An acute ICU in a maximum secure hospital. Psychiatr Bull 20: 306–311

Bullard H, Bond M. 1988 Secure units: why they are needed? Med, Sci Law 28(4): 312–318

Carton G, Larkin E. 1991 Reducing violence in a Special Hospital. Nurs Standard 5(17): 29–31

Cohen S, Khan A. 1990 Antipsychotic effect of milieu in the acute treatment of schizophrenia. Gen Hosp Psychiatry 12: 248–251

Coid JW. 1991 A survey of patients from five health districts receiving special care in the private sector. Psychiatr Bull 15: 257–262

Coldwell JB, Naismith LJ. 1989 Violent incidents on special care wards in a Special Hospital. Med, Sci Law 29(2): 116–123

Cope R, Ndegwa D. 1990 Ethnic differences in admission to a regional secure unit. J Forensic Psychiatry 3: 368–378

Cope R, Ward M. 1993 What happens to Special Hospital patients admitted to medium security? J Forensic Psychiatry 4(1): 13–24

Crighton J. 1995 A review of psychiatric inpatient violence. In: Crighton J. (ed) Psychiatric Patient Violence: Risk and Response. London: Duckworth

Cripps J, Duffield G, James D. 1995 Bridging the gap in secure provision: evaluation of a new local combined locked forensic/intensive care unit. J Forensic Psychiatry 6(1): 77–91

Department of Health. 1992 Report of the Committee of Inquiry into Complaints about Ashworth Hospital. Cm-2028-1 and 2. London: HMSO

Department of Health and Home Office 1992. Review of Health and Social Services for Mentally Disordered Offenders and Others Requiring Similar Services, Final Summary Report. CM2088. London: HMSO

Department of Health and Social Security. 1974 Revised Report of the Working Party on Security in NHS Psychiatric Hospitals (Glancy Report). London: HMSO

Department of Health and Social Security. 1980 Report of the Committee of Inquiry into Rampton Hospital. Cmnd. 8073. London: HMSO

Faulk M, Taylor J. 1984 The Wessex interim secure unit. Issues Criminologic Legal Psychol 6: 47–57

Ford I, Whiffin M. 1991 The role of the psychiatric ICU. Nurs Times 87(51): 47–49

Gordon H, Hammond S, Veeramani R. 1998 Special care units in Special Hospitals. Journal of Forensic Psychiatry 9(3): 571–587

Gordon H, Hindley N, Marsden A, Shirayogi M. 1999 The use of Mechanical Restraint in the Management of Psychiatric Patients: is it ever appropriate? Journal of Forensic Psychiatry 10(1): 173–186

Grounds A, Gunn J, Mullen P, Taylor P. 1993a Secure institutions: their characteristics and problems. In: Gunn J, Taylor PJ (eds) Forensic Psychiatry: Clinical, Legal and Ethical Issues. Oxford: Butterworth-Heinemann

Grounds A, Snowden P, Taylor P, Basson J, Gunn J. 1993b Forensic psychiatry in the National Health Service of England and Wales. In: Gunn J, Taylor PJ (eds) Forensic Psychiatry: Clinical, Legal and Ethical Issues. Oxford: Butterworth-Heinemann

Harding T. 1993 A comparative survey of medico-legal systems. In: Gunn J, Taylor PJ (eds) Forensic Psychiatry: Clinical, Legal and Ethical Issues. Oxford: Butterworth-Heinemann

Higgins J. 1981 Four years experience of an interim secure unit. Br Med J 282: 889–893

Higgo R, Shetty G. 1991 Four years experience of a regional secure unit. J Forensic Psychiatry 2(2): 202–210

Home Office and Department of Health and Social Security. 1975 Report of the Committee on Mentally Abnormal Offenders (Butler Report). Cmnd. 6244. London: HMSO

James A. 1996 Suicide reduction in medium security. J Forensic Psychiatry 7(2): 406–412

James DV, Hamilton LW. 1991 The Clerkenwell scheme: assessing efficacy and cost of a psychiatric liaison service to a magistrates' court. Br Med J 303: 282–285

Kaul A. 1994 Interim hospital order – a regional secure unit experience. Med, Sci Law 34(3): 233–236

Kennedy J, Wilson C, Cope R. 1995a Long stay patients in a regional secure unit. J Forensic Psychiatry 6: 541–551

Kennedy J, Harrison J, Hills T, Bluglass R. 1995b Analysis of violent incidents on an RSU. Med, Sci Law 35(3): 255–260

Larkin E, Murtagh S, Jones S. 1988 A preliminary study of violent incidents in a Special Hospital (Rampton). Br J Psychiatr 153: 226–231

Maden T, Curle C, Meux C, Burrow S, Gunn J. 1995 Treatment and Security Needs of Special Hospital Patients. London: Whurr

Mason T, Chandley M. 1995 The chronically assaultive patient: benchmarking best practices. Psychiatr Care 2(5): 180–183

Mohan D, Murray K, Taylor P, Steed P. 1997 Developments in the use of regional secure unit beds over a 12 year period. J Forensic Psychiatry 8(2): 321–335

Mortimer A. 1995 Reducing violence on a secure ward. Psychiatr Bull 19: 605–608

Munetz MR, Peterson GA, Vandershie PW. 1996 Safer houses for patients who need asylum. Psychiatr Serv 47(2): 117

Murray K. 1996 The use of beds in NHS medium secure units in England. J Forensic Psychiatry 7(3): 504–524

Parker E. 1973 An Inquiry into the Reliability of Special Hospital Case Records with Reference to the Recording of Previous Psychiatric Hospitalisations and Criminal Histories. London: Special Hospitals Research Unit, Department of Health and Social Security

Rix G, Seymour D. 1988 Violent incidents on a Regional Secure Unit. Journal of Advanced Nursing 13: 746–751

Special Hospitals Service Authority. 1991 Advisory Committee on Facilities for Married Patients within Special Hospitals. Interim Report. London: Special Hospitals Service Authority

Special Hospitals Service Authority. 1993 Report of the Committee of Inquiry into the Death of Orville Blackwood and a Review of the Deaths of Two Other Afro-Caribbean Patients: Big, Black and Dangerous? London: Special Hospitals Service Authority

Special Hospital Service Authority. 1995 Service Strategies for Secure Care. London: Special Hospitals Service Authority

Sugarman P, Collins P. 1992 Informal admission to secure units: a paradoxical situation? J Forensic Psychiatry 3(3): 477–485

Taylor PJ, Maden A, Jones D. 1996 Long-term medium security hospital units: a service gap of the 1990s. Criminal Behaviour and Mental Health 6: 213–229

Taylor PJ, Swan T. 1999 Couples in Care and Custody. Oxford: Butterworth-Heinemann

Tidmarsh D. 1974 Secure hospital units (letter). Br Med J 2 November: 286

Torpy D, Hall M. 1993 Violent incidents in a secure unit. J Forensic Psychiatry 4(3): 517–544

Zigmond A. 1995 Special care wards: are they special? Psychiatr Bull 19: 310–312

SECTION 3:
STRUCTURE AND
MANAGEMENT

14

SETTING UP A NEW PICU: PRINCIPLES AND PRACTICE

Andrew W Procter

INTRODUCTION

Throughout the history of mental health care, the methods of managing patients with disturbed and aggressive behaviour have always been important and contentious. This has been particularly the case over recent decades which have seen major changes in effective therapies and the style of delivery of psychiatric care. Since the 1950s the majority of mental hospital wards have been unlocked and there has been a shift in the philosophy (if not practice) of care towards the community. However, with the increasing development of effective and evidence-based models of community care, it has become apparent that there remain a group of patients whose symptoms and behaviour require special care in a dedicated inpatient unit, often referred to as a Psychiatric Intensive Care Unit (PICU).

During the 1970s there were a number of descriptions in the literature of psychiatric intensive care units (PICUs) mainly from North America and Australia. The Royal College of Psychiatrists (1980), in its document 'Secure Facilities for Psychiatric Patients: a comprehensive policy', recommended a range of secure facilities that were necessary to support local mental health services, including local intensive care units.

In 1991, Dr John Reed led a complex review of services for mentally disordered offenders. By this stage, Government policy had been clearly articulated in the Home Office Circular 66/90. Offenders suffering from mental disorder should receive care and treatment from the health and personal social services rather than in custodial care. This policy of diversion of such offenders from the criminal justice system to health and social services, put increasing pressure on the medium secure units, whose inpatient population changed from a heterogeneous group of primarily offenders with some non-offenders, to an almost homogeneous high risk offender population. This 'squeezed out' any admissions from local mental health units of non-offenders, and also made it more difficult for special hospital patients to be rehabilitated through a medium secure unit.

The Reed Report (1992) set out five guiding principles for the care of such patients, who should be managed:

- With regard to the quality of care and proper attention to the needs of individuals.

- As far as possible, in the community, rather than in institutional settings.

- Under conditions of no greater security than is justified by the degree of danger they present to themselves or others.

- In such a way as to maximise rehabilitation and their chances of sustaining an independent life.

- As near as possible to their own homes or families, if they have them.

These five guiding principles should govern the provision of mental health services and are also embodied in the National Service Framework for Mental Health (Standard 5) which proposes that each service user should have 'timely access to an appropriate hospital bed . . . which is in the least restrictive environment consistent with the need to protect them and the public, and as close to home as possible'.

In the UK there has been increasing recognition of the need for a range of secure services. This has been identified in a number of national and regional documents and initiatives. Even so the National Service Framework for Mental Health recognises that 'there are gaps in . . . local intensive care provision' and 'there is a need for more intensive care beds in some inner city areas' (Department of Health, 1999).

The closure of large psychiatric hospitals has led to a degree of decentralisation of inpatient facilities to smaller units, often in district general hospitals, each of which requires access to intensive care. As a result of these types of forces, in the UK, many new PICUs are being designed, commissioned and opened. This chapter will address some of the issues which need to be considered by all those who may be involved in the development and opening of a new PICU.

DEFINITION OF PSYCHIATRIC INTENSIVE CARE

For the effective function of any unit, but particularly in intensive care, it is essential that there is clarity about the purpose of that unit and clarity about the treatment plans of the clients.

PIC has been defined elsewhere as care in a highly staffed unit for those who are mentally ill and behaviourally disturbed. This is often in a secure setting, and ideally by a multidisciplinary team. However such a definition encompasses a wide variation in types of units with a variety of patient groups. These can be most easily described when the functions of the unit and treatment regimes are considered according to the patients' needs.

One of the major functions of any treatment is the management of risk associated with the mental illness. That includes risk to the patient's own health or safety, and that of any risk the patient may present to others.

Although there are a number of ways of assessing risk, one way of describing the risk presented by an individual is to consider three distinct aspects of this. These are:

- The **seriousness** of the act which the individual is at risk of committing (i.e. a postulated dimension from minor public order offenses, through physical assaults to murder).

- The **immediacy** of the risk (i.e. a dimension of probability of that action occurring within a given time period).

- The **duration** of the risk (i.e. how long the individual will remain at that level of risk).

These aspects of risk translate into the characteristics of the environment and treatment for the individual. Seriousness roughly relates to the level of perimeter security required. Immediacy relates to the intensity and quality of supervision the patient requires and the skills of the clinical team. Duration relates to the prognosis of the mental condition and the anticipated duration of the treatment regime. These three dimensions can be varied independently and serve to describe a range of the components of a comprehensive psychiatric service (Figure 14.1).

In this way the purpose and characteristics of a PICU can be defined according to the needs of individual patients.

NEEDS ASSESSMENT

PICU is part of a comprehensive mental health service and even with clear definition need will be in part determined by the range and completeness of the rest of the service.

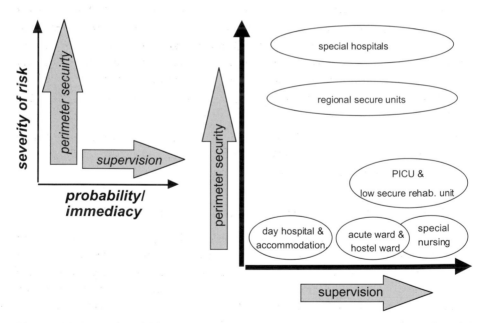

Figure 14.1 – Relationship between components of risk and characteristics of secure units. The three dimensions of risk – seriousness, immediacy and duration – roughly translate into the perimeter security, supervision and duration of treatment. At each level of security and supervision there are various types of service for different lengths of treatment, i.e. acute day hospitals and supervised accommodation, acute wards and hospital hostel wards

The first step in the commissioning and opening of a new PICU is the recognition that such a service is required. This frequently involves some form of local population needs assessment. While there are formulaic predictors of population need these are often not as useful as more local *ad hoc* methods. This is because the requirement for a PICU in a certain area is dependent upon the capacity of other parts of that service to deal with the disturbed mentally ill. Thus measures such as the number of patients in PICUs distant from the local acute inpatient unit or those patients requiring special nursing on general wards probably serve as the best local indicator of the need for a PICU. However future trends and envisaged changes in service configurations need also to be considered in order to address future demands.

PROPOSED SERVICE DESCRIPTION

The population based needs assessment serves to define target patient group and from this it is possible to derive all other features of the proposed service. This applies in particular to the characteristics considered above (perimeter security, intensity and quality of supervision, duration of treatment). With this information a detailed service description can be derived. Such a service description must include detailed information regarding admission and discharge criteria and the processes involved in this, as well as the relationship of the PICU to other parts of the general psychiatry service (acute wards and alternatives to hospital admission), rehabilitation services and specialist accommodation for those with severe and enduring mental illness. Particular attention must be paid to the relationship with services for mentally disordered offenders, including local forensic psychiatry service.

The description of the service also must address the types and duration of treatment and care plans which are likely to be required by the target patient group. This in turn will inform the planning of the staffing of the unit.

THE PROPOSAL: A PLANNING PARTNERSHIP

Once the need for a PICU has been recognised, a partnership between the commissioners of health services and those who provide them is needed to ensure the effective implementation of a plan. While commissioners have responsibility to ensure comprehensive services are provided, it is the responsibility of providers to ensure optimum use of resources. At one extreme, a wholly new service may be commissioned while at the other a provider may reconfigure existing services to create a PICU service within existing budgets. In reality the situation is likely to be somewhere in between these two options. However, it is essential at this stage that the development should take place with a sound financial plan.

This plan will include the consideration of the various options for the PICU. Equally effective PICUs may have very different physical environments and configurations determined according to local need. Thus the first determinant is likely to be the size of the required unit. This can range from an isolatable area within a ward, to a ward or complex accommodating 20 or more patients. The physical size of the unit will determine the possible sites for the unit. The proximity to referring services will affect the operation of the unit especially with regard to admission and discharge procedures. The possibility of a unit serving more than one acute admission unit can be considered here and a service which is shared may have advantages in some circumstances over a small, independent unit when demand is low and infrequent. However this economy of scale and potential for development of specialism among staff, must be balanced against the Reed principle that patients receive care 'as near as possible to their own homes or families', as well as the potential difficulties of transporting acutely disturbed individuals to a separate and possibly distant unit.

The development of the various options to be considered will involve discussion with architects and/or estates departments. The earlier the dialogue can be started between the planners and clinicians the more satisfactory the outcome is likely to be.

THE PROJECT MANAGER OR MANAGEMENT TEAM

One way of establishing a dialogue between the clinicians and architects or designers, is to establish a project management team to do this and implement other necessary tasks. While the project management team may have a wide representation of key stake holders drawn from commissioners, providers (both clinicians and managers), users and others, this group is likely to be too large and unwieldy to successfully oversee the day to day management of the project. A solution to this is the appointment of a single project manager. This may be either a senior member of the staff who will work in the unit, or someone seconded from other duties for the duration of the project. Each has its advantages and disadvantages. A member of clinical staff may not have previous experience of this type of work and the skills necessary, but will have the understanding of the purpose and function of the planned unit. Conversely, someone who will not work in that particular unit in the future may have previous experience of opening similar units or of project managing the other services. The important consideration is that the project manager has the necessary skills to complete the work or has access to appropriate support systems to develop these skills throughout the duration of the project.

The project manager must define timescales for each task in discussion with the relevant groups such as architects and builders. The tasks to be achieved include the building design and other estate issues, staffing of the unit, recruitment and training, and the development of policies for the operation of the unit. This latter issue needs to be considered in conjunction with other agencies with which the unit will have operational links as well as addressing meaningful user involvement.

Estates issues

The importance of a dialogue between architects/contractors and clinical staff from an early stage and throughout the entire process cannot be overemphasised. While there are guidelines for the construction and physical characteristics of medium secure units, no similar agreed guidance exists for PICUs, probably because of the variation in what constitutes a PICU throughout the country. From the preceding discussion about risk and the dimensions of risk, it is apparent that the security of the perimeter of a PICU is of less importance than the safety of the internal environment. This concept may be difficult for architects and designers to grasp without an understanding of the patient group.

The design of the unit therefore presents a series of compromises. The fittings (door handles, lights, sinks, etc.) are chosen balancing robustness and aesthetic qualities. The internal layout of the ward provides potentially a balance between ease of observation and supervision and the patients' needs for privacy.

The treatment plans and ward based activities will determine the rooms and spaces required on the ward. While the number of separate and isolated spaces determines the staffing levels required satisfactorily to supervise these activities. Elsewhere in this volume (Dix 15) more details of the physical environment of a unit are described, however at the planning stage there is real opportunity to determine these. It is these features and the nature and number of the patient group which determine the staffing requirements of the unit.

New or converted buildings frequently require contractors to return to correct faults which have only come to light once the unit is in use. This is usually anticipated at the time the contract for the work is agreed, and this contract will describe what access the builders will have to the unit after completion to correct such faults ('snagging'). Once the PICU is in operation, it can be very difficult for builders to have safe access to the unit. The presence of the builders and associated noise can exacerbate patients' arousal levels. Tools and other equipment provide a source of potential weapons for either self-harm or against others. While it is not impossible for building work to be carried out in an operating PICU, the difficulties of this must be made known to the contractors from the outset, and the extent of access after completion specified in the contract. This is often referred to as a 'no snagging' clause.

There are a number of stages in the planning design and construction of a new building. At each stage the involvement of clinical staff is important. At each stage the involvement of clinical staff is possible and will contribute to the successful outcome of the project. How clinical staff can contribute at different stages in the process is indicated in table 14.1.

Table 14.1 – Desirable clinical involvement at different stages of a building programme

STAGE	ACTIVITY	CLINICAL INVOLVEMENT
Proposal to develop PICU	Size of unit confirmed	Recognition of clinical need
Hospital estates department involved	Initial options considered: • new build versus • conversion • site • size possible	Feasibility of patient transfers access to unit, etc. Outline operational policies to address these points
Architects involved	Confirm space required and layout including perimeter and gardens Detailed room plans developed	Confirm spaces match activities of unit layout ensures safe observation Fitting secure and safe
Initial costings produced	Budget renegotiated	Revised plans still appropriate for activities and safety
Plans agreed and tenders sought		Proposed contract includes clauses regarding site access which allow clinical activity in adjacent areas
Contractors appointed		
Preliminary meetings	Confirm contract agreement	Confirm on site arrangements
Building work commences		
Regular progress meetings between contractors and other parties	Monitor progress	Amend plans in line with unforeseen changes and clinical need
Building work finished		
Pre-handover check	Confirm satisfactory completion of contract	Confirm building meets clinical needs
Handover of building to clinical service	Formal acceptance that work has been completed satisfactorily	Involve local estates in preparing building for occupancy
Post-completion correction of problems		Ensure any works do not interfere with safe and effective running of unit

Staffing issues

From the preceding sections it can be seen that the assessment, care planning and treatments required by the target patients will determine the staff required in the unit. It is necessary to consider the professions which need to be represented, and related to this, the skills required. The size and activities of the unit will determine the absolute numbers of staff of each discipline.

Multidisciplinary team approaches are widely accepted in other sub-specialties of psychiatry as providing effective care delivery for patients with complex needs. The multidisciplinary team is equally effective in the PICU setting. The disciplines of importance include nursing, medical, occupational therapy and other activity-based therapists, psychology, as well as social work. For those patients with severe and enduring mental health problems the involvement of community based staff in the ward activities is likely to promote long-term engagement after discharge. This may be achieved by, for example, involvement of the community staff as patients start having short periods of leave from the PICU prior to transfer.

How each of the disciplines is provided in the PICU may be a matter for a local solution. However an identifiable team of the same nurses, doctors and therapists to work with all patients in the PICU will help promote a consistency of approach which may be beneficial in the PICU.

Prior to the opening of the unit the staff identified to work there will require appropriate training in certain areas. This will include general induction into the local service, and training in procedures common to all the parts of the service. These topics are likely to include fire procedures, training in the Mental Health Act, and the Care Programme Approach (UK Government Policy that certain patients have a care plan which is maintained in hospital, in the community and when they cross geographical boundaries. As well as these general topics there are specific skills which are of particular importance in PICU, such as dealing with violence and techniques of physical restraint.

Having identified a set of core skills required for all staff before the PICU opens, there must also be some process for subsequent appraisal and further training to engender staff development. This will contribute to enhancing staff morale, as well as recruitment and retention of staff. Other factors should be identified at this stage which may improve recruitment and retention and be incorporated into a policy, possibly in line with other units in the organisation, to provide a variety of clinical experience.

The operational policy

When this includes a mission statement and a statement of the strategic objective of the unit, this is a crucial document to provide all staff with a clear understanding of their role in the care of an individual patient who may present unattractive or antisocial behaviours. As such the operational policy is therefore a key document in promoting staff morale, provided all are aware of its content. The document should include not only the procedural details regarding admission, treatment and discharge, but importantly a description of the philosophy of the unit.

In this planning stage the following topics need to be considered and addressed:

- Philosophy of care

- Description of service users

- Admission policies

- Referral process

- Assessment methods (considering standardised tools, see below, 'Audit and Evaluation')

- Care planning

- Treatment protocols

- Review including liaison with likely discharge placement

- Discharge procedures

- Audit and evaluation.

User and carer involvement

It is widely recognised that meaningful user involvement is important for the successful running of effective mental health services. Similarly, carers' needs also need to be addressed by these services. The possibility of having user representation on the project management team has been mentioned above; however, this should not stop once the unit is opened but a process for user involvement in the management of the established unit must be considered.

For an individual patient in the unit advocacy is also important, and some formal advocacy arrangement must be organised. Similarly, the involvement of carers in care plans and the needs of the carers (who may also have been victims) must be addressed by the ward team.

POST-COMMISSIONING POLICY

A well-defined operational policy will ensure that a unit is flexible and adaptable, continues to develop according to evidence-based practice, and to the changing needs of patient and society, rather than become institutionalised and stagnant. Thus, it must have in place a continuous evaluation and audit of service and all aspects of practice, in line with the demands of clinical governance. (a UK Government requirement to ensure a system of improving, monitoring and standardising quality of core across the country).

The unit may also have an educational role to enhance practice in other settings and thereby possibly prevent the need for transfer of patient to a PICU.

Any ongoing evaluation of the service should include measures of not only the core clinical functions, but also staff morale and turnover, as a successful unit needs to be sustainable in the long-term.

CONCLUSIONS

From the preceding discussions it is apparent that while there are a large number of small areas which need to be considered when planning and opening a new PICU, the success of this is dependent on the clarity of the identified purpose of the unit based on an assessment of the local need. If this strategic vision for the unit is then applied consistently in all the subsequent activities the unit is more likely to be successful in the long-term. However, the system needs to be flexible and adaptable to respond to changes in local need and developments in practice, and this adaptability must be built into the oragnaisation from the outset.

Acknowledgments

I am grateful to my colleagues Marie LeMaire and Ernie Croft for helpful discussions about the issues raised in this chapter.

APPENDIX: EXAMPLE OF PICU OPERATIONAL POLICY

AW Procter and E Croft, **** Ward, Manchester Royal Infirmary

**** Ward is a 10-bedded psychiatric intensive care unit serving the **** Healthcare Trust. The ward represents a (low level) secure environment with a locked door to care for severely disturbed patients on an acute short-term basis. Its concern is to effect as rapid a transfer of patients to open general psychiatric wards as possible: the single most important facilitator of this is the efficacy of its admission procedure.

Admission policy

The aim of the patient's admission must be clearly established from the outset, in order to determine the therapeutic benefit of such a decision and the outcomes expected before the transfer back to the referring ward.

**** Ward will typically only accept patients on a referral basis (see Referral Procedure) and after the referring ward has exhausted all methods of managing that patient. As a rule newly admitted patients will not be considered as candidates unless they are well-known as having established patterns of creating problems. The decision to refer a patient has also to take into account how that person's overall needs could be best met.

There must be clear therapeutic outcomes sought by the admission rather than solely being one of containment. Where referrals are not regarded as suitable for a PICU, an appropriate plan of care must be formulated with the referring ward which may include the possible re-referral of that patient at a later date.

Patient characteristics

- Patients suffering from a mental illness and aged between 16 and 65.

- Those patients whose behaviour is so disturbed that it jeopardises the progress and well-being of themselves or others by remaining on a general acute ward.

- Those who are severely ill and repeatedly attempting to abscond from the hospital, thereby placing their own or others safety at risk.

- Those who require a degree of privacy and dignity not possible on a general ward.

Patients regarded as unsuitable for a PICU environment

- Those with a history of serious violence (e.g. malicious wounding, homicide and other serious offenses such as rape).

- Admissions solely as a result of alcohol or illicit substance intoxication.

- Those with organic brain damage.

Philosophy of care

The ward's therapeutic milieu places an emphasis upon personally appropriate solutions to patients' problems, focusing in particular upon the relationship between the individual's strengths, problems and beliefs, health or illness status, and his or her world. Intrinsic to this is the view that each person is a unique individual who possesses the potential for maturation, learning and growth in an environment that preserves dignity and fosters mutual respect and acceptance.

Quality care is of paramount importance for severely disturbed patients at the core of which is a multidisciplinary research-based approach, in line with a strict adherence to the mandatory requirements of the Mental Health Act (1983) and the Care Programme Approach.

**** Ward's staffing levels, training and shift patterns necessarily need to enable appropriate, structured responses to acts of violence, self-injury and social disruptiveness.

Patients are regarded with compassion and interactions met by calmness, respect and gentleness. Rules are kept to a minimum since we believe discussion and negotiation to be a more beneficial and appropriate medium to encourage the acceptance of responsibility. Similarly, informality among patients and staff is regarded as an important tool in maintaining tensions fostered by the admission at tolerable levels.

Consultant responsibility

When a patient is transferred to ★★★★ Ward there is a corresponding transfer of medical consultant responsibility for that persons care. ★★★★ Ward benefits from having one dedicated consultant and supporting medical team that works in collaboration with the nursing team and occupational therapist to provide an overall ethos of care.

Nursing perspective

The management of ★★★★ Ward fully accepts the finding of the scoping study by the UKCC on 'Nursing in secure environments' (1999) and will endeavour to incorporate its recommendations into professional practice. In particular:

*   Practice standards and procedures – there will be an ongoing concern to develop standards (current areas being developed include restraining patients, use of rapid tranquilisation, debriefing procedures and clearer identification of professional roles) that are supported by research evidence and incorporated into overall performance indicators.

*   Pre-registration preparation for nursing in secure environments – ★★★★ Ward is available for clinical placements of learners to facilitate knowledge and understanding.

*   With regard to post-registration nursing staff – individuals will be supported in their continuing professional development through clinical supervision, the use of staff appraisal in a facilitative manner, and robust operational policies and procedures which are regularly monitored and updated.

Discharge criteria

Once ★★★★ Ward have accepted a patient, the referring ward must designate a liaison nurse to visit the client and monitor his or her progress. When the precipitating problem(s) that necessitated the transfer are resolved to such a degree that the patient would benefit more from an open environment, then he or she has to be returned to the original ward to facilitate progress towards discharge. At this stage that patient's key nurse on ★★★★ Ward will effect the transfer of care to the ongoing liaison nurse and, if appropriate, may continue to provide some input to care planning to consolidate the patient's progress.

Other policies

There are additional written policies concerning:

- Referrals

- Patient-centred activities

- Commencing leave

- Low stimulus environment

- One-to-ten nursing observations

- Absence without leave

- Searching of patients

- Restraint of patients

- Rapid tranquilisation

- Debriefing following critical incidents

- Preceptorship.

REFERENCES

Nursing in Secure Environments: Summary and Action Plan from a Scoping Study 1999. London: United Kingdom Central Council for Nursing, Midwifery and Health visiting

Reed Committee. 1992 Review of Health and Social Services for Mentally Disordered Offenders and Others Requiring Similar Services. London: DoH/Home Office

Royal College of Psychiatrists. 1980 Secure Facilities for Psychiatric Patients: A Comprehensive Policy. Council Report London: Royal College of Psychiatrists

UKCC Department of Health 1999. National Service Framework for Mental Health. London: Department of Health

15

PHYSICAL ENVIRONMENT

Roland Dix

GENERAL PHILOSOPHY OF PSYCHIATRIC CARE UNIT DESIGN

The role of the psychiatric intensive care unit (PICU) in relation to other in-patient services remains unclear (Dix and Williams 1996). The reasons for this may be two-fold. Firstly, the Reed Committee (1992) recommended that local services improve service provision for mentally disordered offenders. The implication for the design of PICUs is that perimeter security may need to reflect the needs of the forensic patient. Secondly, it is accepted that the PICU will need to accommodate the acutely disturbed patient, whose behaviour is driven by the acute phase of mental illness (Goldney *et al* 1989). A physical environment able successfully to accommodate both the forensic patient, who may be symptom free and also the acutely disturbed general adult patient, is at best, very difficult to achieve and possibly unworkable. While accepting the difficulties in establishing a clear role for the PICU, it is possible to set a number of general principles that form the foundation on which an effective design can be based.

Much of the design, materials and specifications for the construction of psychiatric hospitals will be well known to NHS trusts estates departments. Documents such as the Design guide for medium secure units (NHS Estates 1993) and Accommodation for people with mental illness (NHS Estates 1996) contain detailed guidance for hospital design, much of what is relevant to the PICU. This chapter aims to provide the clinical context within which PICU design should be considered. The location, size, operational policy and patient population will vary amongst PICUs. An effective PICU physical environment needs to be based on broad principles that reflect the type of service one is proposing. For these reasons, it is inappropriate to lay down rigid design specifications. This chapter provides experienced-based principles for an effective PICU design, around which individual units may be tailored to meet their specific needs.

For the purposes of this chapter the following statements will constitute the terms of reference for PICU design.

Table 15.1 – Terms of reference for PICU design

1. The environment will be effective in providing increased safety against aggressive, impulsive and unpredictable behaviour.
2. The design of the PICU will make it difficult to abscond and the methods necessary for absconding will be predictable.
3. The PICU environment will allow a range of therapeutic activities to take place.
4. It will provide adequate space and facilities for a homely environment in which a patient can spend the majority of their day, for up to 6 months.

These broad statements should be relevant to any PICU, including those based in local services, Maximum Secure Units MSUs and Special Hospitals (maximum security).

PICU POSITION AND LAYOUT

The PICU should preferably be on the ground floor. This will assist in the admission of acutely disturbed patients, and facilitate access to the fresh air. One possible benefit of locating the PICU on the first floor is that it may discourage absconding through windows. However, the benefits of locating the unit at ground level are significant and window specifications can prevent absconding. For PICUs that are part of hospitals, an entrance to the unit that does not necessitate travelling through the rest of the hospital should be provided. Multiple corridors should be avoided in order to promote unobtrusive observation. The amount of space to which patients have access has been an important factor. Palmstierna *et al* (1991) investigated the relationship between over crowding and aggressive behaviour in a PICU. They concluded that aggressive behaviour was more likely in areas of higher patient density. Further evidence that PICUs need ample space is provided by Citrome *et al* (1994) who conclude that length of stay in the PICU is not as brief as may be expected. The NHS Estates department (1993) design guidance for MSUs suggested a 6-bedded medium secure PICU should offer 30 square metres of free access space, per patient. When assessing the available space for patients in a PICU, the mistake of including staff areas in the square metreage should be avoided; 6–8 beds is a good number. There should also be access to an enclosed garden (Dix and Williams 1996, NHS estates 1996).

Effective designs share a number of general characteristics e.g. pipes, wires and heating are hidden. Other important characteristics are listed below and illustrated in Figure 15.1.

a) Wherever possible there should be clear lines of sight. This should also be possible around corners, by means of aligned windows or convex mirrors.

b) Corridors are 3 metres wide allowing four abreast comfortably.

c) Ceiling height is 3 metres giving the feeling of space.

d) The ceiling is fitted with sky lights that allow increased daylight into the main corridor.

SECURITY LEVELS

The level of interior and perimeter security is influenced by whether the PICU is serving the general adult population or the forensic population. PICUs within or serving a medium secure unit will have security characteristics consistent with the NHS Estates design guide (1993) for medium secure units. The same applies for units located within a Special Hospital. For PICUs serving the general adult population things become a little less clear. It is easy either to over- or underestimate levels of security for the general adult PICU. Care should be taken to ensure there is a difference between medium security and the general adult PICU. Otherwise a unit

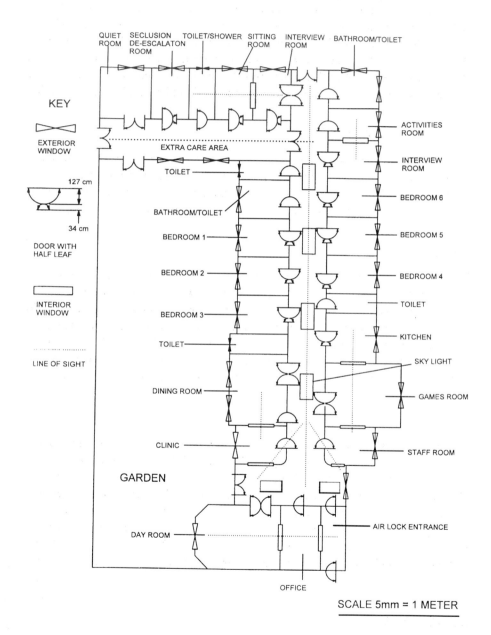

Figure 15.1 – Suggested layout of a PICU

whose expertise and clinical focus is geared towards the general adult population may be placed under pressure to fulfil an inappropriate role, e.g. admit forensic patients. When considering the likely methods that may be used by a patient to abscond, it is a useful exercise to spend at least 2 hours in the unit environment, and ask oneself, 'if I was intending to abscond, how would I go about it?' Following this exercise, many likely methods will become apparent and preventative steps may be employed. Security issues are described throughout this chapter in the specific areas addressed. All security measures, for example, window restrictors, should be as discreet as possible.

SECURE GARDEN

The level to which the garden is secure will largely be a matter for the PICU planning group. Standard operational procedure will generally require a staff presence when the garden is in use. A sensible balance should be drawn between the construction/height of the fence and the oppressive image created by fencing (NHS Estates 1996).

MAIN ENTRANCE

An air lock design is recommended for the main entrance. This means that the entrance comprises of two doors set opposite each other. Once a person has entered through the first door, the second will not open until the first has closed. This may be achieved by means of magnetic lock systems or by synchronised key operated locks. The main entrance should be located away from the main clinical area. This will help in preventing absconding when the entrance is in use. It also helps remove attention from the main entrance which is often the focus of 'drama' with regard to absconding attempts.

FIRE EXITS

Fire safety and security are frequently in conflict. The local fire officer must be involved at an early stage of planning (NHS Estates 1993). It is possible for fire exits to be secured on magnetic locks that become inactive when the fire alarm is activated (Dix and Williams 1996). There can be a number of problems with this arrangement. Firstly, the system will need to be disconnected from the fire alarm test procedure. Secondly, patients may soon become familiar with this system and simply activate the fire alarm in order to abscond. The most reliable method may be to secure the fire exits on a lock and key. This will require a clear procedure for evacuation in the event of fire.

WINDOWS

Dolan and Snowden (1994) concluded that the majority of escapes from a medium secure unit occurred through windows. While windows offer an obvious target for escape, they also help the unit to feel less claustrophobic. Any unit design should aim for as much natural daylight as possible into the main clinical areas. The design suggested in Figure 15.1, includes ample outside windows in all rooms, and where appropriate, interior windows across rooms. Because of the need for clear lines of sight, outside windows directly into the main corridor are difficult to achieve (Figure 15.1). To overcome this, ceiling sky lights may be used, providing the unit is without a second floor.

Polycarbonate, toughened glass and float glasses are recommended. Glass and plastics manufacturers are constantly improving products. Sophisticated glazing panels are available in polycarbonate and glass combinations. The resulting window can be specified as 'bandit proof', shot gun proof, sledgehammer proof and so on (NHS estates 1996). It is also important for the frame to withstand determined attempts at dismantling. Ventilation is also very important (Mueller 1983) and windows should have a restricted opening of no more than 125 mm. In addition to the windows' standard restrictors the inclusion of a camouflaged durable steel bar, fixed to the outside wall is also useful. In some sitting areas, windows should be placed 700–800 mm above the floor to allow seated outside views. In the extra care area (see below), and possibly other areas of the unit, curtain poles should be avoided. Integral window blinds may be used instead. An assessment for the necessity of any fitting that could be used for suicide by hanging should be undertaken.

DOORS

All doors should be of solid core construction at least 45 mm thick. Such doors will be durable against abuse and also offer good sound proofing. Door-frames should also be of sufficient strength to withstand kick and other such forces. Lillywhite et al (1995) pointed out the benefits of interview room doors opening outwards. These benefits include prevention of patients barricading themselves in and promoting easy exit. For the interior of the unit it is most beneficial that as many doors as possible open both ways.

Aggression and access through doors

Areas of high patient concentration are often the location of aggressive incidents (Palmstierna et al 1991). Double doors should provide access to areas from which a patient may require relocation with control and restraint (C & R). This will provide enough width to allow access for a three person C & R team. Several authors have identified the dining area and meal times as a focus point for aggressive incidents amongst in-patients (Fottrell 1980, Kennedy et al 1995, Hunter and Love 1996). Kennedy et al found that of 80 incidents of aggression that took place away from the main residential unit, 74 took place in the dining room. As a general principle double doors should be installed in rooms such as the day room, dining room, activities room and other areas in which more than two patients gather. For bedrooms a half leaf arrangement is useful for allowing access to a C & R team. The measurements are shown in Figure 15.1.

LOCKS

A variety of locks are now available for the modern psychiatric hospital. These include electronic numbered key pads, swipe card locks and the traditional key arrangement. Electronic magnetic locks have the advantage of removing the need for bunches of keys which often have negative connotations in terms of the authoritarian institution. However, they have several practical problems. Locks operated by the combination key pad have a major disadvantage as patients soon become familiar with the combination (Dix and Williams 1996). They require the operator to stand directly in front of the key pad to conceal the combination. Also, they often have a time delay between the combination being entered and the lock becoming re-active. This is also the case for the swipe card lock. The problem here is that once a lock has been activated it is necessary to wait by the door for it to re-engage to prevent a patient following. This becomes a problem when struggles occur in doorways. Unless an electronic lock can be designed without the above problems, the traditional lock and key maybe the most practical. The female part of the lock should be concave in order for the key to be entered quickly in emergencies. The number of different keys should be kept to a minimum reducing the number to be carried.

Where should locks be fitted?

It is desirable to 'lock off' as many of the rooms as possible. Rooms such as the day and dining area will, for the majority of the time, remain open for free access by patients. There may be times, however, when it will be necessary for these rooms to be temporarily restricted. The kitchen area presents particular problems and should always be considered a potentially dangerous place. A clear operational policy should describe the use of the kitchen, including the circumstances in which access may be restricted. Obviously, the bathrooms and toilet will need to be lockable from the inside, staff must be able to override these locks from the outside, with keys held by staff only. Bedrooms may also be locked from the inside with the same precautions as above. It may be useful in promoting responsibility to provide patients with keys to their own rooms, but again this should be with the provision of an override key held by staff. In any room that can be locked from the inside, care should be taken to ensure that the override system will work, even if the interior side of the lock is held.

OBSERVATION

Close observation is a frequently quoted reason for admission to the PICU. One-to-one close observation or 'specialing' is a familiar, and often unpopular practice amongst many PICU nurses. Green and Gatson (1996) found one-to-one close observation to be common practice in 80 psychiatric hospitals in the United States. In their analysis the authors identified several disadvantages including secondary gain and behavioural escalation by the patient. Other authors have also identified one-to-one observation as a problematic procedure lacking clear empirical evaluation of its effectiveness (Duffy 1995, Macpherson 1996, Olakunle *et al* 1997). In their retrospective study, Shugar and Rehaluk (1990) concluded that one-to-one observation in excess of 72 hours was particularly problematic and should be avoided. From the available evidence, and in keeping with the experience of many nurses who have performed this procedure, an effective PICU design should minimise the need for one-to-one close observation.

Figure 15.1 offers a suggestion for design that allows for high levels of unobtrusive observation.

Table 15.2 – Criteria for effective design

1. As many clear lines of sight as possible should be available, avoiding numerous corners and corridors (Figure 15.1). Interior windows should be aligned where possible (Figure 15.1) to allow observation across a number of rooms.
2. All doors (with the exception of the bathrooms and toilets) should be fitted with a polycarbonate observation panel. This will enhance safety when moving around the unit by ensuring that the staff and patients can see the other side of doors.
3. Bathrooms and toilets may be fitted with a 'fish eye' observation lens. This should be covered by a lockable panel.
4. Bedrooms should be fitted with a louvre-type window controlled from the outside.
5. Bedroom lights should be controlled by switches with a dimmer, one inside and the other outside the room. This will allow for night time observation.
6. Where corridors meet, and in other areas without clear lines of sight, convex mirrors can be fitted at ceiling level to allow views around corners.

FACILITIES FOR MANAGING THE MOST ACUTELY DISTURBED PATIENT

Patients who demonstrate extremely unpredictable and assaultive behaviour present particular management problems. Throughout the history of mental health care seclusion was often the solution for this type of behaviour (Renvoize 1991). In recent years the use of seclusion has been questioned for its clinical, ethical and practical value (Hamil 1987, Angold 1989, Tooke and Brown 1992). Kinsella and Brosman (1993) suggested the use of an extra care area (ECA) as an alternative to seclusion. This is defined as a closely supervised living space, away from the main clinical area in which a single patient may be nursed away from the rest of the patients (Dix 1995). The NHS estates building note no. 35 (1996), advises the project group for a new PICU to decide on the need for a seclusion room. If the extra care option is chosen this should be used for the shortest possible time, as extended use is prone to producing the same negative effects as one-to-one observation (Kinsella and Brosman 1993).

Figure 15.1 shows an ECA, which could also include a seclusion room, or, if preferred, a de-escalation room in which staff remain with the patient, rather than the patient being locked in.

EXTRA CARE AREA COMPOSITION

Unless staffing levels will allow staff to be dedicated to the ECA then it should be possible for the ECA to be part of the unit, and not physically separated. In terms of the number of staff needed, there is a danger of creating a ward within a ward. Figure 15.1 shows an ECA separated by double doors, which could be fixed open to allow the ECA to become part of the unit. In the ECA, a higher level of safety is needed than any where else in the unit. Care is necessary to ensure that items which could be used as a weapon are avoided.

The ECA should be able to provide for the daily living needs of a single patient. This will require the following all in close proximity to each other:

Table 15.3 – Contents of extra care area

1. A seclusion/de-escalation room (see below).
2. A toilet and shower facility.
3. A sitting room with simple furnishings.
4. An entrance to the ECA directly from outside the unit, for the admission of acutely disturbed patients.
5. Access to the garden.
6. An intercom system to the main office.

DESIGN OF SECLUSION/DE-ESCALATION ROOM

- Should be located in the extra care area of the unit.

- Furnished with a single moulded vinyl safety bed.

- The size should allow for at least 7 square metres and a ceiling clearance that cannot be reached by jumping or standing on the safety bed.

- The room must be able to withstand determined attack and damage.

- Walls and floors should be lined with a welded seam vinyl surface.

- The door should be of solid core design of a least 55 mm thickness, with an observation panel, double glassed with high-grade 5-mm polycarbonate.

- It should be possible to see into the whole room from the observation panel, without any hidden corners.

- Ventilation/heating is provided through air vents placed at ceiling level out of reach. Noise levels generated by this equipment must also be minimised.

RECREATION AND OCCUPATIONAL THERAPY

The value of planned therapeutic activity amongst patients in the institutional setting has long been accepted (Aumack 1968). There is strong evidence that psychiatric institutions are poor performers in ensuring that therapeutic activity is high on the agenda (Drinkwater and Gudjonsson 1989). Correlations between aggression and inactivity have also been established (Lloyd 1995). With the inevitable preoccupation with safety and containment a PICU maybe amongst the most guilty of psychiatric settings in failing to provide adequate resources for therapeutic activity (Zigmond 1995). Best (1996) dramatically demonstrated the value of activity for bringing about positive changes to disturbed behaviour in the PICU setting. An effective PICU design will have given the provision of therapeutic activity an equal status to safety and security.

Recreation/activity facilities

Figure 15.1 includes

- A games room in which a pool table, table tennis table, exercise bike and punch bag may be placed. This may be more like a gymnasium if there is no gym in the rest of the hospital.

- An activities room in which board games, art equipment and stereo equipment is placed.

- Day room and sitting room equipped with television and video.

- Access to enclosed garden area.

- Agreed policies and procedure for local escorted and unescorted leave.

For the most part, activities will be undertaken with the direct support of staff. Individual assessments will indicate the amount of staff intervention required (Best 1996). When not in use or as clinically indicated these areas may be locked off. Use of activity equipment and facilities should be supported by standard operational procedures (SOP) (see below). Activity programmes must include collaboration between nursing staff and the Occupational Therapist. Electrical sockets in bedrooms are useful for patients wishing to listen to music etc on their own. There should be the provision for the power to be disconnected by staff if additional safety is required.

FURNITURE AND FITTINGS

The unit environment should be made as homely as possible. Wall mounted pictures, pot plants and non-moulded furniture promote a relaxed environment without presenting a major risk to safety. Poster type pictures may be fixed to the wall on a back board covered with polycarbonate. Some units may wish to surround the television and video with a polycarbonate fronted protective case. In the experience of the author, protection of this type may encourage attacks towards the television, rather than deterring them. The unit should be fitted with a pay telephone to which the patients have free access (Mental Health Act Code of Practice Department of Health 1999). This should be on a portable trolley, allowing it to be removed in the event of consistent inappropriate use.

STAFF AND PATIENT SAFETY

Personal alarm systems carried by staff, that when activated, alert others to an emergency are useful. The basic principle of these systems is a signal sent from a hand unit to a wall or ceiling mounted sensor which has an audio visual output. These units operate either by ultrasonic, infrared or radio signals. The technology in this area is rapidly developing and new products are constantly entering the market. When considering which product will be most effective, a demonstration by the manufacturer is a necessary step. The following common problems should be avoided;

- Systems too directionally sensitive resulting in the need to point the hand set directly at the receiver.

- Systems where the hand set is over powered resulting in the activation of several receivers confusing the exact location of the emergency.

- Systems that are under sensitive resulting in the need to press the hand unit several times before the alarm is sounded.

Wall-mounted emergency buttons with audiovisual output are also a necessary fitting. These should be installed in addition to the hand held systems as they also offer protection for the patients. A button should be placed in all rooms and at regular intervals in corridors. There should be the provision for the system to be de-activated centrally in the event of persistent inappropriate use by patients.

COMMUNICATION SYSTEMS

Two way radios are recommended. These are useful for communication around the hospital and on short escorted leave. They are also of particular value in other situations, for example, searching for a patient who has absconded. Again a variety of products are available with new equipment entering the market. For extended range it is necessary for a booster transmitter to be installed on top of the building. Standard industrial units, such as the Motorola Handie-com S 200, are relatively inexpensive and offer reasonable performance (approximately 1.5 miles in a built-up area). For longer distance escorted leave, a mobile phone is recommended, pre-programmed with the numbers of the ward, hospital reception and the police.

STANDARD OPERATIONAL PROCEDURE

The value of equipment and managing the physical environment may be optimised by developing Standard Operational Procedures (SOP). SOPs are widely used by organisations faced with complex management situations. They describe a standard response to situations that commonly occur, and for which contingency plans are needed. They are designed to promote confidence in the staff for dealing with difficult situations, maximizing the therapeutic options that may be considered. The following is an example of an SOP in the event that a patient becomes disturbed, or attempts to abscond while on escorted leave.

1. During every episode of escorted leave, the escort will carry a radio and/or mobile telephone. The mobile phone must also be carried if the destination is over 1.5 miles.
2. Before leaving the unit the escort will ensure a second radio is held by a member of staff and that both radios are switched on and working. The escort will state the intended destination and approximate duration of leave.
3. If there is a deviation from the stated plan or expected duration of leave, the escort will inform the unit.
4. If the patient becomes disturbed or attempts to leave the escort:

    *   Attempt verbal negotiation.

    *   Failing this, contact the unit and assess the appropriateness of physical intervention. Only attempt physical intervention if safe to do so.

    *   If physical intervention is inappropriate, follow the patient at a safe distance, contacting the other staff by radio with situation reports at 5-minute intervals.

SOPs are used to support staff in the use of equipment and maintaining a safe environment. They should be kept as simple as possible and taught to all unit staff (including medical and paramedical team members). In terms of the physical environment, other areas where the development of SOPs should be considered are:

*   Preparing the ward environment for an acutely disturbed admission.

*   Interviewing, or negotiating with, a potentially aggressive patient.

*   Use of the extra care area.

CONCLUSION

In a chapter of this size, it is not possible to describe every detail of the ideal PICU physical environment. The design guidance offered is not overly prescriptive but is intended to provide the principles on which PICU design can be based.

During her study of nurses perceptions of a new PICU, Gental (1996) identified dissatisfaction with the physical environment as a major issue. Taj and Sheehan (1994) also found high levels of dissatisfaction in the architectural design of a new acute unit. After only six months they recommended major design changes. In a statistical comparison of a ward atmosphere and staff attitude between a PICU, MSU and acute ward, Squeir (1994) commented that in the PICU:

> 'Organizational structure and programme clarity were diminished, which indicates the difficulty staff have maintaining order and organization'.

It is essential that the planning of a new PICU involves a detailed and careful analysis of the physical environment. For those planning a new PICU development, it is highly recommended that several visits are made to established units to consider the environments strengths and weaknesses. Once a new unit is operational, it should be considered as an inherent part of planning that the physical environment will be modified and developed.

ACKNOWLEDGEMENT

Thanks to Mr Terence Dix for his expertise with producing the diagram.

REFERENCES

Angold A. 1989 Seclusion, British Journal of Psychiatry 154: 437–444

Ashaye O, Ikkos G, Rigby E. 1997 Study of the effects of constant observation of psychiatric in-patients, Psychiatric Bulletin 21: 145–147

Aumack L. 1968 The patient activity checklist: an instrument and an approach for measuring behaviour, Journal of Clinical Psychology, 25: 134–137

Best D. 1996 The developing role of occupational therapy in psychiatric intensive care, British Journal of Occupational Therapy, April, 59: 161–164

Citrome L, Green L, Frost R. 1994. Length of stay and recidivism on a psychiatric intensive care unit. Hospital and Community Psychiatry 45 (1): 74–76

Department of Health Mental Health Act Code of Practice. 1999 London: HMSO

Dix R. 1995 A nurse led psychiatric intensive care unit, Psychiatric Bulletin, May, 285–287

Dix R, Williams, K. 1996 Psychiatric Intensive Care Units, a design for living, Psychiatric Bulletin, 20: 527–529

Dolan M, Snowden P. 1994 Escapes from a medium secure unit, Journal of Forensic Psychiatry, 5: 275–286

Drinkwater J, Gudjonsson G. 1989 The nature of violence in psychiatric hospitals. In: Howells K, Hollin C (eds) Clinical Approaches to Violence, 287–305, Wiley, Chichester

Fottrell E. 1980 A study of violent behaviour amongst patients in psychiatric hospitals, British Journal of Psychiatry 136: 216–221

Gental J. 1996 Mental health intensive care units: the nurses experience and perceptions of a new unit, Journal of Advance Nursing 24: 1194–1200

Goldney R, Bowes J, Spence N, Czechowicz A, Hurley R. 1985 The psychiatric intensive care unit, British Journal of Psychiatry 146: 50–54

Green J, Grinde C. 1996 Supervision of suicidal patients in adult inpatient Psychiatric Units in General Hospitals, Psychiatric Services 47: 859–863

Hamil K. 1987 Seclusion: Inside Looking Out, Nursing Times, 83 (5): 174–79

Hunter M, Love C. 1996 Total Quality Management and the Reduction of Inpatient Violence and Costs in a Forensic Psychiatric Hospital, Psychiatric Services 47: 751–754

Kennedy J, Harrison J, Hillis T, Bluglass R. 1995 Analysis of Violent Incidents in a Regional secure unit, Med Sci Law 35: 255–260

Kinsella C, Brosman C. 1993 An Alternative to Seclusion? Nursing Times May, 89: 62–64

Lillywhite A, Morgan N, Walter E. 1995 Reducing the risk of Violence to junior psychiatrists, Psychiatric Bulletin 19: 24–27

Lloyd C. 1995 Forensic Psychiatry for Health Professionals, Therapy in Practice, London: Chapman & Hall

Macpherson R, Anstee B, Dix R. 1996 Guidelines for the management of acutely disturbed patients, Advances in Psychiatric Treatment, 2: 194–201

Mueller C. 1983 Environmental stressors and aggressive behaviour. In: Green R, Donnerstein R, Aggression; Theoretical and Empirical Reviews, Vol 2: Issues in research, New York: Academic Press inc.

Musisi S, Wasylenki D, Rapp M. 1989 A Psychiatric Intensive Care Unit in a Psychiatric Hospital, Canadian Journal of Psychiatry, 34: 200–204

NHS Estates. 1993 Design Guide: Medium Secure Psychiatric Units, NHS Estates; An Executive Agency of the Department of Health, Leeds, London: HMSO

NHS Estates. 1996 Accommodation for people with mental illness, Health Building Note 35: Part 1 – The acute unit, London: HMSO

Palmstierna T, Huitfeldt B, Wistedt B. 1991 The relationship between crowding and aggressive behaviour in the Psychiatric intensive care unit, Hospital and Community psychiatry 42: 1237–1240

Renvoize E. 1991 The Association of Medical Officers of Asylums and hospitals for the Insane, the Medico-Psychological Association, and their Presidents, IN: 150 Years of British Psychiatry 1841–1991 Berrios, G and Freeman, H (eds) 29–75, London: Gaskell

Reed Committee. 1992 Review of Health and Social Services for Mentally Disordered Offenders and Others Requiring Similar Services. London: Department of Health/Social Services Office

Squier R. 1994 The relationship between ward atmosphere and staff attitude to treatment in psychiatric in-patient units, British Journal of Medical Psychology 67: 319–331

Taj R, Sheehan J. 1994 Architectural design and acute psychiatric care, Psychiatric Bulletin 18: 279–281

Tooke K, Brown J. 1992 Perceptions of seclusion: Comparing Patient and Staff Reactions, Journal of Psychosocial Nursing 30: 23–26

Zigmond A. 1995 Special care wards: Are they special?, Psychiatric Bulletin 19: 310–312

16

MANAGING THE PSYCHIATRIC INTENSIVE CARE UNIT

Phil Garnham, Debbie Coleman

INTRODUCTION

One measure of effective management is the consistency with which the unit retains its place on the continuum between therapy and custody. The role of the ward manager and the multi-professional team are crucial to this.

The PICU is a place of rapid and constant change, with high levels of arousal, experienced by staff and patients alike. Effective management can ensure that key principles are not lost or compromised by a pressurised environment, and that all actions and care are carried out within the context of safe practice.

Key principles

- A clear sense of purpose for the unit is known and owned by the staff, and communicated clearly to patients.

- The purpose of the unit is to manage acute mental ill health episodes and then return the patient to a more appropriate care setting.

- As far as possible and practicable, patients and their relatives are actively involved in their care and how it is delivered to them.

- Staff at all levels are consulted and involved in the decision-making process with regard to the running of the unit.

- Staff are given full support for career development and the promotion of excellence in practice.

- The functioning of the unit is subject to regular audit and appraisal in order to develop and improve care given to patients.

- Care should be evidence-based.

For any local approach to be achievable and effective, consideration should be given to national approaches. The National Service Frameworks for Mental Health (Department of Health 1999a) sets out standards in five areas to 'reduce variations in practice and deliver improvements . . .'.

Table 16.1 – National Standards and Service Models

Standard one	Mental health promotion
Standards two and three	Primary care and access to services
Standards four and five	Effective services for people with severe mental illness
Standard six	Caring about carers
Standard seven	Preventing suicide

The chapter on 'Effective services for people with severe mental illness', makes frequent reference to psychiatric intensive care and low secure services, e.g. gaps in provision (p. 49); access to hospital (p. 62); monitoring of milestones (p. 68).

DEVELOPMENT OF THE PICU

A fundamental question which must be addressed is where the PICU is situated managerially? That is, does it form part of the acute service, the forensic services, community respite, etc.? The only definite answer is that it probably does not belong in elderly care!

Local services will differ in their function and form, therefore, the decision as to where the unit should be situated is best left to local opinion. However, the authors believe that the acute psychiatric inpatient services are best suited as they will share managerial and philosophical input. Indeed, most of the patients of the PICU will be drawn from these clinical areas.

Policy and guidelines

A PICU will, at times, be a frantic and chaotic place. Staff may have little or no warning of an admission. Invariably, the patient will be experiencing acute psychiatric or drug induced symptoms, or will be expressing feelings of acute anxiety, distress, threat or fear. The nature and definition of the admission will lead to the patient feeling uncertain, frightened and experiencing a loss of control. At times like this the staff may often feel unable to take control of their immediate environment, or frozen by the anxiety of the unknown. It is all too easy, when faced with adversity, to 'batten down the hatches' in a need for certainty and the danger is that patients are forgotten in this crisis, leaving them isolated and uncared for. This can lead to an increase in symptoms experienced by the patient and a subsequent rise in the level of disturbance. Staff will need to feel confident and in control of the admission process, which will then enable a consistent, confident and caring approach.

It is essential then that the ward area can provide a structured, responsive and understanding environment. Patients will respond better to a setting where they feel that their emotions and experiences are contained or held safely. The staff group need to understand clearly what the expectations of their role are and be confident in exercising their ability to care for the individual's needs. An accurate assessment of the patients' needs, often under difficult conditions, is essential to the success of the admission process. The patient may be experiencing a lack of understanding, resentment and occasionally hostility. It is the nurses' role to reassure the patient as soon as possible that they are in a safe, caring and understanding place. Unit policies and guidelines should reflect this approach. Identifying areas where guidance is required, such as search procedures, levels of observation and day-to-day duties, will help the staff to work safely and consistently. These policies and guidelines will also need to provide a degree of delegation to the staff, so that they feel permitted to exercise individual or team decisions within certain previously defined parameters, such as the ability to reduce or increase leave status or adjust individual guidelines.

There are issues relevant to policy and administration and some of the more significant ones are detailed below.

Operational policy

Every unit needs one. It should reflect the local approach to PICU whilst encompassing any larger service frameworks, e.g. Mental Health Nursing: 'Addressing Acute Concerns' (SNMAC 1999a) and Practice Guidance: Safe and Supportive Observation of Patients at Risk (SNMAC 1999b). It should be practical, accessible and realistic.

Working Practice Manual

This document should exist as a wealth of reference for all staff working in the PICU and should remain accessible to health care assistant and consultant alike. It should be relevant and up to date and serve as the main practice area document for induction and on-going practice and development. The working practice manual should be evaluated, reviewed and updated on a yearly basis. Everyone should be made aware of it and the practice laid out within it, adhered to.

The following is a list of some relevant areas that the Working Practice Manual needs to pay particular attention to. The authors have tried to cover the diverse and constantly changing needs of the PICU patient group.

Admission policy

This will reflect the needs of the admitting population as well as any services and agencies that may be involved. It should give clear guidance for staff and be capable of implementation. (see chapter 14 for sample policy)

Visiting policy

This needs to be sensitive to patients and relatives' needs, whilst offering the clinical team a sense of control over access to the unit. Specific attention should be given to the child protection policy and child visitors. (see Appendix A for sample policy No. 1 p. 328)

Restricted items

Patients or relatives may try to bring items onto the unit which, without staff being aware, may cause problems or complicate an already problematic situation. These need to be clearly identified to staff, patients and relatives alike and clear demarcation made between strictly forbidden items and items which may be helpful to a patient's care, but that staff need to know about or have control over.

Table 16.2 – Restricted items

Strictly forbidden	Staff to be informed
Illegal drugs	Money
Weapons e.g. knives (injury/self harm)	Lighters
Scissors/pen knives	Razors
Alcohol	Jewellery
Solvents	Electrical goods
Glass objects	Any medication
Matches	Jewellery
Lighter fuel	

It is important to note that the above is a list of possible options and not exhaustive. What is a safety issue for patient A, may not be for patient B. There is no substitute for a comprehensive individual assessment based on a thorough understanding of the patient's behaviour and need.

Keys

Whether electronic or good old fashioned keys, staff need to be aware of how they work, who can have one and what to do if one is missing, or not working. A common sense but strict policy will enable staff to maintain safety, whilst avoiding a key dominated environment. All new staff should have an agreed, signed induction, before they are allocated a key.

Kitchen/servery

The policy should cover access to these areas, spelling out the criteria, with clear guidelines on how the assessment should be made. Particular attention should be paid to the patient's current and on-going mental state, behaviour, understanding of responsibility and ability to use the environment safely. If sharp knives are to be used, then a full risk assessment should be undertaken and documented using the above criteria and including skill based activities of daily living assessment.

Staff/patient call alarms

The team needs to know how and when to summon assistance and what each individual's responsibility is at any given time. Regular testing should occur and a record of this kept; and as a matter of course all staff should be inducted into the effective use of the alarm system immediately.

Searching patients

As this is a contentious area regarding individual human rights and the responsibilities of professionals, staff will need to be clear on what is permissible and what is not, and to know particularly what other course of action is available to them if a search cannot be undertaken. (see Appendix A for sample policy 2 p. 330)

Clinic checks

Staff need clear direction on what area needs checking and how often. A record should be kept.

Escorts

This policy will need to indicate the balance of responsibility staff have to safeguard themselves whilst providing a safe experience for the patient. Breaking down in table form and clearly identifying who is responsible for what is often helpful, as shown in Table 16.3.

AWOL (Absence without leave)

Clear guidelines, processes and protocols on the reporting and searching of AWOL patients is needed. Police liaison may be of benefit when the PICU suddenly needs to call upon them, or vice versa (see Appendix A for sample policy 3 p. 332).

Table 16.3 – Leave granting

Type of leave	Authorisation
Clinic garden (garden leave)	The team is expected to identify any issues of risk and plan for or implement strategies to minimise risks. This can be given at the discretion of the nursing team.
Internal campus (campus leave) This refers to the central courtyard only and does not include other clinics or the therapies centre	The team is expected to identify any potential risk element as above. However, if this discretion occurs on more than three occasions, then it is expected that the care group will have made representation to the Management Round or Full Review to establish a team view and/or decision. This can be given sparingly at the discretion of the nursing team.
Hospital grounds (ground leave) This includes the entire grounds of the Hospital and all clinics in the area. Subject to visiting hours and any other individual restrictions imposed.	The decision to grant leave should normally occur as part of a Management Round or Full Review. The only exceptions to this would be if attendance to dental or other external service located in the hospital grounds is required. The team are expected to have identified any potential risk element as above (See garden leave).
Leave outside of the hospital grounds (outside leave)	The decision to grant outside leave will always be made by the multidisciplinary team within the context of a Management Round or Full Review. The only exceptions to this will be in the case of emergency medical treatment.

Restraint (see chapter 8)

As there is currently no specific legislation or recommendation governing the use of restraint, the unit will need to make a clear statement on what is permissible, practicable, appropriate and required within the law.

The UKCC Nursing in Secure Environments: Summary and Action Plan (1999) Section 15 on Preparation for the management of aggression and the use of physical interventions found that, 'There are no national standards in relation to physical interventions and therefore professional practice in physical interventions is inconsistent'. Studies are being conducted in this area.

Whatever approach the unit adopts, this should link in clearly with the resources available within the unit, leaving staff with a clear sense of their role and responsibility. Training in Breakaway Techniques is essential and an accepted approach to control or restraint identified. The Royal College of Psychiatrists' (1998) Management of Imminent Violence Occasional Paper OP41 will be of use when agreeing a way forward.

Regular training and refreshers should be provided every six months for breakaways and restraint training and these need to be built into a staff induction package, which is linked to the on-going professional development of the staff team. (see Appendix A for sample policy 4 p. 334)

Seclusion (see chapter 7)

Not all units will opt to use seclusion. Where they have, a clear policy and monitoring statement needs to be made. The Royal College of Psychiatrist's guidelines (1998) on the Management of Imminent Violence can offer a good framework. Where units opt out of the use of seclusion, it must be made clear to staff what alternatives are to be used, along with any resource and training implications. Again the Royal College guidelines can help in the therapeutic management of potential violence and aggression.

Observation/Monitored Supervision

The PICU will be mindful of its approach to close observation. Managing the delicate balance between maintaining a patient's personal safety (at a time when they are usually not able to manage it for themselves), whilst avoiding a custodial or punitive approach to care, is a skill that is developed through supervision, support, education and experience. Poorly implemented observation can produce anger, resentment and frustration, often leading to an exacerbation of the behaviour the observation is trying to prevent.

Given the lack of any evidence towards the effectiveness of observation has led Baxter and Cutcliffe (1999) to propose a move away from 'defensive practices, such as observation' towards the 'human needs of the individual'. However, current practice in many settings is to establish clear criteria for observations in an attempt to minimise inconsistency and maximise safe practice. Any policy must reflect the needs of the patient and give clear/sound guidelines to the practitioner. (see Appendix A for sample policy No. 5 p. 335).

As referred to previously in this chapter – Practice Guidance: Safe and Supportive Observations of Patients at Risk (SNMAC 1999b) is 'intended to be a template for local services to use in developing protocols and practice'.

Risk assessment (see chapter 11)

This will need to follow in line with any trust hospital policy and, whilst providing a framework within the clinical area, should inform staff of the issues around risk assessment. Some way of formally recording any risk assessment should be produced and rigorous evaluation, monitoring and communication of results needs to be encouraged.

It is helpful for any approach to set clear guidelines as to standard risk assessment points which should be addressed in any decision-making process. These areas will include:

- Past behaviour
- Current mental state
- Alcohol and drug use
- History of violence
- History of suicide/self harm
- History of absconding
- Relapse indicators
- Protective factors.

Other factors may be appropriate given a particular individual's circumstances and this should be included and documented in any risk assessment process.

Drug and alcohol use

This area is a sensitive and complicated one. Given our natural reaction to be fearful of drug and alcohol misuse and its potential effects, staff are likely to be defensive about such practices. This is not to suggest that they are right to do so, but to encourage a wider discussion on the realities of the situation. The team should be addressing issues such as 'Why do patients abuse or misuse? How has this developed? Can it be understood? Can it be prevented? If it cannot be prevented, can it be minimised? Can patients be helped to use more appropriately, or do they need to be stopped?' All these issues have differing answers depending on the person who asks the question and the person to whom the question is directed.

Given such a complicated set of issues, a policy will need to balance the need to prevent a crime being committed against the long-term well-being of the patient. A policy which offers clear guidance to staff on what to do in the case of the taking and supplying of non-prescribed drugs or substances, which also encourages a positive and inquisitive approach to the nature of behaviours. The application of the law and boundaries of confidentiality will have to be considered within any policy framework.

Any policy statement will have to balance the therapeutic use of alcohol, e.g. for social or recreation purposes, against its potential for misuse.

If alcohol and drug consumption is to be monitored and the results used as a therapeutic aid, then a rigorous but sensitive process of taking specimens will need to be adopted. Patient's privacy and dignity will need to be maintained, whilst at the same time ensuring that the specimen produced is not tampered with. A good example is a patient who was later found to be negative for cannabis use, but had got a fellow patient to produce a urine specimen for him, which turned out to be positive. Anyone with experience of drug and alcohol care in institutions will know some of the lengths patients will go to, to produce a negative urine specimen. (see Appendix A for sample policy 6 p. 337)

THE WARD ENVIRONMENT

In order to ensure that the environment provides high quality therapeutic interventions balanced against a safe enviroment, the provision of a structured environment is essential.

Of course it could be argued that any combination of effective interventions can, together, make up a safe and structured environment. However, it is often not the case that this occurs by chance. It is not the authors' intention to provide an exhaustive list of possible elements for an effective structure, but to provide a back bone upon which a safe, united, responsive and flexible environment can be created. It is all too easy to settle on a particular approach, which has proven safe, but this cannot always continue to be ensured and can often lead to a custodial and negative approach to patient care. It is essential that the staff team remain alert to all changes that can occur within the environment. They will then remain responsive to the needs of the immediate situation and to those of individual patients.

There will be many other factors that can contribute, but a basic structure is essential. Below are a number of elements essential to the development of an environment that, by its nature, is structured and safe, yet responsive to individual needs.

Buildings should be purpose-built with good observation, preferably the Nursing Office being built as the centre of the unit where all day areas, bedroom corridors, recreation and assessment areas can easily be observed. The unit should be well lit with plenty of natural daylight, providing individual living space, with sturdy, well maintained and decorated rooms.

Management of the ward should be structured, with a clear hierarchy as to who makes decisions, whilst allowing involvement from all staff, with each grade and discipline being clear about their role and function.

The shift system should be clearly defined and the structure adhered to. For example all nursing staff should attend handovers to maintain a consistent care approach with good communication. To assist in this process it would be helpful for the multidisciplinary team to meet before the on-coming shift, to discuss and share observations, check out quality and accuracy of reports and plan for information to be handed over. This will aid team cohesion.

The shift will also benefit from having a co-ordinator, whose duty it is to plan and organise the shift, receive and manage information and be aware of all staff and patient changes.

Crucial to this structure is the consistent and effective use of a Communication Book, Diary and Shift Meeting Minutes and a commitment from all staff to update themselves at the start of each shift.

An individualised handover, where the nursing report is read out to the patient, is a good time for staff to meet and discuss progress with the patient. It will also bring the oncoming staff immediately up to date with the patient's progress.

Regular staff meetings should be facilitated by the ward manager with the intention to include the nursing team in policy and decision-making processes, to foster ownership of the environment and to disseminate any local or national developments. These meetings will need to identify a purpose and direction, to avoid them becoming over critical.

It is desirable to recruit staff with an appropriate attitude and personality and attributes such as the following:

- Non-judgmental
- Patient-focused
- Self-aware
- Reflective
- Able to treat patients with dignity and self-respect
- Committed to self-development
- Demonstrate an understanding of patients' situations.

Lowe (1992) identifies the following categories as suggestions for effective intervention:

- Confirming messages
- Personal control
- Staff honesty
- Providing face-saving alternatives
- Setting limits
- Use of structure
- Facilitating expression
- Monitoring
- Timing
- Calming
- Use of non-verbal skills.

The integration of the above skills into a secure setting where the nursing team manage potentially difficult behaviour, is discussed further in Conlan *et al* (1997).

Staff mix. Wherever possible, the staff group needs to reflect the age, gender and cultural mix of the patient group. However, in reality, this is often difficult to achieve with any consistency and hence concentrating on the above recruitment aspects may compensate for any shortfall.

Internal rotation. Rotas should be organised to maintain consistency and yet mix staff together, e.g. a rota system that enables small teams to work together for the majority of time, but that overlaps with other small teams. This will enable teamwork and a sense of belonging within the staff group, whilst avoiding the development of fixed attitudes and inconsistent approaches.

Therapeutic programme. This will need to reflect the needs of the patient group and be flexible enough to accommodate local changes within the patient group. Any programme will benefit from a focus based plan which enables the ward community to interact together, encouraging socialisation and awareness of the needs of others. Providing occupation can enhance self-esteem, reduce boredom and decrease irritability, minimising the potential for violence and aggression.

Multidisciplinary input. The multidisciplinary team (MDT) will need to adopt a cohesive, consistent and influential position. All disciplines will be represented, provide structured and informative feedback and where appropriate, be prepared to endorse team decisions.

Case-management review system. The PICU requires a space or place whereby the team can reflect on patient care and progress. Given the potential rapid turnover of the patient group it can often be difficult to spend lengthy amounts of time discussing each individual. The team will have to balance the need to review acute symptom management, whilst maintaining a focus on future options. It is easy to become reactive rather than pro-active. This indicates the need for an efficient review system which allows for team discussion and user involvement. A system which allows for monthly reviews of patient care (if longer term care is occurring) whilst enabling weekly management can help. The reviews would be multidisciplinary, concentrating on history, progress, risk management and discharge planning, whilst the weekly management concentrates on day to day issues.

Empowerment of nursing via assessment and decision-making schemes. There should be weekly summaries of patient progress, and wherever possible pre-admission nursing assessments thus primary nurse responsibility is supported and respected by effective delegation, with multidisciplinary team responsiveness.

Effective multi- and interdisciplinary working. The care team needs to be able to agree on risk assessment factors and communicate this to the patient, relatives and professionals such as social workers, probation officers, GPs, the community psychiatric nurse, and other members of community teams. Regular attendance from any or all of the above at case reviews and discharge meetings will greatly enhance the consistency and effectiveness of follow-up treatment.

Evidence-based practice and research. The care team must ensure that their practice is based upon contemporary research and is subject to clinical audit. The audit process has to be viewed in the wider context of Clinical Governance set out in The New NHS (Department of Health 1997) and A First Class Service: quality in the new NHS (Department of Health 1998), whilst taking into account the needs of the local service. This is very important in order to ensure that high quality care is delivered, and the unit strives toward being a 'Centre of excellence' whilst meeting the needs of its patients and staff.

To focus on incident monitoring, use of seclusion, restraint and staff sickness will give a picture of the current atmosphere within the environment, but will only be of use if this is looked at within the wider context of staff recruitment and retention, induction, professional development and job satisfaction, whilst evaluating ward milieu, patient resources and patient satisfaction.

The unique placement of the PICU suggests that key areas of research could be the use of seclusion and the variables of race, gender and time of day of incidents. All incidents, or reports of 'near miss' incidents that occur in the unit should be routinely analysed on a quarterly basis. This will start to build up a picture of where flash point areas occur and will enable ward managers to prioritise resources and target educational areas.

EDUCATION AND TRAINING PLAN

It is important that education and training focuses upon the needs of the patient group which, by definition, will also meet staff needs. When planning training sessions, thought must be given to the symptoms experienced by patients, both from their illness and their treatment. Evidence-based interventions and sociological issues such as lifestyle and coping responses should be included. The training approach needs to be responsive to issues not often experienced or particular diagnoses that staff do not work with regularly. In this way the PICU can provide training that enables the staff to do their job better, feel that they are supported by their organisation in what they do and demonstrate the same sensitive and responsive approach to its staff training needs as it hopes to do with its patient group. The use of a Personal Development Review will assist in identifying the training needs of the staff group as well as of individuals.

Wherever possible training should be interdisciplinary to share and amalgamate different experiences and skills. In fostering reflective practice, significant service carers can be encouraged to present case reviews with the team, to encourage appraisal of care and promote good practice.

As educational needs are many fold, it is useful to attempt to systematise the service's response to its need. It is important that the PICU is clear about its approach to education.

Risk assessment

This will need to reflect the type and nature of admissions, be realistic as to what can be achieved and encourage the development of a format in which information can be managed effectively.

Risk management

Linking risk assessment material into the latest care planning and Care Programme Approach (Department of Health 1999) documentation will enable the multidisciplinary team to look at the patient in a dynamic and objective way thus enabling a care management approach which can be pro-active and responsive to individual needs.

Staff inter-personal skills

Training opportunities which offer the team the opportunity to role-play symptom experience, understand and use effective and appropriate communication skills, whilst enabling the sharing of experiences, feelings and responses can enable a team to develop into a more coherent unit, which will have a positive impact on the quality of care delivery. The Association of Psychological Therapies (APT) workshops on the 'Reinforcing Appropriate, Ignoring Difficult behaviour (RAID)' system for working with Challenging Behaviour or APT: 'How Not to Get Hit – preventing face to face violence', can be of great use to team confidence and sense of cohesion.

Management of violence and aggression

The ability to deal with face to face issues and de-escalation techniques are just as important as an understanding of the theoretical origins of violence and aggression. Also, the ability to appreciate the use of therapeutic milieu and the impact of structure and environment upon the ward atmosphere will greatly enhance the team's attitude to the workplace and influence the unit positively (Royal Coll of Psychiatrists, 1998).

Breakaway techniques/Control and restraint/Care and responsibility

The approach to physical restraint and containment is a difficult area which generates more discussion than there is room for here. The PICU will need to establish an approach that is mindful of its patients' needs and rights, whilst offering the staff group some autonomy and control over their environment. A training strategy that empowers its staff group to approach potentially dangerous situations in a positive and confident manner is less likely to rely upon the use of seclusion and restraint. Enabling the staff to utilise Breakaway techniques and Control and Restraint techniques will remain viable only whilst adequate refresher training and staff resources are present. However, a cohesive and robust attitude to this area will inevitably produce a team that is comfortable in its abilities whilst prepared to reflect upon its actions. This can lead to a positive approach to the treatment of a potentially difficult patient group.

Team building

Although often not cheap, team building and empowerment training can contribute to a team's sense of identity, purpose and cohesiveness. Team empowerment training or away days can offer value for money if set in the context of a wider strategy.

Individual, group and family work

Concentrating on providing a broad but basic level of understanding in the above areas, linked to a treatment philosophy encompassing the same, can provide and maintain effective staff interventions. The team will often be balancing the roles of care-giver and custodian. Having confidence to provide information with a preparedness to listen to concerns and issues from patients and their relatives, linked to a clear treatment goal can enable the staff group to convey warmth and understanding, whilst feeling in control.

Advocacy and empowerment

Advocacy and empowerment are areas recognised as essential to the feeling of involvement (Sang 1999) and a sense of being listened to, that will assist greatly in the patient's recovery.

Empowerment can allow the patient access to information about their rights and treatment and can facilitate the patient having a degree of control over treatment received.

Advocacy can enable users of services to influence practice and give the patients a voice that can be heard, to support them through difficult times. The issue of advocacy and nursing, is stated in the UKCC guidelines as follows:

'5. Work in an open and co-operative manner with patients, clients and their families, foster their independence and recognise and respect their involvement in the planning and delivery of care.'

This is not often as straightforward when applied to PICU nursing. Given the increasing likelihood that some patients detained under the 1983 Mental Health Act will have used illegal substances, often in an attempt at self-medication prior to admission, issues of confidentiality may make nurses' experience an apparent conflict between policies and guidelines on the one hand and the patient's best interests on the other, leaving them unable to remain objective or independent at times.

Exploration, training and reflection will be essential if the nurses are able to pick up on the nuances and subtleties of advocating for this patient.

Formal advocacy may well be served better when provided by outside agencies who are seen as separate from the local service structure such as MIND groups or the National Schizophrenia Fellowship. The PICU would do well to encourage and invite such groups into its organisation to agree local protocols and assist in improving access and feedback.

Mental Health Act 1983

With the increased use of the Mental Health Act and particularly the practice of admitting some patients detained to low secure facilities and the current policy for transfer of patients from prison to NHS facilities under criminal sections, the PICU will require a comprehensive package of Mental Health Act, 1983, Code of Practice (DoH 1999c) training to enable its staff to be confident and competent in these areas. In increasing the staff's confidence the service will enable the team to spend more time concentrating their efforts on assessing and nursing the needs of their patients.

N.B. The current review of the Mental Health Act 1983 (DoH 1999d) may propose changes to existing doctors' and nurses' holding power and these will need to be kept under review. A more detailed discussion of the implications to nursing practice can be found in Ashmore and Carver (2000).

High-dose neuroleptics, emergency medication management and atypical antipsychotics

Input from pharmacy staff on the increasing developments and changes within psycho-pharmacological treatments will enable the team to offer the most effective and appropriate treatment regimes, enhancing the quality of patient care and creating positive experiences for staff and patients.

Evidence-based interventions

Access to medication management training, early warning signs, cognitive interventions for schizophrenia (Wykes *et al* 1998), relapse prevention (Marlatt and Gordon 1985), motivational interviewing (Miller and Rollnick 1991), compliance therapy (Kemp *et al* 1997), KGV symptom scale assessment (Krawiecka *et al* 1977), social functioning scale (Birchwood *et al* 1990), amongst others, will enable the staff to gain a better understanding of symptomatology, to choose more effective interventions to disseminate them throughout the team.

Formal training

The organisation will need to maintain strong links with its Health Care Training provider or local Nurse Training University, to ensure that the education provided remains appropriate to the context of the health care area and provides practitioners that are best equipped to deal with the demands of the day. The PICU service should endeavour to offer its experience and involve itself in the provision of training.

For post-registration staff the current English National Body for Nursing, Midwifery and Health Visiting approve a number of courses that would be relevant to the PICU nurse.

The following are some of the more relevant ones:

ENB 612, 616 and 620	Drug and Alcohol dependency for Nurses, Midwives and Health Visitors.
ENB 769	Coping with violence and aggression: Effective prevention and management techniques for practitioners. Stage 2.
ENB 770	Nursing within controlled environments.
ENB 953	Developments in psychiatric nursing.
ENB 955	The care of the violent or potentially violent individual.
ENB 956	Coping with violence and aggression: Effective prevention and management techniques for practitioners. Stage 1.
ENB 998	Teaching and assessing in Clinical Practice.
ENB A61	Acute Psychiatric Nursing.

It is important for the service to remain aware of the skill and experience mix of its staff group and, whenever possible, utilise them as a training resource to develop any areas of team inexperience. This will enable the core staff group to influence and facilitate improvements in the quality of care given.

Table 16.4 – Summarising a training approach

Safety & Security	Therapeutic intervention	Patient empowerment	Legislation and statutory requirement
Team empowerment	Individual work	Advocacy	Mental Health Act
Risk assessment	Group work	Empowerment	Health and safety
Care and responsibility training	KGV symptom scale assessment	Daily living skills	Fire evacuation training
Use of environment and structure	Inter-personal skills	Motivational interviewing	Control of Substances Hazardous to Health (COSHH)
Induction	Family work	Compliance therapy	Cardiopulmonary resuscitation (CPR)
Management of violence and aggression	High-dose neuroleptic usage	Relapse prevention	First Aid
Risk management	Atypical anti-psychotics	Substance misuse	Care Programme Approach (CPA)
Breakaway	Early warning signs Cognitive symptom intervention		Mental health law
Relevant further and higher education			

Of course this is not able to cover all areas and resource management will be an on-going issue in the prioritisation of training needs, but the use of a focused approach can aid management. It is important that the service remains aware of the skill and experience mix of its staff group and utilise them as a training resource to develop areas of inexperience, whilst empowering its core staff group to influence the quality of care given.

To aid recruitment and retention the service should ensure that the staffing budget has taken into account sufficient provision to enable staff to undertake further education at local or higher level from education providers to enhance skills confidence and understanding.

STAFF SUPPORT

In an environment that is turbulent, constantly changing and very stressful, there is a clear need for structures that offer staff support and the opportunity for staff to explore their practice (Minghueue and Benson 1994). These structures can take various forms, they can be informal or formal, but there must be a forum that all staff recognise as being consistent and safe for them to express their views. The role of the manager is to ensure that these meetings take place and to encourage as many staff as possible to attend. There will be occasions when the manager and members of the multi professional management team should attend and be part of the team, but there will also be times when the rest of the team needs space away from 'management'.

One of the most useful and difficult to achieve skills of a manager is knowing when to attend and when to allow space. This facilitates the balance between a supportive manager and an overcontrolling one. The unit itself and how it is allied to the needs and dynamics within the staff group will affect whether the manager should be present or not. There are no hard and fast rules. Perhaps one of the best ways of getting it right as often as possible, is to make a habit of asking the staff group what their expectations of you, as the manager are. If these expectations are unreal, this should be gently highlighted to the staff group and then the whole team can explore and identify more realistic expectations. These should be achievable and will not then lead to the staff team feeling let down by the manager, or to the manager feeling frustrated or as having let down the team.

Some mechanisms for staff support are detailed below.

Induction and mentoring

This is vital for all new staff to the unit. The PICU can be an alarming place; it has already been stated that there is a need for consistency and the process of induction and mentoring will enhance this, as well as supporting new staff in the environment. It is useful to have a formal record of the induction process, which the individual can refer to and which can be tailored according to the individual's need based on their experience, grade, etc.

The role of mentor or preceptor for newly qualified staff is a very meaningful one and it is vitally important that the person assuming the role is equipped to do so, and elects to assume such a role, rather than having it thrust upon them. Support and ancillary staff also need support, structure and induction.

Reflective practice

All staff should be encouraged to maintain their professional portfolio to enable them to reflect upon their practice (Palmer *et al* 1994).

Shift meetings

The authors believe that every nursing shift should have a space set aside for a shift meeting. This should be at the same time each day, for each shift. All staff on duty, from all disciplines should attend, and the patients should be informed that staff are not available for this period. The content of the meeting is informal and should concentrate on the business of the day, but will inevitably allow staff to reflect on recent incidents and the strategies employed to deal with them. It will also allow a space for ventilation of feelings about current patients and their behaviour, which will assist the staff in going back to face the patients again, and engage in therapeutic interactions. Informal staff support may also occur.

Facilitated staff group

Where possible, the unit should employ an outside facilitator, brought in on a monthly basis, to chair an open session for staff. This is designed to allow staff the opportunity to explore current issues that may be causing division in the care team.

The facilitator may have a psycho-dynamic or psycho-therapeutic background and no clinical experience of the environment. A different strategy would be to employ a clinician with relevant experience who could act as advisor and reflect on the team's practice from an objective perspective.

Both these options have relative merits and disadvantages, but the crucial point is that an outsider comes into the staff group on a regular basis and assists with some of the criticisms of insularity and isolationist practice that may be levelled against staff in a PICU.

Team building

For a newly developed PICU with a brand new team this is an imperative. However, even well established teams can benefit from space away from the unit, facilitated by a team-building expert to assist them to examine how they function as a team.

Clinical supervision

The issue of clinical supervision is of great importance to all staff who are involved in the day-to-day care of patients. It is particularly important in areas of high stress where patients may be difficult to treat, such as the PICU. Various models for clinical supervision have been proposed (Butterworth *et al* 1998); the chosen model should reflect the views and wishes of the majority of staff. With a relatively small staff, there is merit in debating whether the clinical supervision should be offered by external staff. This allows for free expression thus not allowing staff to feel inhibited by talking to their work colleagues. The suitability of the supervisor is important as this prevents the potential clash with the annual staff appraisal. The operative phrase here is 'suitability' of the supervisor. It should be possible to make a reciprocal arrangement with another local team. Even if they work in another specialised field, e.g., elderly care, they may be able to offer a useful focus to the PICU team members.

Post-incidents debrief and support

The link between untoward incidents and incidence of staff sickness and absence is well documented, allied with the increasing recognition of post traumatic stress disorder (PTSD) amongst health care staff. This indicates that a strategy for dealing with serious incidents in a structured way may be advantageous (Wykes 1994, Ch.11).

The strategy for this must include some or all of the following:

- Immediate post-incident debrief for all staff involved, facilitated by a senior clinician who was not directly involved.

- Immediate debrief for patients and opportunity to discuss their concerns.

- Structured post-incident debrief within 3 days for all staff involved. This is from two clinicians who are not from the PICU, and who have skills in such work.

- Individual sessions, fixed term for staff most closely involved or who request such input. This is again from an outside clinician and is totally confidential.

Stress busters

The operating trust/hospital may wish to consider offering an activity for the staff group that will assist in reducing stress, e.g. discounted local gym membership or a similar approach which has been identified as beneficial by the staff group.

Annual appraisal and review

Every employee should have an appraisal at least annually. This should, if possible, be a self-appraisal and should focus on identifying practice deficits and developing a training package to overcome these. Annual appraisal or personal development will enable the manager and his or her staff to have face to face dialogue and identify a training plan.

AUDIT OF STRATEGIES

The manager of the PICU should ensure that there are in place methods of auditing the quality of care given to patients and the quality of staff support available in the unit.

To audit care effectively, it is important to have a clear structure and purpose for the unit, with particular areas of demarcation mapped out. It is then straightforward to audit against them. Any subsequent changes can be measured against initial results, demonstrating whether a change has produced a positive or negative result. The use of staff and patient satisfaction questionnaires should be used widely and also a system set up whereby cross-audit occurs, e.g. one unit auditing another along agreed criteria, to enable comparison and the sharing of knowledge.

Methods for evaluating the quality of staff support should include confidential leaving questionnaires for staff who resign. An analysis of numbers of leavers, as a proportion of the staffing establishment, is a useful measure. Areas such as PICUs do have a high staff turnover, and in order to continually develop the unit needs, new staff will always be required. However, there should be a balance in turnover and stability to ensure consistency. Recruitment to PICUs can be difficult and a high level of staff vacancies can lead to escalating stress, and increasing sickness. Staff satisfaction questionnaires that are anonymous and administered by an outside agency can be a useful gauge of that nebulous but so important staff morale. The canvassing of existing staff on education and training issues, service structures and local decisions can also increase staff well being.

STAFF PATIENT RATIOS

Although there are no nationally agreed criteria for PICU staffing and there are different ways of providing psychiatric intensive care, certain common sense rules need to be applied. Whether provided within the acute psychiatric unit or in a purpose built unit, practicalities of staff and patient safety should remain high on the agenda. If adopting Control and Restraint values a minimum of four staff will be necessary on each shift, all trained and kept up-to-date with refresher courses. Therefore to staff a unit with 24-hour cover will require a ratio of two staff to one patient, the minimum cut-off point being a team of 20 nursing staff. This is regardless of the number of beds. A proviso would be that this limit would only extend to 10 beds; staffing would have to increase proportionately at a 2:1 ratio if there were more than 10 beds. However, a strong argument can be made to suggest that any therapeutic efficacy may be compromised if bed state increases above 10.

CONCLUSION

Obviously many of these proposals have a cost implication, but they should not be discounted. In the long run, many of these strategies can have a cost saving factor. For the PICU to avoid being cited as a place of abuse to the patients most in need of care, a modern, well trained and supported workforce with positive attitudes and an open minded approach to their work can do much to remove the myths and taints of the past.

REFERENCES

Ashmore R, Carver N. 2000 Mental Health Practice (Feb) 3, No 6

Baxter P, Cutliffe J. 1999 Mental Health Practice (May) 2, No 8

Birchwood M *et al*. 1990 The social functioning scale. Br J Psychiatry 157: 853–859

Butterworth T, Faugier J, Burnard P. 1998 Clinical supervision and mentorship in nursing, 2nd edn. Cheltenham: Stanley Thomes

Conlan L, Gage A, Hillis T. 1997 Managerial and nursing perspectives on the response to inpatient violence, 7, In: Crichton J. Psychiatric Patient Violence: Risk and response. London: Duckworth

Department of Health and the Welsh Office. 1983 Mental Health Act 1983. London: HMSO

Department of Health. 1997 The new NHS: modern, dependable. DoH London: HMSO

Department of Health. 1998 A First Class Service: Quality in the new NHS. DoH London: HMSO

Department of Health 1999a National Service Frameworks. 1999 Mental Health. Modern Standards and Service models. London: DoH

Department of Health. 1999b Effective Care co-ordination in Mental Health Services: Modernising the care programme approach – A policy booklet DoH London: HMSO

Department of Health. 1999c Mental Health Act 1983: Code of Practice. London: HMSO

Department of Health. 1999d Reform of the Mental Health Act 1983. Proposals for consultation. London: HMSO

Kemp P, Hayward P, David A. 1997 Compliance therapy manual. Institute of Psychiatry, London

Krawiecka M, Goldberg D, Vaughan M. 1977 A standardised psychiatric assessment scale for rating chronic psychotic patients. Acta Psychol Scand 55: 299–308

Lowe T. 1992 Characteristics of effective nursing interventions in the management of challenging behaviour. Journal of Advanced Nursing 17: 1226–1230

Marlatt GA, Gordon RG. 1985 Relapse Prevention. London: Guildford Press

Miller WR, Rollnick S. 1991 Motivational interviewing: Preparing people to change addictive behaviours. London: Guildford Press

Mingheue E, Benson A. 1994 Developing reflective practice in mental health nursing through critical incident analysis. J Adv Nurs 21: 205–213

Palmer A. Burns S, Bulman C. 1994 Reflective practice in nursing. Oxford: Blackwell Science

Royal College of Psychiatrists. 1998 Management of imminent violence. Occasional paper OP 41 London: Royal College of Psychiatrists

Sang B. 1999 The customer is sometimes right. Health Service Journal, 19 August

SNMAC Standing Nursing and Midwifery Advisory Committee. 1999a Addressing acute concerns – report by the Standing Nursing and Midwifery Advisory Committee, London

SNMAC Standing Nursing and Midwifery Advisory Committee. 1999b Safe and supportive observation of patients at risk, London

UKCC 1999 Nursing in secure environments: Summary and action plan from a scoping study. London United Kingdom Central Council for Nursing, Midwifery and health Visiting

Wykes T. 1994 Violence and health care professionals. Chapman and Hall, London

Wykes T, Tarrier N, Lewis S. 1998 Outcome and innovation in psychological treatment of schizophrenia. Wiley, New York

USEFUL INFORMATION

The Association For Psychological Therapies
APT, PO Box 3, Thurnby, Leicester LE7 9QN.
Tel: 0116 241 9934
www.apt.co.uk

MIND
Tel: 0345 660 123
web: www.mind.org.uk

National Schizophrenia Fellowship
Tel: 0207 330 9100
web: www.nsf.org.uk

NHS Careers Post-Registration Studies Programme
Pre and Post-Registration can be obtained from:

>NHS Careers
>PO Box 376
>Bristol
>BS99 3EY

>Tel: 0845 60 60 655
>www.enb.org.uk/carsect.htm

17

GOOD PRACTICE ISSUES IN PSYCHIATRIC INTENSIVE CARE UNITS

Stephen M Pereira, M Dominic Beer, Carol Paton

INTRODUCTION

By the very nature of its practice, psychiatry today is being increasingly influenced not only by various mental health professionals, e.g. psychiatrists, nurses, psychologists, occupational therapists and social workers, but also by the framework within which care is delivered. This includes legal (e.g. Mental Health Act, Mental Health Act Commission), social (e.g. family), political (e.g. Department of Health guidelines) and user involvement (e.g. user groups). Given the rights of patients enshrined with Statute, e.g. Mental Health Act, and in other government guidance, e.g. Care Programme Approach, Patient's Charter, etc., in no other subspecialty is the interface with legal, ethical, political and social issues more acute than with locked psychiatric intensive care. Yet, astonishingly, it is the one area within which these issues have been most neglected. This is partly because intensive care psychiatry is still in its infancy and has yet to attain a cogent force and status as a subspecialty in its own right and partly due to custodial attitudes and other vestiges of institutional care that still prevail. Zigmond (1995) outlines various problems that have been endemic in this type of unit. Only recently, have there been moves to establish a national network of intensive care units in the UK. This has given rise to discussion regarding standards of care, definitions of these units, the patient group and ethical issues.

UK NATIONAL SURVEY FINDINGS

Summarised below are some of the findings relevant to good practice issues from a national survey (Beer et al 1997) of 110 units.

- 88 units locked their doors at all times.

- 46 of those units accepted informal patients.

- 48 of the 89 units accepting prison transfers also accepted informal patients.

- 72 units accepted a mix of intensive care and chronic or challenging behaviour patients.

- 65 units had a male-to-female ratio of 4:1 and a further 25 units a ratio of 5:1 or more male patients to every female patient.

- Eight units had a ratio of at least 10 male patients to every female patient.

- 76 units did not have a policy for administration of high-dose neuroleptics either for rapid tranquilisation or longer-term in 'treatment resistant' patients.

- 22 units did not have a policy for the practice of control and restraint and 15 did not have a policy for seclusion.

- 32 units had no policy for searching patients or visitors.

- 20 units did not have an admissions/exclusions policy.

- 14 units did not have a junior doctor.

- 58 units were covered by junior doctors of the Senior House Officers grade.

- 29 PICUs did not have a dedicated consultant for that unit, providing overall clinical responsibility.

SOME GOOD PRACTICE ISSUES

Informal or formal status

General clinical impressions have so far suggested that all patients admitted to locked wards should be formally detained under the Mental Health Act. This is certainly borne out by observations of, e.g. Zigmond (1995), amongst others. However, a significant number of units do accept informal patients. Whilst there may be sound clinical reasons for this, it does raise the issue of the rights of informal patients in locked units, e.g. their autonomy in terms of leave off the ward, possessions, visits from relatives, etc. Continuing consent to residence and treatment in such patients is often assumed. However, for such implied consent to be valid, the patient must be accepting treatment voluntarily, i.e. not under coercion. Sugarman and Moss (1994), in their survey of 207 informal psychiatric patients in general wards, found that almost half did not know they had a right to refuse treatment. A substantial number anticipated being instructed, pressurised or restrained if they tried to refuse treatment or leave the ward. One might strongly argue that these figures are likely to be much higher in informal patients in locked psychiatric units. Various other studies (Olin and Olin 1975; Grossman and Summers 1980; Appelbaum *et al* 1981; Wolpe *et al* 1991), have found that psychiatric inpatients frequently did not understand their basic rights and issues relevant to informed consent.

Long- and short-term admissions

A majority of units accept long- and short-term admissions. This unsatisfactory mixture of patient groups, with different clinical needs, treatment and clinical regimens often leads to a poor compromise for all groups of patients. The treatment plans and needs of the acute group of patients are reviewed more regularly than longer-term patients, leading to the care of the latter group of patients being compromised. It is clinically well accepted that the longer-term disturbed, or complex needs patient (see Chapter 9) and the acutely disturbed patient require a completely different philosophy of care. It is impossible to deliver appropriate psychiatric care in a unit that accepts the acute informal, acute detained, longer-term informal, longer-term detained and prison transfer/forensic patients. This places an enormous burden on the staff looking after such groups of patients.

Forensic patients

Due to a more proactive approach to identifying psychiatric disturbance in the penal system, e.g. the court diversion scheme and hospital prison wings, a greater proportion of patients with either past histories of violence or with exposure to it are being admitted to PICUs (Atakan 1995). Prison transfer patients by virtue of their sections have different leave arrangements. These units very often also accept informal patients. This again is unsatisfactory. Care delivery to the patients from the penal system is compromised and especially so is the therapeutic environment in which informal and female patients find themselves; higher rates of violence, substance abuse and sexual harassment give rise to a substantially changed ward milieu. Issues of security also become relevant with restriction orders placed on remand patients. This invariably compromises the 'informal' status of the other non-detained patients in these units. Conversely, with a prison regimen, inmates have basic rights to fresh air, exercise, visitors and other privileges. Owing to staffing shortages on PICUs they may actually lose these rights. Interestingly, from Beer et al's (1997) survey this situation is also common in units that do have admissions and exclusion policies, probably reflecting local pressures to accept all categories of difficult patients.

Male/female issues

Most would consider it unacceptable that, within the locked confines of a PICU, females find themselves in a very small minority. Besides practical difficulties, e.g. shared use of toilet, bedroom, bathing, corridors, facilities and the lack of privacy, intrusion or sexual harassment can be potentially more likely. In a survey by Barlow and Wolfson (1997) of female psychiatric inpatients in open acute and rehabilitation wards, most (76%) had experienced sexual harassment and a few had been the victims of sexual assault. The majority felt that female-only wards and higher staffing would improve safety. Another study by Thomas et al (1995) reported that a similar proportion (71%) of female inpatients had experienced unwanted physical and sexual experiences and a significantly higher incidence of minor and serious sexual discrimination. These findings are not surprising given that in addition to disturbed behaviour, 67% of male patients admitted to PICUs are in the under 30-year age group and 96% of male patients were either single, separated or divorced (Mitchell 1992). Also, there may be a tendency to neglect the needs of female patients. This aspect requires to be especially highlighted in newly built Intensive Care Units, where provision can be made for grouping male and female bedrooms, toilet, bathing and living areas separately. Some thought also needs to be given to redesigning such facilities in existing PICUs. Indeed, there is pressure from the British government to move towards separate wards for male and female patients.

The Patient's Charter has incorporated the right of female patients to be admitted to female-only wards (DoH 1995) but unfortunately extra resources will not be made available to implement this.

Clinical leadership

In our survey (Beer *et al* 1997) a third of PICUs do not have a consultant with overall responsibility for the PICU. This partly reflects the confusion of the role of a PICU within general adult services. Most would argue that if specific and clear guidelines were in place for the use of a PICU, then clear clinical leadership would ensure efficient and appropriate use of the facility. This has implications for the type of patients occupying PICU beds. It is also inappropriate to have a majority of PICUs staffed by junior doctors. Given the high levels of disturbance, the high dose medication and complicated legal issues such as consent that arise, doctors with a greater level of experience, e.g. MRCPsych and above, should provide input. Indeed, Zigmond (1995) recommended that junior medical staff must have training before being 'on call' for such a unit. This is not least because very often, junior doctors, in practice, do as they are told by the nursing staff in these units, e.g. where use of emergency or high-dose of medication is concerned. This is more likely to occur in the absence of a dedicated consultant for the PICU. If the unit is nurse led, as described by Dix (1995), then clear lines of responsibility need to be agreed with local management and doctors.

Policies

It is inappropriate for a PICU not to have a policy for high-dose medication, either for rapid tranquilisation or longer-term treatment. A significant number of the PICUs do not have a policy for the practice of control and restraint and seclusion. This clearly has implications for clinical practice. The regulations for management of health and safety at work (Health and Safety Executive 1992) require hospitals to assess health and safety risks to employees, patients and visitors. Measures resulting from this risk assessment, including adequate safety training, must be recorded. This is impossible if clear policies do not exist for standard practice of procedures such as seclusion or control and restraint. It may also result in difficult situations such as acutely disturbed informal patients in these units finding themselves in seclusion. Lack of policies may also lead to unsafe and substandard use of control and restraint procedures. Clear policies for assessment and observation with appropriate training in control and restraint procedures have a significant role in the reduction of violence in these units (Mortimer 1995). Along with the lack of consultant responsibility, it may be suggested that such PICUs are being used inappropriately by referrers, and show lack of uniformity in the application of care to individual patients. (see Chapter 16 by Garnham and Coleman for further details of policies.)

Factors affecting good practice in PICUs

Lack of a clear operational definition is the most important impediment to the efficient running of a PICU. Within the constraints of delivering a locally sensitive service, it is crucial to define the role to the PICU. Failure to do so is an invitation to bad practice. There are no national guidelines regarding definitions. Some may argue that this is not essential. Forensic units have their role defined by the courts in the type or category of patients they accept. This has lead to consistency in the running of these units, planning services, research, audit, policies, procedures, etc.

An acceptable working definition for a PICU might be:

'Provision of intensive/comprehensive multidisciplinary treatment and care by trained staff for severe or consistent disturbance exhibited by mentally disordered patients, over a time limited period, usually within conditions of security. This is according to an agreed philosophy of unit operation, underpinned by principles of containment and risk reduction. The ability of staff to respond to situations is immediate'.

It could be argued that this broad definition could equally apply to any locked or even an acute inpatient ward environment, or indeed forensic units. Further research is necessary to derive meaningful operational definitions. This is essential to clarify the interface between open acute, intensive care, long-term low secure, intensive rehabilitation and forensic units. Other factors that can affect good practice relate to the following categories:

Clinical criteria

- Levels of disturbance
- Levels of dangerousness
- Diagnostic considerations

Operational criteria

- Staffing levels
- Fabric of accommodation
- Philosophy of unit operation

Containment criteria

- Legal requirements, e.g. Criminal Part of Mental Health Act
- Level of observations required
- 'Out of control' patients

Other criteria

- Previous knowledge of patient history
- Staff training, experience in coping
- Idiosyncratic factors

Good practice in a PICU should be based on the following processes derived from discussion with local services:

Processes relevant to admissions, discharges

- Clear admission criteria
- Clear discharge criteria
- Clear referral systems
- Clear and transparent assessment system with response times
- Clear feedback forms
- Discharge information forms
- Good liaison with referrers

Processes relevant to operational functioning

- Locally derived, clearly understood operational policy
- Central, well understood philosophy of unit functioning
- Dedicated medical/clinical leadership
- Policies, procedures covering all aspects of PICU practice

Processes relevant to clinical functioning

- Dedicated, regular slots for multidisciplinary team clinical reviews/ward rounds
- System of clear communication within the team and with referrers
- System of dedicated interventions from:
  - medical staff, e.g. reviews
  - nursing, e.g. care plans, keyworking sessions
  - occupational therapy, e.g. regular programme
  - psychology, e.g. short-term therapy, assessments

- pharmacology, e.g. medication reviews

- social worker, probation, art therapy, etc.

- Clear documentation of interventions, decisions taken

- Regular clinical and objective risk assessment measures

Processes relevant to updating practice

- Clinical databases, e.g. admissions, discharges, adverse incidents

- Regular audit, e.g. control and restraint, rapid tranquilisation episodes, seclusion

- Staff support, e.g. regular multidisciplinary team forum to discuss relevant issues, teambuilding

- Staff training, e.g. assessments, control and restraint, de-escalation

Processes relevant to good liaison

- Advocacy services for patients

- Links with forensic services

- Regular meetings with referrers

It is crucial that any PICU as part of good practice should watch out for and act upon:

- Patient complaints

- Staff complaints

- Referrers' complaints

- Increased sickness rates, low morale in staff members

- Any increase in number of adverse incidents

- Signs of institutionalisation in patients and staff.

CONCLUSION

A clear and defined system of operating a PICU fosters good practice. This demystifies the role of the PICU, leads to a transparency of practice and encourages self-critical and innovative methods of working rather than reinforcing traditional views of what constitutes PICU practice.

ACKNOWLEDGEMENTS

Special thanks to the Publications Department of The Royal College of Psychiatrists for permission to use the article on 'Good practice issues in PICUs: findings from a National Survey' (Pereira et al 1999).

REFERENCES

Appelbaum PS, Mirkin SA, Bateman AL. 1981 Empirical assessment of competency to consent to psychiatric hospitalisation. Am J Psychiatr 138: 1170–1176

Atakan Z. 1995 Violence on psychiatric inpatient units: what can be done? Psychiatric Bulletin 19: 593–596

Barlow F, Wolfson P. 1997 Safety and security: a survey of female psychiatric inpatients. Psychiatric Bulletin 21: 270–272

Beer MD, Paton C, Pereira S. 1997 Hot beds of general psychiatry. A national survey of psychiatric intensive care units. Psychiatric Bulletin 21: 142–144

Department of Health. 1995 The Patient's Charter and You. London: HMSU

Dix R. 1995 A nurse led psychiatric intensive care unit. Psychiatric Bulletin 19: 285–287

Grossman L, Summers F. 1980 A study of schizophrenic patients to give informed consent. Hospital and Community Psychiatry 31: 205–206

Mitchell GD. 1992 A survey of psychiatric intensive care units in Scotland. Health Bulletin 50: 228–232

Mortimer A. 1995 Reducing violence on a secure ward. Psychiatric Bulletin 19: 605–608

Olin GB, Olin MS. 1975 Informed consent in voluntary mental hospital admissions. Am J Psychiatr 132: 938–941

Pereira S, Beer D, Paton C. 1999 Good practice issues in psychiatric intensive care units: findings from a national survey. Psychiatric Bulletin 23: 397–404

Sugarman P, Moss J. 1994 The rights of voluntary patients in hospital. Psychiatric Bulletin 18: 269–271

Thomas C, Bartlett A, Mezey GC. 1995 The extent and effects of violence among psychiatric inpatients. Psychiatric Bulletin 19: 600–604

Wolpe PR, Schwartz SL, Sandford B. 1991 Psychiatric inpatients knowledge of their rights. Hospital and Community Psychiatry 42: 1168–1169

Zigmond A. 1995 Special care wards: are they special? Psychiatric Bulletin 19: 270–272

APPENDIX A

POLICY NO. 1

VISITING

1. The Unit operates an open visiting policy, but it is considered helpful to organise visiting along the lines of 'a working day', so as not to interfere with a patient's 'therapeutic programme'. Numbers of visitors, at any one time, are at the discretion of the shift team, depending on the individual patient and the climate of the ward.

2. It is suggested that there should be an induction of a patients' nearest relative or carer, by the primary nurse or member of the care group, to the unit and other areas of the Unit. During this induction, various issues should be explained to the person including visiting times, where visits are held and which items are permitted on the unit.

Visiting times:
Monday – Friday   5pm – 9pm
Weekends and Bank Holidays   9am – 9pm

3. The day area should generally be used for visiting, but group rooms may be used after agreement of the Care Group and with permission of the shift team.

4. Visitors should not be allowed to wander, unescorted, around the unit. The visitors' toilet is to be used by visitors.

5. All property brought in by visitors should be channelled through the nursing staff. All visitors should be made aware of articles that patients are unable to keep. In general, visitors' bags should not be searched unless there are grounds to suspect they may be deliberately bringing contraband onto the unit. Visitors may be given the option of leaving their coats and bags in the care of staff during their visit or of leaving them outside the unit.

6. The patient or nearest relative should be asked to provide a list of visitors, including addresses, prior to those individuals visiting. Special consideration must be given to any visitor who may also be a victim of the patients' previous attack or crime.

All visitors, including official visitors such as solicitors, social workers etc., will be asked to sign the visitors' book kept at reception. Visitors who refuse to give required information will be referred to the shift co-ordinator for a decision to be made regarding entry.

7. All children's visits must comply with the Child Visiting policy. Staff should first check the CPA documentation to ensure that the child is on the nomination list.

8. Decisions regarding supervision of visits should, where possible, be made at multi-professional reviews but should nevertheless be made using a common sense approach.

9. Workmen on the Unit:

   a) Any workmen carrying out repairs must bring the minimum number of tools and equipment onto the unit. (They may leave surplus in the care of the nursing staff).

   b) At all times whilst on the unit they will remain under the observation of staff, being escorted as necessary.

10. Visitors from other wards should make a prior appointment with permission gained from the specific ward concerned.

N.B. The nurse-in-charge of the unit may at any time refuse admission to any visitor if it is felt not to be in the visitor's interest to or to the detriment of unit safety.

Last reviewed   date

Next reviewed   date

POLICY NO. 2

SEARCH PROCEDURE
(Individual Patients and Patient's property)

FOREWORD

The searching of an individual patient or patient's property is a delicate procedure and should be managed with the utmost integrity and highest professional standards. It must be emphasised that it is a potentially provocative procedure and will be construed as degrading by the individual. Therefore, the following guidelines are offered to facilitate the greatest practicable attention being paid to the dignity and welfare of patients at all times.

1. Guidelines

1.1 Searching an individual or an individual's property may only be implemented at the request of a shift team should they have reasonable grounds to suspect that the patient is in possession of items which present a potential or immediate risk to their safety or that of others (including drugs or alcohol) with the approval of the Senior Nurse-on-call for the Unit.

1.2 The implementation of a search must demonstrate that all previous measures utilised have proved fruitless in providing a satisfactory solution to the apparent problem. It should therefore be termed a 'last resort measure' and not utilised as a possible primary solution.

1.3 Talk to the patient at all times during the procedure, provide a forum for them to express their anxieties, but do not become complacent in the effectiveness of the exercise.

1.4 In the event of a search, the permission of the patient should be sought whenever practicable, but is not required, in order to carry out the search. The patient may wish to remain present, staff numbers should be taken into consideration, in order to maintain safety.

1.5 If the Search Procedure is implemented for the loss of unit equipment, see relevant policy in manual and follow accordingly.

2. Procedure: Individual Search

2.1 Patients will be searched individually in the privacy of their own room, unless extenuating circumstances are apparent.

2.2 Patients will be searched by a minimum of two staff members at all times. The staff will be of the same sex as the patient – one of the staff will be a trained nurse, although consideration of urgent necessity might very occasionally dictate otherwise.

2.3 The patient must be informed of the circumstances resulting in a personal search (if not already aware), and an opportunity will be given for imparting any relevant information to the staff prior to the search procedure.

2.4 Any items of clothing to be removed by the patient under the supervision of staff and searched in conjunction with their body.

2.5 INTIMATE BODY SEARCHES ARE NOT PERMITTED.

2.6 The staff are responsible for ensuring that the patient is properly clothed before removing them to another location.

3. Personal Property Search

3.1 The searching of patient's property to be implemented with the patient in attendance whenever appropriate.

3.2 Property to be searched by two members of staff at all times, one member of staff should be the same sex as the patient, one of the staff should be a trained nurse (although consideration of urgent necessity may occasionally dictate otherwise).

3.3 All property to be replaced as it was found and the utmost care to be used to prevent accidental damage to personal effects.

3.4 The search and the results of this must be recorded in the patient's notes.

Last reviewed   date

Next reviewed   date

POLICY NO. 3

ABSENT WITHOUT LEAVE (AWOL) POLICY

1. The particulars and physical characteristic sections of the AWOL form should be completed upon admission and kept in the patient's notes.

2. If it is suspected or known that a patient has gone AWOL, the Nurse-in-Charge must be informed immediately.

3. Unless the patient is known to have left the grounds, an immediate search should be made quickly to confirm this.

4. Remainder of the AWOL form should be completed. It is essential that where 'WARNING SIGNALS' have been highlighted on the form, the police are informed of these.

5. Ensure all necessary parties are informed – Nurse-on-call, Responsible Medical Officer and persons considered to be at risk, having considered issues of confidentiality in advance.

6. Unit staff, as available, should be sent to search outside the grounds and additional staff, as required, should be called upon to assist.

7. Staff searching for the patient should not take any risks and should ensure they have sufficient numbers if they find and are to return the patient.

8. Notify the Home Office (C3), if required, normally within 24 hours.

9. When the patient is found and has been returned to the Unit, ensure all relevant personnel are informed.

10. The Nurse-in-Charge must complete an Incident Form and ensure that full details are recorded in the patient's notes.

11. A new AWOL form should be commenced for future use.

12. A Team debrief is held to examine the cause and effect and implications for future practice.

POLICY NO. 3

Actions to be taken if a patient is suspected to have gone AWOL

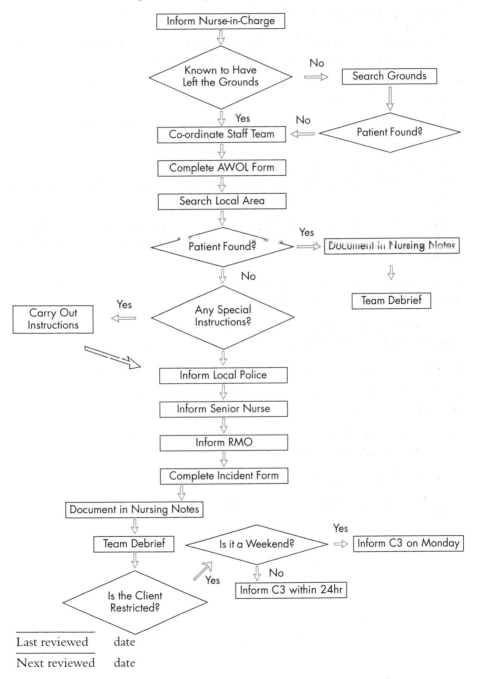

Last reviewed   date

Next reviewed   date

POLICY NO. 4

USE OF RESTRAINT POLICY

- All staff should be aware of Chapter 18 of the Mental Health Act Code of Practice: 'Patients Presenting Particular Management Problems'.

- The levels of restraint may vary. The essence of the restraint is to contain or limit another person's freedom. When restraint is used, particularly physical with or without seclusion, it must always be 'the last resort' when all verbal avenues have been exhausted and when it is obvious that there is real danger of physical assault, destructive behaviour or over-activity likely to cause exhaustion and disruption.

- Where restraint is thought necessary, assistance should be sought by the call system or verbally.

- One team member should assume control of the incident. Where possible, the patient should be approached and agreement sought to stop behaviour or to comply with a request.

- The Team should be trained in C&R techniques and use these to safely and effectively restrain the patient and minimise a risk to all involved with the incident.

- Any restraint must be 'reasonable in the circumstances'. It must be the minimum necessary to deal with the current situation.

- All incidents should be recorded in the patient's notes and on the Incident Report Forms.

- Any patient who has been physically restrained should be seen, as soon as practically possible, by a doctor.

- Any injuries to the patient or to staff must be recorded and appropriate medical attention sought.

- In the event of patients receiving injuries which require hospital treatment, the unit manager, senior nurse and consultant, having investigated the matter thoroughly, will decide whether the Mental Health Act Commissioners need to be informed.

- Following an incident, the staff involved should meet as soon as possible as a group in order to discuss and offer support to all involved.

Last reviewed   date

Next reviewed   date

POLICY NO. 5

PATIENTS WHO REQUIRE MONITORED SUPERVISION

From time to time members of staff will be confronted with a patient who makes comments or performs actions indicating they intend to seriously harm themselves or other people. In many instances, the patient is merely reacting to feelings of frustration, anger or despair. However, in some circumstances, the threat could be real. Any member of staff confronted by such behaviour or comments should take the following initial steps:

1. Inform the Nurse-in-Charge of the shift as soon as possible.

2. Record details of comments made, or the general behaviour which has given rise to concern, in the nursing notes.

3. The Nurse-in-Charge should in turn consult with the Responsible Medical Officer or his deputy as soon as is practicable and agree on the level of supervision necessary.

4. The RMO or his deputy and the Nurse in Charge should record details in the nursing notes.

• The Nurse-in-Charge will always be expected to take interim measures based on professional judgement until the RMO or his deputy can be contacted.

• When deciding on the level of supervision, the term 'specialing' should never be used. Levels of supervision should be in accordance with those described in the policy manual.

• It is the responsibility of the allocated nurse, in the absence of the responsible Keyworker, to update the care plan. The following should be considered:

1. The nature of the problem must be clearly defined.

2. The purpose of the supervisory level indicated.

3. Nursing care plan must clearly state the level of supervision required.

4. The care plan should be reviewed on a 24 hourly basis.

LEVELS OF SUPERVISION

1. Nominal supervision:

The whereabouts of the individual is known at all times and visual checks are made half-hourly whilst on the Unit (in accordance with the role of the Allocated Nurse). *Escorted or unescorted leave as appropriate.*

2. Close attention:

Continual awareness of a patient's location for the purpose of assessment and observation of his/her needs. To be seen and checked at regular intervals, agreed by the Nurse-in-Charge and RMO or his deputy. *Escorted leave only.*

For Level 2 **(Close Attention)** only: If the implementation of Level 2 supervision (Close Attention) was by nursing staff, then a decision may be made by a Charge Nurse to adjust the frequency of the regular checks or to reduce to Level 1.

If the Level 2 supervision was implemented jointly by medical and nursing staff, then it can only be reduced by the Responsible Medical Officer or his/her deputy. The Nurse-in-Charge can increase the frequency of the checks but not reduce them.

3. Constant care:

Continual presence of nursing staff for observation of the physical and mental condition of the patient. Visual observation should be maintained, but privacy may be granted for the purposes of bathing, toileting or undressing. *No leave, with the exception of the garden at the discretion of the RMO or his deputy and the Nurse-in-Charge.*

For levels 3 (constant care) and 4 (intensive observation) only the RMO or deputy can either discontinue or reduce the level of observations.

4. Intensive observation:

The patient must be in the continual presence of nursing staff and constant direct visual observation maintained at all times. *No leave, with the exception of the garden at the discretion of the RMO or his deputy and the Nurse-in-Charge.*

For the purposes of observation in 2, 3 and 4 ABOVE, an hourly rota should be organised by the shift co-ordinator. It is wholly inadvisable for a member of staff to engage in such demanding observations for more than one hour at a time.

N.B. Staff should make themselves aware of the:

SNMAC Standing Nursing and Midwifery Advisory Committee. 1999b Safe and supportive observation of patients at risk, London.

_____

Last reviewed   date

_____

Next reviewed   date

_____

POLICY NO. 6

DEALING WITH THE TAKING OR SUPPLYING OF NON-PRESCRIBED DRUGS/SUBSTANCES.

The Need

It is not seen to be in the best interests of individuals to condone their taking of non-prescribed medication/substances as this could:

- Have serious side-effects (physical/mental).

- Affect the individual's ability to make informed choices.

- Could create disinhibition to an extent which compromises the safety of the individual, or others.

- Promote questionable habit forming behaviour.

- Lead to 'difficult situations' on the Unit.

- Mean the law is being broken.

Aims of Policy

1. Educate.

2. Encourage healthy living.

3. Minimise the use of non-prescribed substances.

4. Adhere to legal/professional guidelines.

5. Maintain the safety of the individual.

6. Minimise risk to others.

The Policy Statement

The use of or supplying of non-prescribed drugs/substances on the Unit is not allowed.

Achieving the Aims of the Policy

1.

a) A shortened version of the Policy to be supplied to each Patient's Room, preferably on the wall.

b) A discussion related to the Policy to take place and be recorded in the Patient's notes.

2.

a) A draft letter to all Visitors discussing the reasons for the policy.

b) Staff member to ensure that this is done and recorded.

3.

a) Educational sessions for both staff and patients related to the use of non-prescribed substances.

b) Develop links/liaison with other clinical areas.

To minimise usage

Our course of action related to the taking or supplying of non-prescribed substances is that where staff suspect an individual is not abiding by the rules, they may, after informing the patient:

i) Ask for a urine sample.

ii) Be involved in the searching of an individual.

iii) Be involved in the searching of the Unit or any part thereof.

iv) Take the required legal steps. In the event of possession or supply, the local Police will be informed and necessary steps taken.

v) Inform the patient of the possibility of future spot checks which could involve all, or any of the above, as well as continued checking of visitors.

Adhere to Legal/Professional Guidelines

Consult and liaise, as appropriate, with local Police Force, Mental Health Act Commissioners, Oxleas NHS Trust Management and the Home Office.

Maintain safety and minimise risk

Discreet personal searching will take place with respect for dignity. Searching of property and rooms will take into account the number of staff required to maintain safety.

The permission of a patient is not required in order to carry out a search of their room. This may be done with the agreement of the Nurse-in-charge with the proviso that staff have reasonable grounds to take action.

Refusal

Refusal to give a urine sample will be taken as indicative of the individual having broken the rules and staff will proceed as if the sample were positive.

Awaiting Results

Certain substances can be detected by ward urinalysis kits. The patient may be present whilst this test is performed. If there remains any doubt after ward testing, the sample should be sent to hospital labs for confirmation. Whilst waiting for the results of a urine sample, action may be taken related to the leave status, or other conditions of residence of the individual.

Positive Result or Possession or Supply

Any sanctions related to a positive test will be discussed within the Care Group and the Clinical Review where further screening, spot-checks, or other course of action may be authorised. The following may happen:

– Leave status halted/reduced/stopped.

– Visits monitored/supervised/stopped.

   Reduced access to clinical areas.

– Reduced use of facilities.

– Programme reviewed/halted.

Discovery

Discovery of a substance of 'questionable' nature could involve any or all of the steps outlined in the policy document. The substance will be retained and sent to the Pharmacy Department for disposal. The substance should be placed in a sealed envelope labelled 'Unknown Substance – Please Destroy'.

Last reviewed   date

Next reviewed   date

OTHER POLICIES WHICH CAN BE FOUND IN THIS BOOK

INDEX